Napoleon's Doctors
The Medical Services of the Grande Armée

NAPOLEON'S DOCTORS

THE MEDICAL SERVICES OF THE
GRANDE ARMÉE

by

Dr Martin R Howard

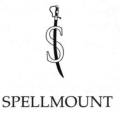

SPELLMOUNT

British Library Cataloguing in Publication Data:
A catalogue record for this book is available
from the British Library

Copyright © Dr Martin R Howard 2006

ISBN 1-86227-324-3

First published in the UK in 2006 by
Spellmount Limited
The Mill, Brimscombe Port
Stroud, Gloucestershire GL5 2QG

Tel: 01453 883300
Fax: 01453 883233
E-mail: enquiries@spellmount.com
Website: www.spellmount.com

1 3 5 7 9 8 6 4 2

Printed in Great Britain by
Oaklands Book Services
Stonehouse, Gloucestershire GL10 3RQ

Contents

Maps

Acknowledgements

I am much indebted to the following for their help in locating books: Bibliothèque Nationale de France, Paris; Wellcome Library for the History and Understanding of Medicine, London; The British Library, London; York District Library; Librairie Historique Clavreuil Fabrice Teissèdre, Paris; Le Livre Chez Vous, Paris; Jeffrey Stern Antiquarian Books, York. I am very grateful to Professor Alan Forrest who generously shared his extensive knowledge of the armies of Revolutionary and Napoleonic France. Many thanks to Jamie Wilson and all at Spellmount for giving me the opportunity to write a second book on the military and medical history of this fascinating period.

Glossary

Administration: The administrative department of the *Grande Armée* which exerted considerable influence over the *service de santé*.

Aide-Chirurgien (Aide-Major): Surgeon acting as an assistant to a *chirurgien-major*. Equivalent to second class.

Ambulance: A term variably used to describe an ambulance wagon or ambulance organisation (e.g. flying ambulance) or a small field hospital (see Chapter IV).

Ambulance volante: A mobile ambulance attached to the advanced parts of the army. Sometimes used to describe Larrey's flying ambulance.

Antiphlogistic treatment: The use of drugs such as emetics and purgatives and other strategies (e.g. bleeding) to 'rid' the body of the impurities thought to be causing disease or inflaming wounds.

Apothecary: An archaic term for pharmacist.

Bark (Quinine): Peruvian bark, the source of quinine. Useful in the treatment of malaria.

Bistoury: A long surgical knife with a narrow blade.

Blistering: The intentional blistering of the skin as part of disease treatment.

Brancardier: Stretcher-bearer. Also termed *'despotat'*. Probably little used in practice.

Caisson: A small wagon sometimes used as an ambulance or a chest possibly used for surgical instruments and medical supplies.

Cauterisation: The application of heat to a wound.

Chirurgie de bataille: A comprehensive system of battlefield surgery proposed by Percy but not instituted.

Chirurgien: Surgeon.

Chirurgien de pacotille: A pejorative term, probably coined by Percy, for French army surgeons of low calibre.

Chirurgien-Major: Senior surgeon of a regiment. Equivalent to first class.

Commissaire de guerre: Agent of the army's administration. They often had an uneasy relationship with the *officiers de santé*.

Conseil de santé: A senior body of the *service de santé* composed of a surgeon, physician and pharmacist. Created in 1800 and abolished in 1803.

Contagion: A more modern theory of disease spread (than miasma) based on transmission from one man to another.

Cupping: The placing of a warm cup on the skin to facilitate bleeding by creating a vacuum.

Despotat: See *brancardier*.

Directoire Central des Hôpitaux Militaires: Organisation founded in 1800 and composed of five members taken from retired army officers and senior administrators.

Disarticulation: Removal of a limb by separation at the hip or shoulder as opposed to amputation.

Dysentery: A debilitating and potentially fatal infectious disease characterised by diarrhoea.

Effusion: The collection of fluid in a body cavity (e.g. pleural effusion in the chest).

Epaulette: A formal mark of military rank and prestige not worn by the *officiers de santé* despite lobbying by Percy and others.

Femur: Major bone of the upper leg.
Field hospital: Small temporary hospital created near to the fighting. Often referred to as an 'ambulance' in French accounts.

Fourgon: A long covered wagon sometimes used as an ambulance.

Fourniture (demi-fourniture): Units of military bedding.

Gale: A very common skin disease among soldiers. Probably scabies.

Grognard: Veteran soldier of the *Grande Armée*. Literally a 'grumbler'.

Hôpitaux d'instruction: Military hospitals with a training role.

Hôpitaux Militaires: The military hospitals of the army (see Chapter VII).

Hôpitaux temporaires: Hospitals formed in time of war to receive evacuations from the army – divided into first, second and third lines and including special hospitals for skin and venereal diseases (see Chapter VII).

Hospital employees: Non-medical staff giving assistance in the hospitals.

Humerus: Major bone of the upper arm.

Imperial Guard: The elite military formation of the *Grande Armée* eventually divided into Old, Middle and Young Guards. It had its own medical service.

Infirmier: Medical orderly used to give help to wounded in the field and assist in the hospitals. Organised into companies under Percy's direction (see Chapter V).

Inspector General: Senior doctor of the *service de santé*. In 1803 six inspector generals (Coste, Desgenettes, Heurteloup, Larrey, Parmentier, Percy) were appointed as a supervisory committee.

Intendant-Général: Senior administrator ultimately responsible for all the needs of the *Grande Armée* including the medical services. Pierre Daru held the post from 1806 to 1812 and again in 1815.

Invalides (hôtel): Large hospital in Paris for wounded, sick and infirm soldiers.

Lazarets: Hospitals for infectious diseases (e.g. plague hospitals in Egypt).

Légion d'honneur: An order of civilian or military merit instituted by Napoleon in 1802.

Ligation: The tying off of a blood vessel.

Médecin: Physician.

Miasma (miasmata): Atmospheric pollutants exuded from vegetable matter. Thought to be a major cause of disease but challenged by the newer 'contagion' theory.

Moxa: An ancient form of cauterisation favoured by Larrey.

Nostalgia: The depression experienced by soldiers on campaign. In modern parlance, most probably a combination of post-traumatic stress disorder, shellshock and malingering.

Officier de santé: A term very loosely used to describe the doctors of the French army and lesser qualified doctors in civilian practice (see Chapter II).

Ophthalmia: General term for a variety of infectious eye diseases. Prevalent in Egypt.

Ordonnateur: Senior grade in the army's administration.

Pharmacien: Pharmacist.

Plague (bubonic): An infectious disease transmitted to man via rat fleas. Prevalent in Egypt and the same disease as the 'black death' of the Middle Ages.

Round shot: A spherical solid cannon ball of cast metal varying in weight according to the calibre of cannon.

Scurvy: Disease caused by deficiency of vitamin C.

Service de santé: The medical service of the French army.

Shock: A medical term which now refers specifically to the state resulting from loss of blood but which in the Napoleonic period was more generally used to describe the systemic impact of severe wounding.

Smallpox: Highly contagious viral disease characterised by a skin rash. Vaccination was introduced during the Napoleonic era and sparingly used in the *Grande Armée*.

Solde: Soldier's pay.

Sous-Aide-Chirurgien: Lower surgical grade equivalent to third class.

Suppuration: Infection. More literally, the formation of pus.

Tetanus: Disease of contaminated wounds characterised by intense muscle spasm and a high mortality. Also called 'lockjaw'.

Tourniquet: A device for constricting the arteries of arm or leg to slow bleeding.

Trepanning (trephining): The operation of creating a hole in bone (usually the skull).

Triage: A system for dividing up wounded men and prioritising treatment on the basis of severity of injury and likelihood of successful intervention.

Typhus: A potentially fatal infectious disease spread by the human body louse.

Wurst: Early mobile ambulance system designed by Percy.

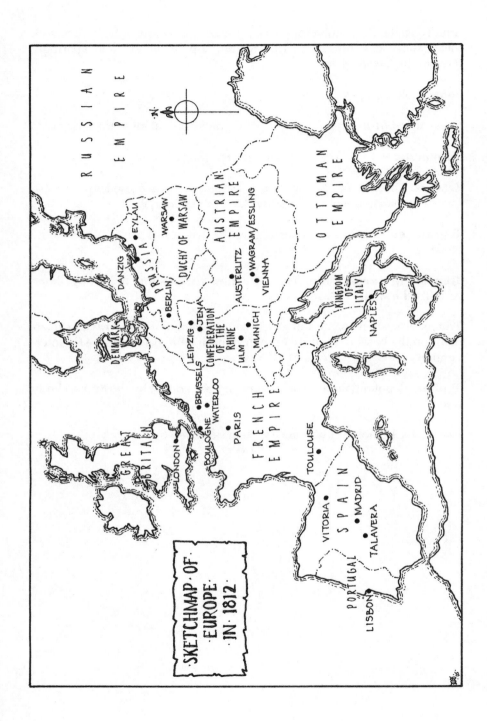

SKETCH·MAP·OF·
·EUROPE·
·IN·1812·

CHAPTER I
Service de Santé

In his account of his experiences in the Peninsular War, Pharmacist Sébastien Blaze draws some conclusions regarding his status in Napoleon's *Grande Armée*. Blaze neatly divides the French army into four classes. In the first class were men who had both glory and riches. These were the marshals and generals of the Empire. They 'harvested in the fields of Mars'. In the second class were those with glory but no riches. Blaze decided that most soldiers belonged to this category. Even the officers were usually denied their fortune by the accidents of war. In the third class, described in some detail, are the miscreants who obtained riches without glory. Here we have the employees of the despised administration and corrupt senior officials, men who feathered their nests while others sacrificed their lives. In the fourth and final category were the unfortunates who could expect neither glory nor riches. Blaze is in little doubt that this is where he belongs. He includes all the army's *officiers de santé*, the physicians (*médecins*), surgeons (*chirurgiens*) and pharmacists (*pharmaciens*). Blaze gloomily notes that the army's doctors 'often share the dangers of the soldiers but not their glory.'[1]

Blaze implies that Napoleon's doctors were relegated to a lower league of the army's hierarchy, under-appreciated and under-rewarded. However, other contemporary accounts by French army doctors paint a subtly different picture. Perhaps the average doctor would not win medals for heroism in battle or become fabulously rich but there were more intangible rewards. Louis Kerkhoves, an army physician, followed Napoleon into Russia, quite possibly the nadir of Napoleonic campaigning. As the miseries of the retreat multiplied, the double veneer of civilisation and army discipline was stripped away and more fundamental sentiments and loyalties were all that was left. Kerkhoves relates his experiences around the bivouac fires.

> More often than not there was nothing to burn but green wood which would not ignite despite every effort and when we were fortunate enough to have a good fire it was necessary to do everything possible not to be grilled on one side and frozen on the other. At these sad fires,

where there was no shelter against the wind and the snow and where one sometimes saw men sitting on dead bodies, some among us were roasting scraps of horseflesh whilst others were making thin gruel with a little flour. When people not belonging to the bivouac approached they were sent away. To get a place at the fire it was necessary to supply some means of warmth or a little brandy or food. It was especially the *commissaires de guerres*, the employees of the administration, whom the soldiers would not tolerate at their bivouac. They showered them with abuse and chased them off mercilessly. They had, perhaps, done nothing wrong ... but if, in these awful circumstances, the soldiers showed their feelings with respect to people of whom they had complaint, they, in general, showed kindness and sometimes gratitude to the physicians and surgeons even though at this disastrous time they had no hope of a medical service. They often said, 'the doctors are always interested in us. They have done only good for us.' During the retreat some physicians and surgeons owed their lives to the soldiers.[2]

For a typical soldier's view of the army's doctors we can turn to Elzéar Blaze, brother of Sébastien, a captain in the *chasseurs à pied* of the Guard. In Elzéar's eyes the doctors are either at the top or the bottom of the pile. He acknowledges that many of the more senior regimental surgeons (*chirurgiens-majors*) were 'expert practitioners' who could amputate an arm or leg with equanimity and a high success rate. 'These gentlemen were full of zeal. You often saw them on the battlefield risking their necks while they cared for the wounded ... From having to constantly treat wounds of all sorts they had learned as much as they needed to know.' On the other hand, Elzéar was familiar with another type of army doctor.

> We were always getting young men from France who – through patronage and to avoid joining the army with packs on their backs [being conscripted as combatants] – had obtained, I don't know how, an appointment as a junior regimental surgeon (*sous-aide*) after a three month course at the school of medicine. Thereafter they learnt by on-the-job training in the army at the expense of their patients. Woe to the poor devils who fell into their hands; escaping the cannon they faced their scalpels.

The latter doctors were often referred to as the *chirurgiens de pacotille*, a term coined by Pierre-François Percy, the army's senior doctor, to describe draft-dodging doctors of minimal quality and experience. In Elzéar Blaze's world the only use of such doctors was to be the butt of endless practical jokes, which he describes in excruciating detail. His schizophrenic attitude to the army's medical personnel persisted throughout the war, 'but don't make too much fun of the army doctors, I owe my life to one of them'.[3] Such anecdotes paint a tentative picture of Napoleon's doctors. Already we can start to see that any status that they held was uncertain and fragile. Some were respected, whilst others were held in contempt.

We will return to the worth and role of individual army doctors in more detail but it is necessary to first understand the system in which they worked – the army's *service de santé*. There has been no comprehensive account of the medical services of the *Grande Armée* in English. This is unsurprising as even Alain Pigeard, an eminent French Napoleonic historian, has to acknowledge, in a recent concise review of Napoleon's *service de santé*, that although a 'noble institution' it had previously been described in an anecdotal manner and that its organisation was particularly complex, '… a true imbroglio of regulations changed without decree, its functioning remaining obscure.' Pigeard lists fifty-eight different pieces of legislation pertaining to the *service de santé* issued between 1792 and 1813.[4] Nevertheless, it is feasible to give a simplified and coherent overview of the *Grande Armée*'s medical system, stressing the few key decrees that ultimately dictated its workings on campaign, whilst being a little economical in describing the remainder. It is helpful to start with the army medical service of the 18th century as Napoleon, in his evolution from General Bonaparte, inherited not only an army but also its doctors.

Louis XIV created the *corps de santé militaire*. An edict of 1708 established military hospitals in fifty-one French cities and an associated infrastructure where sick and wounded soldiers were managed by physicians, surgeons and apothecaries under the supervision of the First Physician, First Surgeon and the Minister of War. A training programme for young surgeons was established in the hospitals, which were in turn subject to detailed regulations. This degree of control brought considerable benefits and for much of the 18th century the military medicine service was superior to its civilian equivalent. However, there were underlying dissensions with conflict between the physicians and surgeons and a constant three-cornered tug of war between army doctors, professional soldiers and administrators. Unfortunately, this was to remain the case throughout the Revolutionary and Napoleonic eras. Much of the good work was undone by reforms in the 1780s, which were undertaken for economic reasons – another recurring theme of army medicine. In 1788 all but eight of the military and naval hospitals were closed and the educational role of the 'teaching hospital amphitheatres' was terminated.

Regimental hospitals were to be opened in large numbers to provide a cheap alternative to central hospital care in the military and civilian facilities. The outcome was chaos with the administrators of the army corps having neither the knowledge nor the funding to set up an alternative hospital in each regiment. In the event, many sick or wounded soldiers had to be referred to inadequate civilian hospitals. On the eve of the French Revolution the morale of army medical personnel was low. With pay seriously in arrears many army doctors returned to civilian practice;

3

the number of *officiers de santé* with the army fell from 1,200 in 1788 to around 200 in 1789–90. This was at a time when the planned increase in military forces was 169 battalion companies, a total of 101,000 men. Although the actual figure raised was nearer to 50,000 there was evidently a sizeable discrepancy between the newly formed revolutionary army and the number of its doctors.[5]

ₐIf the Revolutionary Wars brought severe logistical difficulties for the army's doctors they also brought new attitudes to war and military medicine. War itself had become more terrifying. Revolutionary generals had to win at all costs and used inexperienced troops indiscriminately. Those who survived battle often succumbed to epidemics of disease sweeping the ranks. This nightmarish scenario was an entirely new experience for the army medical service. Whilst these horrors cannot be expunged, and resources were totally inadequate, there were also positives for the army's doctors. Primarily for reasons of expediency doctors became more autonomous. Freed from the threats of the *commissaires des guerres* they were left to arrange an admittedly haphazard medical service themselves. The democratic element of the Revolution tended to blur distinctions between medicine and surgery bringing all doctors together as *officiers de santé* or 'health officers'.

There was also a heroic aspect to the military proclamations pertaining to the sick and wounded. Although, as is the case with many of the decrees of the Revolution, implementation may have been variable, there was at least intent to emphasise and elevate the status of wounded men and the care they received. Thus, decrees of the mid 1790s stated that when soldiers wounded in battle were carried to receive medical help, all stationary corps that they passed were to give them military honours, all the drums to beat and the men to present arms. Similarly, all sentries were to give special acknowledgement to all uniformed soldiers with severe limb injuries who passed in front of their post. At public fete days a special place was to be allocated to the wounded warriors. Under the Ancient Regime only officers had been admitted to the *Hôtel des Invalides* in Paris. The revolutionaries, in contrast, insisted that 400 places in the hospital be allocated solely on the basis of severity of wounds. Citizenship implied equality. This spirit of altruism was also extended to foreign prisoners of war who were to receive in the military hospitals of France the same care as its own. A decree of 1793 states, 'where the *officiers de santé* do not understand the language of the foreigners they will find an interpreter for them.' The uniform buttons of the *officiers de santé* bore witness to this ethos, carrying words such as *humanité* surrounded by the inscription *Hôpitaux Militaires*. French historians have reasonably claimed that this type of legislation put in place the first principles of the Geneva Convention.[6]

The organisation of the medical services of the revolutionary armies was determined by a number of major decrees appearing between 1792 and

1800.[7] Whilst it is important to acknowledge the legislation it is equally pertinent to note that ambitious objectives were not always achieved and that many directives were only temporary or even immediately contradicted. In 1792 there was little formal organisation and very few resources. Vess has aptly described French army medicine of this period as being a 'grand and desperate innovation' with a handful of veteran army officers and experienced doctors of the old regimen hanging on to the tiller.[8] The 'Terror' invoked by the Central Committee of Public Safety at least brought the ruthlessness needed to provide additional manpower and supplies for the impoverished service. The committee's representatives on mission had considerable authority over the army's affairs and senior doctors looked to them for their immediate needs. Decrees now emanated at short intervals from the more rigidly centralised authorities in Paris. Legislation in 1793 and 1794 organised the army's hospitals. We will consider hospitals in more detail in a later chapter but, essentially, by 1794 each army had attached to it a senior surgeon, physician and pharmacist and there were four categories of hospital. The first of these categories, the military hospitals (hôpitaux militaires) was divided into two groups. The 'fixed' hospitals were subdivided again into those of the 1st, 2nd and 3rd classes and served both the army and the garrisons. The 'ambulant' or 'mobile' hospitals (the precursor of the ambulance) were to follow each army division. The second category of hospitals was educational (hôpitaux d'instruction) providing courses of instruction and situated wherever was decreed to be most convenient. Finally, there were the 'special' hospitals for venereal and skin diseases and the 'spa' hospitals (hôpitaux d'eaux minérals) that catered for both soldiers and civilians.

With respect to the supervision of the service, three separate groups of staff shared the key administrative work: the medical professionals (surgeons, physicians, and pharmacists), purely administrative staff, and the commissaires des guerres, agents of the administration, who also had a policing role. This division was unhelpful and carried the risk of demoting the officiers de santé to the role of simple and expendable military employees. However, in the early years of the Revolutionary Wars, it appears that the regulations were adhered to in spirit rather than applied literally and the army's doctors were not subjugated in the way that was to occur under the Consulate.

At the head of the service de santé, an administrative committee, the central conseil de santé was formed, reconstituted by the decree of April 1793. It was composed of three physicians, three surgeons and three pharmacists. These were senior army doctors, all having at least twenty years of high quality military service behind them. The members were nominated by the Minister of War. The duties of the conseil were 'the direction and supervision of all things relating to the health of the troops and medicine in the military hospitals ...' Members were expected to pay visits to the armies in the field and make appropriate inspections of hospitals. Their authority was strictly controlled. For instance, they had no right to dismiss incompetent *officiers de santé*. In this event they had to consult with local medical administrative bodies more closely attached to the armies (so called auxillary *conseils de santé*) and the Minister of War alone could take the final decision. Later in the year, the *conseil de santé* was replaced by the *commission de santé* but this appears to have been a nominal change with the duties of the new commission unchanged and only a small increase in its members to twelve. It continued to play a key role in communicating with the senior *officiers de santé* of the army, making inspections, examining new medical recruits, and delivering verdicts on the quality of food and medical treatments.

It was a characteristic of the revolutionary *service de santé* that change in administrative structure – what is now commonly referred to as 'modernisation' – was incessant. By 1796 the *commission* had gone, replaced by the 'Inspector Generals'. These were six *officiers de santé* of at least twelve years' service nominated by the Minister of War. Again, the actual duties of this senior administrative body were much the same as before and it continued in the same vein as the *commission de santé*. Two decrees of 1800 heralded a new era of more real and substantial change in the army's medical service and initiated a series of events which were to prove both unfortunate and demoralising for the *officiers de santé*.[9] The first re-established a *conseil de santé* of just three senior army doctors, one from each of the professions. The particular functions of the new body were to submit candidates for *officier de santé* posts in the army and hospitals, to correspond with the army doctors on medical matters, to write instructions on the treatment of diseases, and to select and distribute medicines and surgical instruments. It was accountable to the Minister of War. This all seems more of the same, but, crucially, another body was now created – the *directoire central des hôpitaux militaires* – made up of five non-medical members. These men were picked from unemployed general military officers and senior military and civil administrators. Apart from the *conseil* and *directoire* more local equivalents were set up in the permanent hospitals and close to each army.

Inevitably, the presence of this additional body impinged on the influence of the purely medical *conseil de santé*. The extent to which this occurred is revealed in a telling article of the decree of 4 *germinal* year VIII (1800).

> The *conseil de santé* will be under the immediate orders of the Minister of War: it will be called upon, to a greater or lesser degree, by the *directoire central des hôpitaux militaires* to give advice on subjects on which the *directoire* judges it appropriate to consult it.[10]

At a stroke the authority of the army's most senior medically constituted body had been reduced to a degree that it could only give an opinion when it was asked. The *officiers de santé* were now strictly controlled, subjugated to purely administrative forces. Free spirits among the army's doctors, such as Pierre-François Percy, could only revolt as he saw the service into which he and others had invested such effort delivered into the hands of mediocre officers. He was particularly outraged that the low quality members of the *directoire*, mostly dredged from retirement, were given equal or more credence than the senior doctors of the *conseil*. Percy, a character who figures large in subsequent pages and chapters, offered his resignation but was refused.

The *conseil de santé* itself appeared naïve and lacking in foresight. Its three members at this time were Physician Jean-François Coste, already an old man, Surgeon Nicolas Heurteloup, and Pharmacist Antoine-Augustin Parmentier. They were overly optimistic with regard to the new administrative arrangements and, more forgivably, were distracted by what appeared to be real hope of a lasting peace. In peace, the shortcomings of the new system would be easily accommodated. In this spirit of optimism they recommended a number of initiatives to the Minister of War, establishing the relative strengths of the 'corps' of *officiers de santé* in peace-time and in war and particularly the means of transferring from one footing to another. Simultaneously, the uniform of the *officiers de santé* was simplified, a further indication to some that their prestige was being relentlessly eroded. The next blow fell in the decree of 15 *nivose* in the form of large-scale redundancies of army doctors. The articles of the decree largely refer to redundancy payments but the most damaging legislation is explicitly stated in an attached circular.

> … The *service de santé* of the armies will be formed only on a temporary commission; that is, in peace, the *officier de santé* who has never been appointed with tenure in a military hospital will not be kept by the service: that the title of those that the government retains will be purely individual and, effectively speaking, there will not be a *corps de santé*.[11]

The underlining is mine. It can hardly have been the intent of the *conseil de santé* to create a 'disposable' army medical service and leave the redundant *officiers de santé* in destitution. However, this is effectively what had occurred. The later pleading of the *conseil* for these unemployed officers has the sound of a stable door being slammed shut. The army's senior council was reduced to alerting the local municipal authorities, the local *prefects* and *sous prefects*, as to the high abilities of the ex-army *officiers de santé*. But the return of these men to their home villages was fraught with difficulty. Whilst they had been fighting for the Revolution and liberty their civilian colleagues had been establishing reputations and developing a clientele.

Throughout the years of the Revolutionary Wars the number of *officiers de santé* in service varied widely determined by need, attrition and redundancies. In 1793 doctors were in short supply with over 600 of the 1,400 men enrolled in 1792 having perished from wounds or disease. Many simply departed for home as the theatre of operations moved from their home soil into Belgium and Germany. A few were dismissed for incompetence and perhaps more were harassed out of the army by overly zealous Jacobins denouncing their lack of patriotism. Of the further 2,700 *officiers de santé* enrolled in 1793 nearly 1,000 would be lost on the battlefield or in epidemics of disease.[12] Any respite in hostilities was used to try and fill the gaps. By 1799 there were 1,907 *officiers de santé* in the service at a total budget of 3,218,000 francs.

We have seen, with reference to the senior ranks, that there were distinct medical specialities: the physicians (*médecins*), surgeons (*chirurgiens*) and pharmacists (*pharmaciens*). Regulations in 1793 subdivided the specialities into grades dependent on merit and the nature and length of previous service. Subsequently the training needs for the grades were more specifically defined. For instance, in 1796 surgeons and pharmacists of the third class (the lowest grade) had to be at least 25 years old and show 'some knowledge' in an examination. To qualify for the second class they needed two years' experience at the lower grade and to have more stringent testing. The first class required two years at the second class and the demonstration of practical knowledge in front of a jury of professors.[13]

Regimental surgeons had their own specific ranks in addition to the above grades. Their role under the Revolution appears to have been limited by the closure of many regimental hospitals. From 1793 each *demi-brigade* of infantry had to have only one *chirurgien-major* and another surgeon for each battalion. These men were nominally chosen by the *conseil de santé* but, in reality, they were often selected haphazardly by military officers. Their role was to make daily visits to barracks and tents and also to the local hospitals to treat the sick of their corps. They were entrusted with funds to cover their duties and were expected to keep senior military and medical officers informed of the state of health of the troops. A regulation of 1795 put *chirurgiens-majors* into the second class and made them equivalent to captains with respect to rations and incidentals. Subsequently, sixty selected regimental medical officers were admitted to the first class and titled *officiers de santé des corps*. By 1799 each *demi-brigade* of infantry included three *officiers de santé* and each cavalry regiment one *chirurgien-major*. These medical officers were allowed the same food and fodder as military officers of the same grade.

The following inventory of what may be loosely termed the 'corps' of the *service de santé* in 1801 gives a good overview of the numbers of *officiers de santé* in different specialities and in the hospital and army corps.

Members of the *conseil de santé*	3
Secretary to the *conseil*	1
Professors (in *hôpitaux d'instruction*)	25
Hospital physicians (*médecins*)	30

Physician of the Guard	1
Available physicians	9
Surgeons (*chirurgiens*) with the corps	489
Surgeons in the Guard	11
Surgeon in the *gendarmerie*	1
Surgeons in the hospitals	90
Available surgeons	59
Pharmacists (*pharmaciens*) in the hospitals	90
Pharmacists in the Guard	4
Available pharmacists	31

This was a total of 844 staff. Relatively more surgeons and pharmacists of the higher grades (first and second classes) were found in the hospitals than in the army corps.[14]

What quality of service did these men provide throughout the wars of the Revolution? There was unrelenting demand for new doctors to replace those lost. A combination of war, desertion and disease had removed perhaps three quarters of the *officiers de santé* enrolled since 1792. Under such duress it was inevitable that compromises were made with respect to the quality of new medical recruits. As early as 1793 a contemporary document criticised the *officiers de santé*, stating that they had no knowledge of either medical or military life. The *aides* and *sous-aides* were admitted to the army without examination. Many were of 'mediocre talents' and the author concluded that it would be difficult 'to make them love their duties'.[15] There are numerous anecdotes of poor medical services during the Revolutionary Wars. Medical care on the battlefield was either non-existent or arrived twenty-four to thirty-six hours after the action. Wounded and sick men rotted in filthy hospitals, often lying on straw crawling with vermin. Others could find no medical provision at all. A soldier of the Army of the Rhine suffering from fever presented himself at a hospital in the Haute-Saône but the hospital's nuns were unable to receive him. He then experienced similar refusals in the hospitals at Luxeuil and Remiremont. From there he gradually made his way to Besançon. During a bout of fever he lay down in a ditch at the side of the road waiting for it to resolve. By the time he arrived at Besançon he was not so sick and following return to his corps he sought refuge in the ambulance of his regiment.[16] We can only presume that many died in similar futile journeys seeking basic medical help.

The failings of the revolutionary army's medical services have to be viewed in the context of the wars. All was chaotic and deficient. There were never enough horses for transport. Food was so short that doctors had to slaughter their own horses to feed the sick and wounded. Shoes were viewed as a luxury. All equipment and supplies were insufficient and drugs were largely unavailable. Thus, it would not be fair to attribute all the deficiencies of the *service de santé* to the incompetence of its doctors.

There is evidence that, particularly in the early years of the wars, the doctors were enthused with revolutionary fervour. Surgeon Jean-Pierre Gama describes his young colleagues:

> They sought out the wounded on the battlefield, stripped off their own clothes to cover them, used their own food to nourish them, then bandaged them and had them taken or carried them themselves to the ambulances … in these patriotic acts they often attracted the fire of the enemy and were killed.[17]

For all its shortcomings, the French army's medical service was probably the best of the revolutionary period. Accounts of the Prussian hospitals and ambulances are damning.

The year 1803 marked the end of the Revolutionary Wars and the start of the Consulate and Empire. It also brought fundamental change in the *service de santé*. The new autocracy ushered in a different view of the role of the army's doctors. The beginning of the Consulate appears a watershed between the years of republican rule when the welfare of citizens and soldiers, including their health, was of genuine concern, and the fifteen years of Napoleonic domination when medical considerations were submerged by the stringencies of military strategy, administrative authority and economy. The Emperor thought only of the health of the Empire.

The first crucial legislation under the Consulate was the decree of *frimaire* year XII (December 1803) which dictated major organisational change in the *service de santé* including the abolition of the *conseil de santé*, some reorganisation of military hospitals and redefinition of the regimental medical arrangements. The *conseil* was replaced with a return to six inspector generals: two physicians, three surgeons and one pharmacist. At the outset these were Pierre-François Percy, Jean-François Coste (*médecin en chef de Val-de-Grâce*), Nicolas Heurteloup (*chirurgien en chef d'armée*), Dominique Larrey (*chirurgien en chef de la garde des consuls*) and Antoine-Augustin Parmentier (*pharmacien en chef de l'armée de Côte*). Undoubtedly, the previous *conseil* had been too small and had been elderly and ponderous. However, it had wielded some power. The newly elected inspector generals were younger and more dynamic but they tended to be isolated and were unable to act together in the interests of the service. This was despite the heroic individual efforts of Percy, Larrey and others. The overall impact of the new legislation was to allow the senior officers of the *service de santé* to fall further under the tutelage of the *commissaires des guerres* of the administration. The simultaneous closure of the hospitals of instruction exacerbated recruitment problems. Historians of the French Army have gone so far as to say that the legislation of *frimaire* XII was the 'decree of destruction of the *service de santé*'.[18]

If the decree was damaging to the service as a whole it did however bring some gains. The regimental medical staffing was better defined and organised. On a war footing, two surgeons were to be attached to each battalion and one to each cavalry squadron. Only one of the regimental surgeons was to be a *chirurgien-major*, the others being either *aides-majors* or *sous-aides* as shown below.

Regiment of 4 battalions
War footing: 1 *chirurgien-major*, 3 *aides-majors*, 4 *sous-aides*
Peace: 1 *chirurgien-major*, 1 *aide-major*, 2 *sous-aides*

Regiment of 3 battalions
War footing: 1 *chirurgien-major*, 2 *aides-majors*, 3 *sous-aides*
Peace: 1 *chirurgien-major*, 1 *aide-major*, 1 *sous-aide*

Cavalry Regiment of 4 squadrons
War footing: 1 *chirurgien-major*, 1 *aide-major*, 2 *sous-aides*
Peace: 1 *chirurgien-major*, 1 *aide-major*, 1 *sous-aide*

These surgeons were employed both with their corps and in local military and civil hospitals. *Chirurgiens-majors* and *aides-majors* were now required to have a medical doctorate and the *sous-aides* had to at least have passed some form of examination.[19]

The final indignity for the *officiers de santé* came in the form of a decree of November 1811. In fact it simply formalised a growing reality – the subjugation of the army's doctors to the *commissaires des guerres* and other agents of the administration. The *officiers de santé* were 'for that which concerns the service, the administration and execution of regulations, under the supervision of the *intendants genereaux* of the armies, the *commissaires ordonnateurs* and the *commissaires des guerres*'. Explicit details are provided as to appropriate punishments for the misdemeanours of senior and junior *officiers de santé*. For instance, 'All *commissaires des guerres* who have to punish an *officier de santé* of a lower grade, attached to an ambulance or hospital under their supervision, must immediately return a justification to the *commissaire ordonnateur* of the district.'[20] Senior *officiers de santé* might be subjected to suspension or even arrest on the orders of senior administrative staff such as the *intendants genereaux* or senior *commissaires ordonnateurs*. Predictably, the legislation was unpopular among the army's doctors as it removed any possible illusion as to their real position in the army's hierarchy.

If the uneasy relationship with the administration was one problem that the officers of Napoleon's *service de santé* had inherited from the revolutionary period, another was the lack of a true 'corps'. Their status remained low – a subject to which we will return – and their commission was only temporary, allowing them to be summarily dismissed with minimal notice. This lack of security also served as a disincentive for other employees in the *service de santé*. Following the Battle of Eylau in 1807, Percy recalls his conversation with the Emperor.

> 'Have you got a lot of wounded?'
> 'Sire, I believe that we have dressed 4,000.'
> 'Are they severely wounded?'
> 'There are a thousand who are in a very serious condition.'
> 'How many of the wounded will you lose?'
> 'A third, because the grapeshot and bursting shells have caused great destruction.'
> He asked Monsieur Lombard [*ordonnateur en chef*] if he had had a lot of people to assist. He replied that there were no hospital employees or *infirmiers*, but that there was no shortage of linen or lint or instruments.
> 'What organisation!' said the Emperor; 'What barbarism!'
> 'Sire,' said Monsieur Lombard, 'when one is sure of dismissal at time of peace, whatever good conduct one has given during the most miserable and perilous war, it is difficult to maintain enthusiasm and to commit oneself to follow an army as an employee or *infirmier*.'

Percy seized the moment to remark that service was good in the Imperial Guard because the medical personnel were entirely military and he pressed Napoleon to adopt a proper corps of surgeons for the rest of the army. The Emperor made a few platitudes but was shortly interrupted by an aide-de-camp of Marshal Davout and another opportunity was lost.[21] Percy's continuing efforts to gain his colleagues military status and some feeling of permanency were ultimately unsuccessful.

Despite the lack of real organisation under the Empire, the number of *officiers de santé* in the field gradually increased from a nadir of 1,085 in 1802 to 5,112 in 1812 (see Appendix I). With respect to the three specialities, the number of physicians increased from sixty-two to 277, surgeons from 842 to 3,762 and pharmacists from 171 to 1,011.[22] The remaining staffs were the inspector generals and other very senior officers. Although apparently inadequate for Napoleon's enormous armies, maintaining even this number of *officiers de santé* was a constant challenge. The disastrous Russian expedition of 1812 destroyed the *service de santé* as much as the rest of the army. All figures must be approximate but it appears that of over 800 surgeons registered in February 1812 fewer than 300 were alive in early 1813. The number of physicians was reduced from around a hundred to only thirty.

Despite relentless new legislation, the three basic medical specialities remained unchanged through the Revolutionary and Napoleonic Wars and it is appropriate to consider each in more detail. As the above figures demonstrate, the surgeons were the most numerous of the army's *officiers de santé*. Although their competence varied, they were in many ways the doctors most suited to the business of war, being practical men who could apply the necessary first aid on the battlefield and perform the subsequent surgery in the ambulances and hospitals. Their role was certainly less ambiguous than that of the physicians and pharmacists and, accordingly, requires less explanation. Surgeons were employed not only with the regiments, but also in the hospitals, with the army's ambulances, and at headquarters. There were generally more surgeons with the army than in the hospitals although the disparity varied year by year. In addition to the three grades of surgeon attached to regiments there were more senior ranks such as *chirurgien en chef* who would oversee the army's surgical service and supervise or perform more major operations in the field hospitals. A surgeon of the first class would often be responsible for the surgeons of a division. Within the hospitals, surgeons were divided into first, second and third classes equivalent to *chirurgien-major*, *aide-major* and *sous-aide* respectively. Surgeons were often frustrated in the hospitals, particularly the civil institutions, where they found themselves outranked by military and local physicians. Regimental surgeons fulfilling duties in such hospitals were not only limited in their authority but also sorely missed by their own units.

Surgeons appear more in their element on the road or the battlefield and Pierre-François Percy's memoirs give many helpful insights into their routine duties. Percy carried a considerable entourage of surgeons with him, forty-six in the campaign of 1807, and he gave considerable thought to their optimal distribution. As a single example, during the campaign of 1806,

> I have already sent three surgeons to Kronach and as many to Koenigshoffen ... Surgeons have left for Nuremberg, Anspach and other destinations. There remain only six surgeons at Branau and three at Augsbourg.

He was determined that his surgeons should all be put to optimal use and in Spain in 1808 we find him writing to Chief of Staff Berthier requesting that regimental surgeons remaining inactive at the regimental depots be sent to headquarters. He was fiercely proud of most of his surgical staff and when Napoleon criticised the hospital employees after the Battle of Eylau he was quick to jump in: 'Your Majesty, I am sure, will never confuse the surgeons with such men.' Yet even Percy had to acknowledge that the unstinting demand for more surgeons was compromising quality. Thus, in 1807 he writes: 'The majority of the young surgeons sent from Paris since 12 May have fallen sick. They are children of nineteen years who have no other vocation than removing themselves from conscription.'[23] The number of surgeons was often entirely inadequate for the task in hand. The Legion of the North in 1808 had only eighteen surgeons for over 5,000 men. As the Legion was short of trained military officers one of the *chirurgiens aide-majors*, Belhomme, took command of a company and showed great bravery. Sous-aide Dietrich was at the head of another. According to Lazare-Claude Coqueugnot, the Legion's major: 'I had nobody to dress the wounded because the surgeons were fighting as company commanders.'[24] This was evidently unacceptable and what was needed was a formal surgical corps to provide well regulated care on the battlefield. As we will see in a later chapter, Percy made just such a plan – his *chirurgie de bataille* – but like many of his laudable initiatives it was destined to fail in the face of Napoleon's indifference.

The profession of physician (*médecin*) was poorly represented in the army. Physicians were ultimately accountable to the *médecin en chef* who was responsible for their placement in the hospitals and the quality of the treatment administered to the sick. There were physicians of the first and second classes and also assistant physicians (*médecins-adjoints*), the latter being attached to the larger hospitals. The physicians generally receive a poor press, but this is perhaps partly because most of the medical accounts of the wars are the work of surgeons. Percy was not well disposed to physicians regarding them as potential competitors to his beloved surgical colleagues. When a failing Coste was replaced by another *médecin en chef*, Percy struggled to hide his disappointment, no doubt hoping that the post would become obsolete.[25] In his journal, he rarely misses a chance to criticise the hapless physicians. Thus at Tilsit in1807, 'We have 600 sick. Seven or eight physicians, of whom three are principals, just go for walks and it is our surgeons who do all the work. None of them [physicians], except those of the reserve, ever put a foot in our hospitals; tomorrow I will force them to do some work or will throw them out of town.' Later, we meet a physician 'who will abandon the service at the first migraine' and again it is the surgeons who save the day.[26]

Although Napoleon retained the post of *médecin en chef* he appears to have shared the disdain of the surgeons for the physicians. In December 1806, following a rant against the absent Coste in the presence of Percy, Napoleon turned his invective on all physicians. 'These are not the men that I need. I want young active men who are a little coarse and have balls.' We may conclude that he was thinking of surgeons and, indeed, he promptly dictated a note limiting the physicians to the hospitals and then for good measure, 'A *médecin en chef* in an army corps is absurd and useless – the *chirurgien-major* must also do the duty of the physician.'[27] Whenever the immediate concern was with battlefield surgery it is understandable that the physicians appeared at best supernumerary and at worse useless. However, they had a vital role to play in the control and management of disease and senior men such as Coste and Desgenettes did much good. Some of the more junior physicians also exceeded their duties suggesting that not all were intellectual fops conversing in Latin. Dutch physician, Salomon-Louis Laurillard-Fallot, one of the many foreign doctors who fought in the *Grande Armée*, overcame initial hostility from the French surgeons. At the Battle of Wagram in 1809 he stayed on the sidelines, 'the nature of my duties did not call me onto the field of suffering.' But in Germany in 1813,

> I assisted at the Battle of Bautzen. On the second day of this battle our ambulance was exposed to the fire of the enemy for a long time. I did not stop rendering treatment to the limit of my surgical knowledge although, strictly, my status as a physician exempted me from staying there. The presence of my black collar in the middle of the crimson collars [worn by surgeons] was noted by Monsieur Larrey. He remembered this at the end of the campaign when he was asked to make recommendations for honours.

At Waterloo, he was still more involved. Initially, he bandaged the wounded, but when he saw that his surgical colleagues were no more dexterous than him, he proceeded to perform several amputations.[28]

The third of the medical specialities, the pharmacists, had been previously referred to as apothecaries. At the outset of the Revolutionary Wars it was intended that there should be a pharmacist for every fifty sick men. This was certainly not achieved and under the Empire their number in the *Grande Armée* varied between 200 and 1,000. Just as for the surgeons and physicians, there was a senior *pharmacien en chef* directing the service with subordinate staff divided into three classes. It was their duty to manage the medicines both in the hospitals and with the army. Generally, one pharmacist would be attached to a hospital and several to an army division. In many campaigns both pharmacists and drugs were in short supply and the army's doctors were forced to deal directly with local apothecaries who were often 'miserable speculators'. As considerable amounts of money were used in the purchase of drugs the pharmacists themselves were not above suspicion. Percy writes in his journal at Danzig in 1807:

> The pharmacists have rushed here to request drugs; they are going, they say with a contented air, to purchase them for one hundred thousand francs; but I understand that their statement will be seen and signed by me and this disturbed them a little; I also understand that one of our surgeons will assist at the payment for the items.[29]

Unfortunately, there had been several well documented cases of corruption by pharmacists. In Egypt in 1799, the senior pharmacist was entrusted with five camels to bring medicines to the army. Instead he substituted sugar, coffee, wine and other foods for his own benefit. When his cheating was discovered he was ordered to be shot but he was reprieved following representations by other *officiers de santé* who felt that the honour of the service would be irredeemably damaged.[30] In Spain, Chief Pharmacist Flamand was dismissed after being found guilty of pillaging the pharmacy in the hospital at Burgos. Such anecdotes should not obscure the vital service provided by the pharmacists. Accounts by men such as Antoine-Laurent-Apollinaire Fée, Sébastien Blaze and Pierre-Irénée Jacob demonstrate that many were honest and capable. When the need arose, they were also prepared to step outside their usual role. At the Battle of Haslau in 1805 Jacob helped the surgeons at the ambulance, dressing the wounds and holding limbs during amputation.[31]

Napoleon's Imperial Guard had its own autonomous medical service. As befitted an elite unit this was well resourced and organised. Indeed, it was the only part of the *service de santé* that consistently functioned well and, ideally, it should have served as a model for the whole army. When first formed in 1800, the Guard had a general staff, an infantry corps, a cavalry corps and an artillery train. The infantry corps was composed of two battalions of *grenadiers* and one of *chasseurs* and included two surgeons of the first class and one of the second. The cavalry corps contained three squadrons of *grenadiers* and one of *chasseurs* and had one surgeon of each class. The Guard also had its own hospital at Gros-Caillou in Paris. This was overseen by the *commissaires des guerres* suggesting that even this privileged part of the medical service had not escaped the grasp of the administration. The precise number of medical personnel varied through the years of Empire depending on the size of the Guard. In 1804 it was as follows: one *chirurgien en chef* (Dominique Larrey), one surgeon of the first class (Paulet), two surgeons of the second class (Poirçon, Zinck), two surgeons of the third class (Ferlut, Vergès), one *médecin en chef* (Sue), one *pharmacien en chef* (Sureau), one pharmacist of the first class (Alyon), one pharmacist of the second class (Lagarde) and two pharmacists of the third class (Barbès, Foucy).[32]

These men were appointed by the Emperor following recommendation by senior generals. Staffing levels were increased at intervals although at times the service became hard-pressed with the hospital able to accommodate up to 500 sick and wounded. The Guard's medical service was 'militarised' with *infirmiers* (medical orderlies) taken directly from the battalions and the necessary transport and equipment being an integral part of the Guard's train. The relative efficiency of this service is likely to account for the more optimistic account of the wars given by Dominique Larrey compared with that of his colleague Pierre-François Percy. In his privileged position at the head of the Guard's service Larrey was to some degree protected from the realities of the remainder of the *service de santé*. Percy, in turn, was well aware that something similar to the Guard's medical service would have been an incalculable benefit to the soldiers of the line. When he does refer to Larrey and his service there is more than a hint of regret. For example, at the Battle of Jena in 1806,

His Majesty reviewed his Guard; I saw the Guard's surgeons, all well dressed with Monsieur Larrey at their head, and the *infirmiers,* commanded by a decorated officer, having their uniforms presented to them on the field.[33]

A more detailed account of the functioning and deficiencies of the *service de santé* in the hospitals and on the battlefields of the Empire is the subject of later chapters but we will complete this initial overview with some more general comments regarding the quality of the service. The following, written by Jean-Pierre Gama, who campaigned in Spain, is likely to represent the views of many doctors.

The Republican government which had sustained itself in the name of liberty had disappeared; that which had succeeded it took the path of love of glory, which is natural in France, but it did not retain the example of altruism so remarkably demonstrated in the welcome the wounded received on leaving the battle … already everything was haggled over … also it was necessary to call up the worst students found in the schools and even those from hospitals which were not approved for training. So-called doctors without experience or talent were admitted into the higher ranks of the army's *service de santé,* a sad necessity in view of the need to organise the service for the campaign of Austerlitz and the likely subsequent campaigns. The shortage of men destined primarily for a military career was a real misfortune for the army; but this misfortune would have been greater still if, at this time of glory and conquest, the enthusiasm with which each man tried to show himself worthy of his position had not made up for the knowledge which most of them lacked.[34]

It can be argued that the *service de santé* reached its peak during the last years of the 18th century in the Egyptian campaigns, stagnated between the years 1800 and 1809 and then collapsed in the final years of the Empire. This is contestable as there are undoubted examples of poor medical care throughout the years of Revolution and Empire, and equally, some instances of excellent medical provision at the end of the era. However, the combination of the Emperor's indifference to the service, unhelpful legislation, administrative incompetence, increasingly desperate medical recruitment and escalating casualties far from France's borders ensured that the deficiencies of the army's medical service became more obvious with each campaign. No longer were a few very competent and enthusiastic senior doctors and military officers able to paper over the cracks. The increasingly brutal nature of warfare, particularly in Spain and Russia, also played a role, removing the local help upon which the army's doctors had relied in earlier years. Undoubtedly, many of the *officiers de santé* were of mediocre quality but even those of exceptional merit were likely to sink beneath the growing sea of sick and wounded, hampered as they were by the grinding shortages and unhelpful administration. In these circumstances the medical service itself became dehumanised. One doctor writes of the Russian campaign:

> Everyone had the same idea; get rid of the wounded. Whenever the soldiers stopped to camp or to rest and these unfortunates needed to get out of the carriages or to have their dressings changed they were abandoned.[35]

This is not an isolated viewpoint. It is symptomatic of the declining years of an Empire that was born in the quest for glory and conquest but ultimately came to scorn humanity itself.

Notes

1. Blaze, S, *Mémoires d'un apothicaire sur la guerre d'Espagne*, Vol. II, pp. 220–30.
2. Brice, Docteur and Bottet, Capitaine, *Le Corps de Santé Militaire en France*, p.xxiv.
3. Blaze, E, *Military Life under Napoleon*, pp. 138, 146.
4. Pigeard, A, *Le Service de Santé de la Révolution au 1er Empire 1795–1815*, pp. 3, 73.
5. Vess, D M, *Medical Revolution in France 1789–1796*, pp. 24, 34, 38, 56, 65.
6. Brice, Bottet, pp. 53–5.
7. Pigeard, p.73; Brice, Bottet, pp. 53–8.
8. Vess, p. 68.
9. Brice, Bottet, pp. 57–9, 112.
10. ibid., p. 112.
11. ibid., p. 119.
12. Vess, pp. 85, 153.
13. Brice, Bottet, pp. 96–7.
14. ibid., pp. 98–9, 121.
15. Tissot, C J, *Observations générales sur l'administration des hôpitaux*, p. 6.
16. Morvan, J, *Le Soldat Impérial*, Vol. II, p. 297.
17. Kouchnir, S L L, *Considérations sur l'évolution du service de santé militaire de 1789 à 1814*, p. 19.
18. Brice, Bottet, p. 125.
19. ibid., pp. 126–7.
20. ibid., pp. 172–3.
21. Percy, Baron, *Journal des Campagnes de Baron Percy*, p. 168.
22. Brice, Bottet, p. 171.
23. Percy, pp. 75, 421, 371.
24. Brice, Bottet, p. 187.

25. Lemaire, J-F, *Coste: Premier Médecin des Armées de Napoléon*, p. 295.
26. Percy, p. 360.
27. Lemaire, J-F, *Napoléon et la Médecine*, p. 130.
28. Laurillard-Fallot, S-L, *Souvenirs d'un Médecin Hollandais sous les Aigles Françaises 1807–1833*, pp. 24, 33, 93, 111.
29. Percy, pp. 310, 267.
30. Brice, Bottet, p. 85.
31. Jacob, P-I, *Le Journal Inédit d'un pharmacien de la Grande Armée*, p. 86.
32. Brice, Bottet, pp. 148–50; Pigeard, p. 35.
33. Percy, pp. 91–2.
34. Brice, Bottet, p. 134.
35. Weiner, D B, *French Doctors Face War 1792–1815*, p. 70.

CHAPTER II
Officier de Santé

In describing the *service de santé* over the course of the Revolutionary and Napoleonic Wars we have relied largely on published regulations and other formal sources. To understand better the professional life of the ordinary army doctor – the *officier de santé* – it is necessary to resort to more anecdotal accounts. Only a review of the memoirs of doctors and soldiers allows an accurate portrayal of Napoleon's doctors. Only in these first-hand accounts can we plot their progress through early education, conscription, promotion and eventual dismissal from the army and also begin to understand their competence, status, rewards and disappointments.

We are using the term *officier de santé* to refer to the army's doctors. This requires explanation. During the revolution, zealous political correctness meant that the term 'doctor' could not be used. This might have implied inequality of the citizens of the republic. Any person engaged in treating the sick, whether properly qualified or not, and whether in military or civil capacity, would be addressed as *officier de santé*. In the first few years of the 19th century it was apparent that France required a structured legal framework for the orderly practice of medicine, surgery and midwifery. Particularly, training requirements needed to be more precisely defined. In 1803 Antoine François de Fourcroy, a doctor of medicine, chemist and teacher, created the legislation which underpinned medical practice in France for almost a century.

The major article of Fourcroy's Law made it unlawful to practise medicine in France without proper qualifications and created a two-tier system. Fully qualified doctors had to complete a conventional course of secondary education followed by studies at a medical faculty of a university leading to the degree of doctor of medicine. However, there were also medical practitioners of a lower calibre, the *officiers de santé*, with a more limited secondary education and the requirement for only a medical apprenticeship. The *officiers de santé* were effectively second class practitioners. For instance, doctors could practise anywhere in France but they were restricted to the *départements* in which they were registered. It was possible to move from the lower to the higher grade. In the army, physicians and surgeons who had been employed in a position of command or as a more senior *officier de santé* for two years could obtain the degree of doctor by presenting themselves to one of the medical schools and undergoing the last stage of the qualifying examination or by submitting a thesis. As we will see in subsequent pages, some army medical men did aspire to this promotion. The creation of the lower medical grade was an attempt to provide medical care for the enlarging army and the poorer sections of France.[1]

It is quite clear from contemporary documents that, in reality, there was considerable confusion regarding the terminology of medical practitioners. Thus, at the start of a document the term *médecin* might be used generically to describe the surgeons (*chirurgiens*) and physicians (*médecins*) and *officiers de santé* but, at the end, the term *officier de santé* suddenly appears as a description of all physicians, surgeons and pharmacists. Percy decried this general use of the term *officier de santé*. In 1806 he writes in his journal,

> I took this opportunity to ask Monsieur Intendant General to refer to us as *chirurgiens* and not as *officiers de santé*, a vague and generic denomination in which we are reluctant to be included and which causes us to be held in contempt.[2]

Nevertheless, there was a tendency to use the term to describe all the army's doctors, surgeons included, and this is reproduced in many later historical accounts of the *service de santé*. In this work, in the interests of simplicity, *officier de santé* refers to the entirety of Napoleon's doctors, irrespective of speciality or rank. Similarly, the English term 'doctor' is also used in its most general sense and does not imply anything more than *officier de santé*.

For the *officiers de santé*, the first step on the road to Austerlitz, the Berezina and Waterloo was their early education and their choice of medicine as a career, or at least as a way of avoiding conscription. Undoubtedly, the education of many was modest and ill prepared them for the later duress of army medicine. However, some had a prestigious medical training which, in different times, would have qualified them for a potentially lucrative and rewarding career in civil medicine. Surgeon Louis-Vivant Lagneau joined the army in 1803 and fought in the campaigns of Poland, Spain, Russia, France and the Hundred Days. Born in 1781, his earliest education was with a personal tutor and then in the college of his native town where he was taught Latin and grammar by the monks. At 16 years old he attended the local civil and military hospital at Chalon-sur-Saône under the tutorship of the hospital surgeon. Here, Lagneau says, 'there were a great number of young men who performed dressings and studied surgery ... The aim of most of them was to avoid conscription and be commissioned into the army as a surgeon.'

Lagneau had more principled goals. In order to improve the quality of his medical education he asked his mother and father to send him to Paris to 'follow the great masters of the art'. This, he acknowledges, was a great financial burden for his parents. At 18 years of age in 1799 he arrived in the capital and commenced an education that was unequalled elsewhere in France. He subscribed to courses in anatomy, physiology and surgery taken by the great medical doyens of the age such as Bichat and Boyer. In his second year, at the *école practique*, he continued these subjects but also studied chemistry, pharmacy, medicine and obstetrics. He notes that the professorial teaching in anatomy, physiology and medicine was excellent. At the end of three years' conscientious work, 'forcing my lazy memory to retain everything to which I entrusted it', he felt ready to attempt his *certificate de capacité*, the title of doctor not then being enacted (Fourcroy's Law being still two years in the future).

A great opportunity then presented itself to the young Lagneau. The so-called grade of *interne* was the most prestigious training post in the Paris hospitals. It had previously been awarded more on the basis of connection and patronage than on ability but, in the new order of things, all students were now able to enter the examination. The competition for the medical student's *'baton de maréchal'* was predictably intense. The few successful candidates would be expected to see all sick patients on their arrival at the hospital and then make evening rounds supervising treatment and dressings and making appropriate notes. It was an unparalleled learning opportunity. Lagneau's industry was rewarded and he was able to answer the examination questions with 'aplomb and sang-froid'. Moreover, his lofty third place entitled him to a place at the desirable *Hôtel Dieu*, a privilege limited to the six most successful students. This honour was denied him by a less able but better connected student, an echo of the past, and he performed the bulk of his internship at the *service des infirmeries et des nourrices* and the *Hôpital du Midi* where he was able to pursue a thesis in venereal diseases. He then left the hospital to assist a successful Paris doctor in his local practice, holding surgeries in the doctor's absence and making home visits to the patients. By the summer of 1803 he had submitted his thesis and obtained the *certificate de capacité*, a qualification which, following the new legislation of the same year, could be exchanged for a doctorate in medicine.[3]

François Poumiès de la Siboutie obtained his internship in 1812 and his memoirs are an evocative account of a Paris medical education later in the wars. He was candid regarding his reasons for studying medicine.

I had always thought the life of a medical man a most enviable one. In the country districts there were very few of them and they were only called in emergencies. On ordinary occasions people were content with the services of the *officier de santé*. Doctors were welcome everywhere

23

and highly paid. They kept fine houses and received numerous presents of early fruit, vegetables, game, and fish and were treated with unusual deference.

When he first arrived in Paris in 1810 he was struck by the number of 'hunchbacks and cripples' among his fellow medical students, nearly all the fit young men having been conscripted into the army. By 1811 he had risen to the position of 'dresser' at the *Hôpital Saint-Louis* and he spent his time dissecting, attending lectures on surgery and taking clinical notes. Although not such a brilliant student as Lagneau, in the following year he came seventeenth out of 120 candidates for the *interne* post and just qualified for one of the eighteen places.[4]

One of the great advantages of the Paris internship was that it attracted 500 francs per year in addition to free board and lodgings whilst on duty. Many medical students of the era struggled to pay for their studies and deeply regretted being a drain on their family. Joseph Tyrbas de Chamberet came from a noble but ruined family and he spent the last few pence of his inheritance qualifying as a doctor. He later entered the army as a physician and campaigned in Italy and Spain and witnessed the disintegration of the *Grande Armée* at Waterloo. His life as a student in the Paris hospitals in 1804 was not an easy one. He had only the miserable sum of fifty francs per month to pay for his food, lodgings, lighting, laundry and new shoes and clothes. In these circumstances, he was forced to plan his expenditure to the nearest centime and resort to the 'most severe and strict economies'. Every evening, he worked with his impoverished fellow students without a fire and reading under a single candle. During the day he frequented cheap restaurants in the Latin Quarter surviving on cheese, milk and dry bread. Concerned that his health might suffer from such a spartan regime he took special care to protect himself, taking walks in the gardens of the Luxembourg and bathing in the Seine. He was especially careful to wash himself after the anatomical dissections, sometimes repulsive, and after prolonged work in the hospitals. Tyrbas de Chamberet's dedication was rewarded as he ultimately obtained an internship with attachment to a number of Paris hospitals including the *Cochin, Saint-Louis* and *Hôtel Dieu.*[5]

Others had to overcome not only physical hardship but an initial dislike of their chosen vocation. Urbain Fardeau served as a surgeon in the armies of Republic and Empire, winning the *Légion d'honneur* for his gallantry in the field. He was initially destined for the priesthood but then changed to medicine and arrived in Paris in the 1790s to further his studies. At first he was revolted by surgery but, by degrees, he accommodated himself to it and resolved to overcome all difficulties to learn 'this beautiful art which makes the lame walk and the blind see'. Fardeau was older and more affluent than most of the Parisian students and, as he also befriended the senior surgeon of the *Hôtel Dieu,* he had a very comfortable life in the city.[6]

Of course, for all the students in whom we have an interest, the future Napoleon's doctors, their studies were a precursor to their eventual entry into the army. A few joined up because they had a true vocation for the military life or out of patriotic fervour, but, for the great majority, the reasons were more pragmatic. To appreciate this fully it is necessary to understand the means by which Napoleon conscripted new recruits into his army. In each local community an alphabetical list of potential conscripts was drawn up. This included all young men of suitable age who were deemed fit for service. A draw was made and those whose number was selected were then destined for Napoleon's legions unless they could afford the hefty sum of six to ten thousand francs to purchase a replacement.[7] For most students of medicine the latter was not an option and joining the army as a doctor appeared a lesser evil compared with the random conscription of an ordinary soldier. Thus, in 1803 at 21 years old, the talented medical student Louis-Vivant Lagneau was called up to join the army.

> My position was becoming difficult. My title of *interne* and even that of doctor did not enable me to ignore the law and if I left I would be saying good-bye to my dreams of advancement in the Paris hospitals. On the other hand, my parents finances were not sufficient to find me a replacement as a soldier. I therefore attempted to join the army as a surgeon of the third class (*sous-aide-major*).

Lagneau heard nothing from the army's medical service and began to fear that he would indeed be enlisted as an ordinary soldier and would lose all the potential benefits of his four years of medical study. Out of desperation he presented himself to Percy, at this time an inspector general of the *service de santé*, showing the senior army doctor his thesis and diploma. He also wrote letters to two of the other inspectors, Larrey and Heurteloup. All this lobbying was ultimately successful and in October 1803 he was attached to the ambulances of the *Armée des Côtes* which was in camp on the northern French coast preparing to invade England.[8]

Ten years later, medical student Jacques Duret joined the *148ᵉ de ligne* as an *aide-major* in identical circumstances. Whilst he was studying in Paris, the draw for conscription was made in his home town of Dijon and he drew the unlucky 'number 3'. He estimated that a replacement would have cost 10,000 francs and that, in any case, this would simply have been a stay of execution. According to Duret, the application for a surgical post in the army was the usual resource of medical students.

Although the avoidance of conscription is a dominant theme in the memoirs of army doctors, some did join for other reasons. However, even in these cases, the reasons were more often prosaic than sentimental. Percy joined the army as an *aide-major* in 1776 simply to avoid being a financial liability to his family. Heinrich Roos, a physician in the *Grande Armée*, was following in a family tradition of military service. In his formative years he accompanied his soldier father in the campaigns of the last decade of the 18th century and was particularly impressed by the military physicians serving in the hospitals of Alsace and the Rhine.[9]

Whatever their reason for joining Napoleon's forces, the new army doctors often had serious reservations regarding their new life. Even those with some sense of vocation were often less than wholehearted. Heinrich Roos remembers that when he marched out of his home country of Württemberg he and many of his friends embraced the frontier post wondering if they would ever again see their birthplace. Those whose medical commissions were effectively obligatory were, predictably, even less enthusiastic. Lagneau bitterly regretted being forced to leave his comfortable and promising career in Paris and, although spared from 'carrying the musket', he viewed the future with deep pessimism. Joseph Tyrbas de Chamberet, short of money and disillusioned with Napoleonic France, later regretted that he had joined the army 'blindly' and had wasted six years of his life. Jacques Duret claimed that his military services ultimately brought him, 'forty francs, pox, misery, the loss of my big right toe, typhoid fever, and the medal of Saint Helena'.[10]

The combination of heavy losses of medical officers and the reluctance of doctors to join up led to inevitable difficulties in recruitment for the *service de santé*. By early 1813 the problem had become acute. To bring the service up to strength there was a need for around 120 physicians, a little over 400 surgeons and a similar number of more junior *sous-aides*. Two circulars, one in April regarding the physicians and surgeons and a second in May concerning the *sous-aides*, were sent to the prefects of each department demanding that they each send to the army's headquarters in Mayence (Mainz) one physician, four surgeons and three *sous-aides*. If all were able to comply this would provide 188 physicians, 472 surgeons and 354 *sous-aides* in total. The less experienced *sous-aides* could still be culled from those students wishing to avoid conscription. For the more senior posts of physician and surgeon the demand was for men approaching 30 years, ideally unmarried, and who had previous service with the army.

A few prefects quickly complied with this order putting the requested doctors on the road to Mainz. However, only around forty prefects replied with perhaps double this number remaining silent. A few expressed their difficulties in writing.

> Our *officiers de santé* who have already served are all old, wounded, fathers of families, and in no condition to serve again. Among the others, the government has requested that we favour those who are unmarried. And there are so few of them suitable that I regret we will not be able to be restricted to this class.[11]

Many who were ultimately selected were old, sometimes over 50 years, and poorly qualified. Following the disastrous retreat from Russia doctors in civil life had little interest in joining the army. This reflected a wider malaise. During the campaign in Germany, the number of deserters from the army as a whole rose to 250,000. Some medical men nominated by the prefects simply disobeyed. Others went to elaborate lengths to avoid the wars. This was a particular problem in 1813 but it was hardly new. In 1807 a medical student named Teisseia was fined five hundred francs and jailed for two years for distributing a powder which could be used to induce an eye disease. In 1810 Percy and Desgenettes toured the hospitals seeking out young men who were simulating illness in the hope of being discharged. Larrey, by dint of his seniority and reputation, received letters from senior colleagues requesting that particular 'deserving' students be excused from military call up. For instance, the following from the senior physician at the hospital of *Enfants de France* on behalf of one of his favourites in 1811.

> He was elected external pupil at the *Hôtel Dieu* in the competition of 1809 and since this time he has worked with great zeal. Unfortunately, his constitution is not as good as one might desire. His chest is narrow and feeble and he only enjoys his current health because of a cautery [heat treatment] he had four years ago. In this situation, he dreads conscription ...[12]

Some of the doctors near to Napoleon also appeared a little reluctant to get too close to the war. The Emperor had a senior physician, surgeon and pharmacist as part of his personal staff. The physician, Corvisart, was hastily summoned to Vienna a few days after the Battle of Wagram. Napoleon promised him further fighting and the spectacle of a great battle. 'Sire,' he replied, 'I am not curious.' The pharmacist, Boyer, campaigned in Spain, where he performed a delicate operation on Marshal Suchet's anus. He lived in constant fear of the Spanish guerrillas and when returning to Paris he vowed never again to go on a similar adventure. When Deyeux, a teacher of chemistry at the Paris Medical Faculty, was offered the post of personal pharmacist to the Emperor it was accepted with one condition – he would not go to the army.[13]

Despite the continued strain of maintaining medical recruitment at the necessary levels, an attempt was made to ensure at least a minimal level of competence. From the earliest years of the Revolutionary Wars, doctors entering the army had had to pass some form of examination although this was often rudimentary. In 1791 a young surgeon called Lombard, the son of the former surgeon-in-chief of civilian and military hospitals, sat the examination which included questions on the methods used for ensuring competence of health officers, the methodology of wound bandaging, and the correct surgical management of aneurysm, the ballooning of an artery. In his eight-page answer sheet he noted in his answer to the first question that too many incompetents were being admitted to the army. He later detailed surgical measures for aneurysm which would have been inevitably fatal. He still passed and was assigned to the Army of the Rhine as a surgeon of the first class.[14]

Ironically, the most talented doctors in the army were also expected to comply with the vagaries of the National Convention's examination system. In 1793 it was decreed that all *officiers de santé*, irrespective of previous service, had to pass an examination to continue to serve in the hospitals and in the army. The *conseil de santé* was entrusted with this undertaking which involved a combination of written and oral tests. Percy, despite his lofty academic qualifications and elevated post in the army, was sent these questions in a sealed envelope. He then had to attend his own municipality of Bouzonville to open the envelope in front of local officials, including the mayor, and answer the questions immediately without books or notes. This must have been a source of irritation to him but he dutifully complied. When Louis-Vivant Lagneau took a similar test in 1797 he thought that the questions were 'elementary'.[15]

Similar practices continued under the Empire, although the implementation was variable. Eugene Fenech, of Maltese extraction, joined the *Grande Armée* in 1807 as a *chirurgien sous-aide* to avoid conscription as a soldier. Initially working in the naval hospital at Toulon, his request for a transfer to the army was made to the *conseil de santé* and he received the following questions to answer: 'Describe the peritoneum and give the names of all the types of abdominal hernias. Describe the bubonocoele [a type of hernia] and discuss the most appropriate time for operation and the method used.' Under the supervision of a doctor in Toulon, Fenech was shut in a room and allowed two and a half hours to write his answers. He was later permitted to make a neat copy under strict instruction to make no alterations. Twelve days later, he was ordered to join the *corps d'observation de la Gironde* as an army doctor.[16]

Although the questions seem little suited to assess ability as an army surgeon, Fenech's examination was well organised and invigilated with little opportunity for cheating. This was not universal. Antoine-Laurent-Apollinaire Fée served as a pharmacist in the Peninsular War and at Waterloo. He originally joined the army in 1809 as a *pharmacien sous-aide* to the Army of Spain.

> Such was the difficulty of securing adequate numbers of *officiers de santé* that the requirement for proper examinations was dispensed with. It was enough to respond in writing to some elementary questions. Called by the Minister of War to fulfil this formality, I found myself by the side of a young man who was planning to be a surgeon. Because our applications were different, they believed it acceptable to leave us together. This was

a mistake because I did both tests, mine and his, and yet I had scarcely any knowledge of surgery at all. He was accepted and much later I saw him again with the army carrying his head high and very proud of his knowledge.[17]

Once in the army, most doctors began to think of promotion. This was poorly regulated and was influenced by a number of factors including merit, seniority and patronage. The support of senior military and medical officers was especially important. Percy took great delight in furthering the careers of his young surgeons, 'my hussars', as he fondly referred to them. When, in 1809 in Spain, Napoleon decorated several surgeons, Percy personally embraced them and pinned the ribbon to their uniforms. He recorded in his journal: 'This day will be among the best days of my life.' Although evidently very protective of his junior staff, Percy was not sentimental and had fixed views as to the type of men whom he wished promoted. As the senior surgeon in the field he rejected appointment on the basis of seniority alone.

> I replied to his Excellency [the Minister of War] that there was no point in sending me an invalid to assist me; that I had already too much to do myself; that he should have been convinced by the example of M. Dupont that old men were out of place in the army of Spain; that, far from thinking like my septuagenarian colleagues, who attribute all to seniority and calculate endlessly the days and years, I prefer to appoint young men …

Percy was keen to impose his own views on the service and made specific suggestions for promotion of surgeons. Thus, late in 1809, we find him writing a long letter to the Minister of War in which he suggests twenty sous-aides for promotion. In general, he seems to have succeeded in his nominations although, on occasion, he was frustrated by apparently random medical promotions. In Valladolid, the Emperor promoted two aides-chirurgiens to chirurgien-major on the recommendation of the colonels of their regiments. Percy was not amused,

> … the second is better than the first. At least he campaigned in Portugal, something for which His Majesty is keen to give reward. However, the other stayed in France and got married, not serving for a whole year. Moreover, he is a repulsive figure with no trace of education or talent. It would be better if His Majesty required proof of competence before approving those that the colonels present to him.[18]

Percy's involvement in patronage is confirmed by the frequency with which his name is invoked in the memoirs of more junior doctors. For example, Louis-Vivant Lagneau received three letters of support from Percy in his quest for promotion from *sous-aide* to *aide-major* in the years 1804 to 1806. In all three letters, Percy, in a very informal style, pledges support to Lagneau, but also stresses that he does not have unlimited powers. On 3 March 1804:

> I have not been able, my dear sir, to get my colleagues in Paris to agree to propose you for the rank of *chirurgien-aide-major*; it is not that they do not, like me, have great regard for your good conduct or your education, but they are afraid to break the rules in promoting to the second rank a young man who has been only five or six months in the first … Your title of doctor and authorship of a very interesting thesis seems to me to be irrefutable. However, all is lost to those terrible words 'don't break the rules'. Camus is an extremely ignorant fool, but having dragged his stupidity through the hospitals for twelve years, he has obtained the title that really I had believed fair and decent to ask for you. They are a fine thing, rules!

Percy reassured Lagneau that there was a good chance of him soon replacing a resigned *chirurgien-aide-major*. He encouraged him to seek further patronage from men such as Larrey and Desgenettes. An educated man like Lagneau was just the sort of doctor whom Percy wished to succeed. In July 1805 the desired promotion had still not materialised and Percy again corresponded with the young surgeon, encouraging him to petition the Minister of War directly as he had such a strong case. 'I assure you that none of your competitors interests me more than you.' By January 1806 the pressure was increased as Percy added a personal note to a letter of Lagneau and sent it on to the Minister of War:

> My dear Lagneau, I have sent to the Minister of War, the letter you have written to me from Lagnago. I have added the words, 'A scandalous injustice has been committed in naming Monsieur Fondretona, the most mediocre of *chirurgiens-aides-majors* and a former hat maker's assistant, as *chirurgien-major* and a disgraceful mistake has been made in not presenting for advancement, Monsieur Lagneau, one of the most distinguished surgeons of our armies and an eminent doctor of the School of Paris.'

One detects a hint of snobbery in the reference to the maligned surgeon's former occupation. Lagneau eventually attained promotion to *sous-aide* and to *chirurgien-major* both because of and despite the influence of patronage. His second promotion to *chirurgien-major* in the Imperial Guard was achieved despite the opposition of Larrey who had his own favourite. Lagneau's application was supported by Napoleon as he had already been awarded the *Légion d'honneur* and because, perhaps surprisingly, the intervention of Larrey carried little weight among the more senior military officers of the Guard. Lagneau was later to miss out on an effective promotion to a more prestigious regiment within the Guard as the general responsible for the appointment selected his own favourite surgeon who had treated his wound at the Battle of Witepsk. This was despite Lagneau's precedence as the most senior *chirurgien-major*.[19]

Percy makes cameo appearances in other memoirs. In April 1812 Pharmacist Pierre-Irénée Jacob obtained his promotion to *pharmacien-major* following 'several visits to Monsieur Percy'. He had previously campaigned in Poland and Spain and subsequently fought in Russia and in the campaign of 1813. In January 1814 Maltese army doctor Eugene Fenech presented a fellow countryman to Percy as a potential *chirurgien-major*. The promotion was promptly expedited but Fenech notes that the recipient 'was not grateful to Monsieur Percy and did not thank him, attributing his promotion to the recommendation of the colonel of the regiment'.[20]

The process of promotion could be complicated and was prone to error. Aide-chirurgien Jean-Baptiste d'Héralde believed his promotion to have been delayed because the senior surgeon supporting him was not favoured by Percy. When he finally did receive his promotion to *chirurgien-major* whilst campaigning in Poland in 1807 it was in Percy's presence and in farcical circumstances. At the army's headquarters, Percy initially apologised to d'Héralde for his lack of advancement and explained the reasons. However, the army's senior surgeon then consulted the orders of the Fifth Corps and it was apparent that a name had been crossed out and d'Héralde inserted as a *chirurgien-major* in the Second Division. According to d'Héralde, 'All my comrades started to laugh and I do not know if I or the *chirurgien-en-chef* was the most embarrassed. I did not know if I ought to thank him.' It was not the correct division but d'Héralde kept the higher rank.[21]

Where patronage was not so prominent, promotion was likely to be driven by seniority. When Heinrich Roos entered Russia in 1812, he was the most senior of the twenty-six physicians in his army corps and he was promised promotion at the first vacancy. In a destructive campaign promotion was likely to be more rapid. This was largely the reason that André Guilmot joined the expedition to St Domingo as a 24-year-old *officier de santé* in 1802. After an earlier dismissal from the army, he regarded this as his best opportunity for advancement as a surgeon. 'In St Domingo I could make my fortune; if things work out well I should obtain at least the second grade and then try to return to France.' As for many others, the West Indies attachment was not so kind and he was soon sick and facing another retirement from the army.[22]

There are examples of officers receiving promotion entirely through their competence and devotion. Hyacinthe Covali, *aide-major* of the battalion of the *tirailleurs de Po*, was said by the members of the *conseil d'administration* of the *11ᵉ léger* to have given high quality care to the soldiers of the regiment for nine years. They requested that the Minister of War elevate him to *chirurgien-major*. This was complied with but the surgeon died the same year at the crossing of the Berezina. If promotion was not forthcoming it was usually attributed to some injustice rather than to any lack of merit. Dutch physician Salomon-Louis Laurillard-Fallot served with the French army on the notoriously unhealthy island of Walcheren in 1808. He says that his failure to progress from *médecin adjoint* (assistant physician) to *médecin ordinaire* was primarily due to unfavourable reports made by the senior physician at Middelburg. 'It was an injustice, if I dare say it, because my service left nothing to be desired.' He had to wait another four years for the promotion. Joseph Tyrbas de Chamberet, who takes a jaundiced view of the army's affairs, sums up the feelings of many in explaining the lack of progress of a talented colleague.

> If rank had been given on the basis of merit and good service he would have filled one of the senior positions in military surgery. However, he was only a simple *aide-major*. It is because to get into the higher ranks of this career, as in others, it is necessary to employ intrigue, slipperiness, and charlatanism and that which is generally known as *savoir-faire* and he was totally lacking in these things.[23]

If promotion was obtained it was all too often insecure and transient. When Jean-Baptiste d'Héralde received his commission as a surgeon of the third class at the military hospital of Saint-Denis in 1802, he was phlegmatic regarding its 'temporary' status as this was regarded as normal for military doctors. The lack of a proper corps of army doctors in the *service de santé* and the temporary nature of the commissions of the *officiers de santé* has already been alluded to. Peremptory dismissal was a constant threat. The first substantial wave of redundancies occurred in 1800 and 1801. This was exacerbated by a decree of 1802 which led to a reduction in both the number of available (*disponible*) surgeons and the surgeons belonging to the corps. Their total number was reduced to little over 500, well below the minimum of a thousand recommended by the *conseil de santé* to the Premier Consul. By 1803 the hospital staff was also under attack with the *hôpitaux d'instruction* closed and the personnel in the remaining hospitals limited to a physician, a *chirurgien-major* and a pharmacist. Not even the presence of the *chirurgien-major* was guaranteed, the Premier Consul suggesting that hospital patients could be cared for by *officiers de santé* of the corps stationed in the vicinity. These measures may have been reasonable in a stable peace but with the constant likelihood of further fighting they appear ill considered.

Percy decried the practice of laying off *officiers de santé* during the short breaks in the war. In 1807, shortly after the Battle of Friedland, he raised it directly with Napoleon.

The Emperor said some very flattering things about the function of our [medical] service; I praised the skill and precious work of our surgeons, who alone did everything that was possible; I made a point of recommending to him this group of doctors so necessary and so devoted and explained to him the danger of dispersing and laying them off in peacetime. Unusually, I took leave of His Majesty without waiting for him to dismiss me with the words 'it is good', as was his custom. In my situation I was always very preoccupied and one can forgive me for having erred in a matter of etiquette.[24]

A further wave of dismissals struck the *officiers de santé* at the two Restorations. After the first fall of Napoleon in 1814, a prolonged peace was anticipated and Percy and Larrey were instructed to take on the thankless task of laying off their colleagues. According to General Marchand, they had to restrict those remaining to the absolute minimum. The process was complicated by the need to reinstate elderly army doctors who had shown earlier loyalty to the Royal Family, for instance those who had served in the Army of the Condé. Dismissals were not unique to the *service de santé* but the army's doctors were particularly poorly treated. Joseph Tyras de Chamberet recalls:

A little later, the allied troops having evacuated the capital, *l'hôpital du Roule* was closed and I was laid off like an enormous number of employees and military officers of the army. But I was not to enjoy the half-pay that was granted to the latter. I found myself, once again, having to consider my future.[25]

The early education of the *officiers de santé* has been discussed. But what did they learn once they joined the *Grande Armée*? In the Revolutionary Wars there had been well-meaning attempts to ensure that young military doctors were trained on the job. One suggestion was that students should learn by helping in the treatment of wounded at first-aid camps near to the armies in the field. This practical type of teaching persisted under the Empire and its importance was extolled by Larrey and Percy. Larrey's memoirs are peppered with references to teachings which were attended not only by the surgeons under his charge but also by civilian doctors and even the enemy surgeons of occupied countries. At Vienna, where he treated the wounded of the Battle of Wagram, he asked the Emperor for a school of military surgery in Paris but this was apparently not followed up. The convent of *Val-de-Grâce* in the capital had been converted to a military teaching hospital by the National Convention but it did not ever properly fulfil this function.[26]

Percy also made time in his busy schedule to educate his younger colleagues but it was not always easy. For instance, at Warsaw, after the Battle of Eylau in 1807:

The town is so dirty and there is so much mud inside and out that it is difficult to walk about. We have gathered to talk about surgery; I have given two long lectures on surgical instruments and tomorrow we will start a course on bandaging. Our young men have not been taught and I believe they are not disposed to educate themselves; they spend half the day foraging up to three or four leagues to feed their horses and to contrive to feed themselves.

The army's senior doctor persevered and, after Friedland, we find him delivering a lecture on botany to a group of surgeons. Percy believed that it was important to use the resources of the surrounding country to stimulate and educate. In Egypt, Desgenettes encouraged the physicians in the expeditionary force to read extensively about the prevailing diseases.[27]

It is easy to understand an army doctor's indifference to further education when he was struggling to survive on campaign. However, when circumstances were more favourable, at least some showed a desire for self-improvement. This was particularly the case in 1804 in the camps of northern France, the formative period of the *Grande Armée*. Here, young surgeons such as Louis-Vivant Lagneau, Jean-Baptiste d'Héralde and Urbain Fardeau showed a real enthusiasm for their new vocation. Lagneau assisted at operations and remembers the surgeons and physicians getting together at Ostend to form a society where they could discuss pertinent points in medicine and science. This was actively supported by Percy. D'Héralde also had plenty of opportunities to learn.

The *médécin en chef*, Monsieur Biron, who showed some interest in me, sent me from the camp to serve as an *aide-major* at hospital number 1 in Calais. This was the happiest time of my life ... It is there that I met Monsieur Chappe, principal surgeon of 4e corps. He gave me the responsibility of delivering courses in anatomy and operations and dressings to all the *aides* in hospitals number 1 and 2; I had to work day and night ... I was allowed to perform all the major operations in the hospital which were a daily occurrence in view of the large number of wounded from the fleet which was involved in bloody fighting nearly every week; there were subluxations and fractures caused by the frequent falls of the soldiers onto the decks and the musket ball wounds that they received all too often.[28]

Urbain Fardeau claims that when he tried to arrange courses of instruction at the hospital in Boulogne, Percy acted to prevent him. This appears a little strange and one can only presume that he had his reasons. In the event, Fardeau appealed directly to Marshal Soult and was permitted to teach subjects such as anatomy, physiology and disease;

his pupils were a diverse group including *chirurgiens-majors*, hospital employees, *commissaires* and young officers from the Paris schools. The determined surgeon was one of a number of army doctors who contrived to further their medical education during the intensive campaigning of the Napoleonic wars.

> During my stay in Paris, I submitted my thesis which I had written, without any books, in a windmill in the small village of Hussowitz on the field of the battle of Austerlitz, near to the famous windmill of Milzée, where the three emperors met.[29]

Despite the attempts at training, many of the doctors of the *Grande Armée* were of low calibre and competence. This reality, like many of the shortcomings of the *service de santé*, was to some degree inherited from the revolutionary period. Shortages of army doctors in the last decade of the 18th century led to very generous assessment of competence. For example, an elderly farm worker was commissioned as a pharmacist because he had been 'apprenticed in pharmacy' in his earliest years. Under the Empire, the combination of a relentless demand for *officiers de santé* and the increasing desperation of young men to avoid conscription as soldiers meant that mediocrity had to be tolerated. Percy coined the term '*chirurgiens de pacotille*' to describe this rump of low quality and uninterested army doctors. 'Pacotille' is literally translated as 'cheap rubbish' or 'junk'. In his journal, Percy frequently shows his exasperation with the behaviour of such men. After Eylau, he describes a 'certain *aide-major*' using a poor saw to clumsily cut through the bone and damaged tissues of the leg of a captain who had been struck by a cannon ball. It was a wholly inappropriate procedure.

> To save this brave officer who had clearly suffered so much it was necessary to amputate at the hip on the same or following day. The *aide-major* is a detestable surgeon and should be sacked for his immorality.

Under extreme provocation, Percy was unable to restrain himself.

> This morning, a man named H......, *sous-aide* to the 44e regiment, where he had murdered an officer and from where he had been driven out, presented himself to me wearing the magnificent uniform of a *chirurgien-major* and an Asiatic sabre etc. I fell upon him with kicks and punches and hit him so hard that I have damaged the ring finger of my right hand.

In addition to the immediate damage caused by these incompetent surgeons, Percy feared that they would bring into disrepute his precious discipline of military surgery when later discharged from the army.[30]

Many ordinary soldiers have left accounts of their encounters with the *chirurgiens de pacotille*. Jean Morvan, in his magisterial review of the soldiers of Napoleon's army, *Le Soldat Impérial*, expresses the common view.

> They had become *officiers de santé* to escape the musket and the haversack; scarcely had the campaign opened than they tried to avoid the fighting. They protected themselves, they clung on to the first hospitals, they stopped near to the first cripples, they did not move beyond the first group of wounded soldiers.

When Colonel de Gonneville became ill at Tilsit in 1807, he says that the *chirurgien-major* was an 'ass' and that everything he prescribed had a completely opposite effect to that anticipated. Lieutenant Heinrich August Vossler, a Württemberger accompanying the *Grande Armée* into Russia, worried about his sick and wounded men, 'for we knew a great deal about the negligence and sometimes downright brutality with which French doctors were in the habit of treating their patients'. Whilst this opinion may have had a nationalistic slant, the French doctors themselves had to acknowledge that some of their colleagues left much to be desired. Assistant Physician Joseph Tyrbas de Chamberet was unimpressed by senior colleagues without instruction or diplomas who, prior to joining the army, he had seen 'dragging their ineptitude and ignorance around the streets of Paris'.[31]

Tyrbas de Chamberet was also quick to point out that not all his fellow army doctors were like this and, indeed, it would be wrong to tar all *officiers de santé* as *chirurgiens de pacotille*. There is enough anecdotal evidence to suggest that significant numbers of military doctors were not only competent judged by contemporary standards, but were also highly principled, displaying selflessness, dedication and, above all, bravery. To practise good medicine and surgery in the face of the constant threats from disease and arms was a considerable challenge. The losses of *officiers de santé* in the Wars of Empire speak for themselves. In Egypt, the doctors were quarantined inside the plague hospitals, dying by the side of their patients. Eighty-two of them perished, a third of all the surgeons failing to survive the campaign. The West Indies was a greater death trap. In St Domingo in 1802, the *officiers de santé* were under siege both from yellow fever and the local insurgents. Refusing to abandon their patients in the hospitals, those who survived infection were indiscriminately massacred when the hospital fell into enemy hands. Sous-aide Guilmot writes that of two hundred *officiers de santé* who had arrived on the island before him, there were only five left alive. This may appear greatly exaggerated but the names of 180 physicians, surgeons and pharmacists who failed to return from the expedition are inscribed on the marble tables of the *Val-de-Grâce*.[32]

The demoralising losses of army doctors continued during the wars of attrition fought in Europe between 1805 and 1815, particularly in Spain and Russia. In the Peninsula, it was commonplace for the *service de santé*'s hospitals to be left in the hands of a few young and wholly inexperienced 'doctors'. In 1812 the *officiers de santé* were not spared the decimation that afflicted the rest of the *Grande Armée*. Pharmacist Pierre-Irénée Jacob's division entered Russia with one physician, eight surgeons, four pharmacists and four hospital employees. In January 1813 he was the only one to recross the Oder river, the remainder already dead or lying sick in the hospitals. Of the latter, he knew of only one who had actually returned to France. The division of Heinrich Roos fared little better, he being the only one of seven physicians to survive the Russian debacle.[33]

Apart from the constant threat of disease, the army's surgeons frequently found themselves working under fire. There are numerous examples in Percy's journal. At the Battle of Eylau in 1807, Surgeon Poussielgue bandaged the wounded in the neighbouring town but was eventually forced to abandon his post by the shells and cannon balls destroying the houses. Later, at the siege of Danzig, the *chirurgien-major* of the 2[e] regiment of infantry miraculously escaped when four cannon balls struck the building in which he was working. On occasions, surgeons deliberately exposed themselves to danger in order to protect their patients. Larrey recounts that in Cairo in 1798 he went to the hospitals to assist the surgeons and was shocked to find at the hospital number 1 gate, 'the mangled and bloody corpses of my two companions, Mongin and Roussel, who were killed together with many of the soldiers, in defending the entrance to the hospital'. At the Battle of Lützen in 1813, 20-year-old surgeon Côme Atoch of the 4[e] line regiment left the relative safety of the ambulance behind the lines to tend the wounded inside his regimental square. The soldiers feared for him as he was seen to be indispensable. When, inevitably, he was hit, he asked for a piece of paper, writing to his father: 'I was struck down by a cannon ball … I am going to die … Do not regret it, I die bravely.' The heroic exploits of Urbain Fardeau became legendary. Indeed, he appears to have spent more time terrorising the enemy than performing surgery. In Italy in 1799, in just one of several similar exploits, he and a handful of colleagues dispersed an entire column of Austrian infantry by charging it fearlessly.[34]

Percy initiated the term *chirurgien de pacotille* and perhaps inadvertently tainted all the army's surgeons. However, his account of the wars contains many allusions to surgical colleagues who overcame all the hardships and dangers of campaigning to perform their duties with devotion and a high level of competence. Thus, at the town of Thorn after the Battle of Eylau, where there were forty patients with complicated fractures and more than thirty amputation cases, Surgeon Tissot battled heroically against all odds, not least the complete lack of surgical instruments. He repeatedly lobbied the *commissaires des guerres* for supplies, dictated laws and regulations for the benefit of the sick, and pinned a list of the surgeon's duties on the door of the hospital. Percy acknowledged that when Tissot had to eventually return to his division he would be a hard act to follow.

During the campaign in the Peninsula in 1808, the Emperor asked Percy for his opinion of his colleagues.

> Sire, in your army of Spain there are 28 or 30 *chirurgiens-majors* so skilful and knowledgeable that they could teach and practise with brilliant success in the greatest towns of your Empire; there are among them men to rival Pelletan, Boyer and Dubois, my esteemed colleagues.

The latter were surgeons well respected in civilian life. Percy was keen to promote military surgery and highlight its achievements. In the course of an ingratiating eulogy to Napoleon intended for publication in a Paris newspaper in 1809, he notes that the Emperor 'showed particular goodwill to military surgery', and suggests that even affluent parents might encourage their sons into a career which offered both the opportunity of scientific prizes and the glories of war. Percy's most illustrious colleague, Dominique Larrey, was also quick to praise the commitment and energy of the surgeons under his command.[35]

It is understandable that the army's senior surgeons wished to publicise the achievements of their most talented officers. But the plaudits also came from senior military officers. General Foy eulogised the medical men of his army.

> *La Patrie* owes recognition without limits to the modest services of the *officiers de santé* ... Situated between the cupidity of the administrators and the ambition of military officers, this respectable class of citizens together showed a devotion of undoubted purity.

Louis-François Lejeune witnessed this devotion of French army doctors at the siege of Saragossa in Spain where, he says, they 'cared with equal solicitude for Spanish and French ... it was impossible not to admire the calm courage with which they came to our help'. Also in the Peninsula, at Coimbra in 1810, Jean Jacques Pelet, aide-de-camp to Marshal Masséna, discovered a group of doctors who refused to abandon the hospital in the face of the enemy. 'The surgeon of the 2e *léger* had shown them a noble example in refusing to leave his colonel, Merle, who had been seriously wounded.' Military officers often viewed hospitals with dread and clear sighted officers like Lejeune recognised the valour of the men who worked there. After Wagram, he was sent to visit the hospitals by Napoleon. Here, he says, 'Percy and Larrey set an example of great courage to their young fellow surgeons compelled to spend whole days in the polluted atmosphere ... I never left the hospitals without admiring their steadfastness and thanking god for guiding me to choose a profession less sad than theirs.'[36]

Such recognition and praise was designed to raise the stock of Napoleon's doctors. What, in reality, was their status in the *Grande Armée*? This is not a straightforward question to address as we need to take into account both their rank and medical speciality and also the nature of those standing in judgement upon them. For instance, they may have been viewed quite differently by disparate groups such as ordinary French citizens, doctors in civilian life, military officers, soldiers of the rank and file, and other army employees including the administrators. We can review the available evidence and draw some general conclusions.

Any respect from the army's military officers had to be earned. The *officiers de santé* were encouraged by their medical seniors to be an advocate for the sick or wounded soldier, irrespective of rank. In Larrey's words:

> The [army] doctor is and must be the friend of humanity. In this quality he must always speak and act in its favour. You must always dress the guilty just as the innocent and you must see only the sick man. The remainder is of no importance. Inspire your colleagues with these ideas and make sure that we never have to reproach ourselves for the death of a single innocent man.[37]

This advice must have seemed daunting for young men fresh to the army but at least some aspired to these lofty principles. At the Battle of Lützen in 1813 26-year-old Eugene Fenech had surgical responsibility for a whole army corps of 13,000 men. He assured the local administrator that, despite his young age, he was well able to cope. This willing acceptance of responsibility frequently brought admiration from the army's military officers. Praise from men such as Foy, Lejeune and Pelet was not isolated. Some officers showed not only respect for the army's doctors but were also reassured by their presence. Pharmacist Jacob notes that Marshal Ney, renowned for his bravery, had so much faith in Jeantet, *chirurgien-major* of the 50ᵉ *ligne*, that he ensured that the surgeon was always close to him on the day of battle. On occasion, this trust was translated into practical help. Percy, writing in 1799, says that there were a number of senior military officers who showed real concern for the army's surgeons and who took every opportunity to support them. He particularly singles out Saint-Cyr and Lefebre. The latter vigorously opposed the decision to deprive the surgeons of *demi-brigades* of their horses. 'Go and see, you wretches [the *conseil de santé*], if a surgeon who has a haversack on his back and who has had to march six leagues, can give help to the wounded with calm and ease.' But this generosity was not universal. Often, the surgeons were largely ignored by military officers and left to fend for themselves. Percy's memoirs are full of accounts of doctors in desperate straits. In 1807 after Eylau, most of his fellow surgeons had no money, their clothes were in tatters, and they were forced to go from door to door attempting to purchase new boots. All Percy received from the military authorities were 'sterile promises and vain compliments'.[38]

This was the other side of the coin, a relationship between the army's doctors and officers based on indifference, misunderstanding and disdain. Undoubtedly, there were army officers who regarded the *officiers de santé* with contempt. Physician Joseph Tyrbas de Chamberet came across a number of these men during his campaigning in Spain. Army doctors arriving at new destinations were not always welcomed by the local military officers. He describes the experiences of a physician who, at short notice, was ordered to attend the military hospital at Aranjuez where the previous incumbent had just died of typhus. When he reached the town late at night and reported to the military commander, he was told peremptorily that he was not needed and that he would not qualify for food or lodgings. The doctor showed his valid papers and pleaded for some accommodation but the commandant lost his temper and threatened to throw him into jail. It was only after the intervention of Desgenettes that the senior officer was reprimanded and the physician allowed to take up his post. In another similar incident, Tyrbas de Chamberet and a group of surgeons, in the mountains near Requena, were forced to report to a military officer who had authority in the area. They found him in a convent, sitting at a table covered with half-eaten food and empty bottles and accompanied by two women with 'low cut dresses'. The officer arbitrarily limited the surgeons to only a half-ration of food and forage. 'Why?' asked Tyrbas de Chamberet, 'because it was his will, his caprice of the moment!' When typhus and dysentery struck the local garrison and the doctors were sorely needed, the rations were suddenly restored.[39]

The most revealing anecdote is that of a young well educated *chirurgien aide-major* who found himself in Spain eating in a bivouac with twenty officers. Unfortunately, there were only seven or eight wine goblets and they had to be shared. The surgeon was sitting next to an officer of infantry who had already drunk several times but gave no sign of passing on the goblet. In answer to a polite request from the doctor for a share of the cup, the officer brusquely refused. The surgeon made a further request and the officer's simmering indignation became apparent. 'You, you want to drink from my glass. I am an officer, me! Nobody has the right to drink from my glass. You are not worthy of eating from the table of officers. It is a dishonour to my epaulettes to be sat next to a surgeon, a civilian!'[40]

It would have taken considerable courage, if not foolhardiness, on the part of the surgeon, to have taken this matter further. There are some instances of doctors standing up to senior military officers but for them to escape severe punishment there had to be exceptional circumstances. Eugene Fenech encountered just such a situation at the Battle of Bussaco in Portugal in 1810. Whilst he was working hard at the ambulance dressing the injured, he received a request from an officer to provide a state of the wounded for the colonel. Fenech reasonably argued that he could not abandon the wounded and refused to comply with the order. After the battle, he was ordered to present himself to his senior officer. The latter laid into Fenech: 'Who has f...... me with an *aide-major* like you! If we were at any other time, I would have you f..... into jail for a month!' Fenech replied that he understood his duties in the regiment. 'I am a surgeon and not a sergeant, secretary, or quartermaster. My time is very precious today and my presence at the ambulances indispensable. If you have nothing more to say to me I will return there immediately. Do you want me to look again at the bruising you received this morning?' 'No' was the colonel's response, 'Go to the devil!' Fenech got on his horse and returned to the field. To his credit, the colonel later relented and invited the surgeon to dine with him.[41]

Only on a day of battle was a medical officer likely to have been excused such insubordination. The gulf in status between doctors and military officers was formalised by the refusal to award *officiers de santé* permanent commissions and also *l'epaulette*, a recognisable status symbol. The lack of the epaulette on the uniform underlined the fact that doctors had only the courtesy status of military officers and no definite military rank or authority. The *officiers de santé* were acutely aware of this. When Chirurgien Aide-major Louis-Vivant Lagneau had an argument with an adjutant-major over accommodation in Austria in 1805, he acknowledged that the officer was a good and brave man, but he also noted that, 'he had a prejudice common enough among military officers. That is, they believe themselves much superior to the *officiers de santé* of corresponding rank because we do not wear the epaulette.' Apart from putting them at a disadvantage in their relationship with officers, the lack of the epaulette meant that the army's doctors all too often had responsibility without authority. Physician Laurillard-Fallot escorted a convoy of twenty sick men from a hospital in January 1814. He noted wryly that he led them but did not command them, 'but it was no less the case that I had full responsibility for them until our arrival at Luxembourg where I handed them over to the commander of the place'.[42]

Percy fully understood that the granting of the epaulette to medical officers would immediately increase their credibility and authority in the *Grande Armée*. He took any opportunity to remind the Emperor of his views and to support his case for elevating the army's doctors. In conversation with Napoleon in Poland in 1807, he extolled the virtues of the young surgeons, many of them of good birth. He pointed out that some were of a calibre to attend military schools such as Fontainebleau but had chosen to become surgeons by vocation. No mention of the *chirurgiens de pacotille* here! Percy noted in his journal that he lived in the hope that all the surgeons would eventually obtain a proper rank in the military hierarchy, something he regarded as politic and fair, and that if he did not achieve this objective it would not be for lack of trying. He was as good as his word, although destined to fail. In December 1807 in Spain, he made an appeal to the Emperor in writing. On this occasion he decided to make the request more specific.

> Sire. I write with regard to the elite surgeons on horseback that belong to the light ambulances of Your Majesty's headquarters and those of the outposts of the army. Although never having received the least incentive, they are mounted and equipped at their own expense and they serve with a shining zeal and a devotion which you have deigned on several occasions to honour with your approval. These military surgeons, whose bravery is no more in doubt than the utility of their profession, do not wish for any particular monetary compensation. They aspire to a reward more noble and more worthy of them. They dare, through the voice of their chief, to beseech Your Majesty to willingly grant them the epaulette of the rank equivalent to that which the law classes them, thus that of *sous-lieutenant* for the *sous-aides* or lieutenant for the *aides*, of captain for the *chirurgiens-majors*, of lieutenant-colonel for the principal surgeons. They should have, on the opposite shoulder, a braid of gold clover. This distinction, which their life in bivouac and among soldiers makes necessary, will be the exclusive privilege of the elite and battle surgeons. It should become for the other surgeons, those on foot who accompany the ambulances, something great to emulate. It will thus be, moreover, a way of removing the decadence of an entirely military state, which more than anything must be sustained and encouraged by Your Majesty.

Marshal Duroc took responsibility for the letter and presented it to Marshal Berthier, Napoleon's loyal and influential chief of staff. Berthier, who Percy says never showed the army's doctors 'the least mark of goodwill', objected to the request, stating that it would need a decree from Napoleon. This should not have been an insuperable obstacle but it was obvious that nothing was going to change.

Why Berthier, or indeed the army's other senior officers, should bear ill will towards the *service de santé* and its staff is not clear. At one point in his journal, in 1807, Percy states that many were jealous of the favour the surgeons received from Napoleon. The surgeons themselves felt that they had little reason to invoke the jealousy of others and some were demoralised enough to transfer to purely military posts. For example, at Koenigsberg in 1809, Percy treated the wounds of a man who had formerly been a *chirurgien aide-major* but had become an officer in the 3ᵉ *cuirassiers*. Some time earlier at Danzig he had noted in his journal:

> My colleagues feared this [dismissal from the service] so much that several took up service as [military] officers and had been received by His Majesty with a mixture of surprise and disaffection. Sixty four among them asked to retire because, in their absence, they had been drawn for

conscription. This affected two thirds of them; eighteen or twenty had been condemned as draft dodgers or deserters.[43]

It seems implausible that serving *officiers de santé* should be treated in this way but a letter of October 1807 to Daru, the *intendant-general* of the *Grande Armée*, from the Minister of War, explains why Percy's account is almost certainly accurate. It is apparent that the authorities had only the vaguest idea of the numbers and identities of the *officiers de santé* with the army.

> In the course of this year I have not received any of the states for the *officiers de santé* of your army. This means that I cannot give their families news of them when they ask and that it is equally impossible to reply in a positive manner to the *prefects* and *M. le directeur général de la conscription* when they consult me regarding those of the officers who are of an age for conscription.[44]

Daru was instructed to ask the senior *officiers de santé* for the relevant information as quickly as possible. One can easily understand the distress of *officiers de santé* giving loyal service to their country who suddenly discovered that their efforts were entirely unrecognised and that they were being branded as cowards and deserters in their home towns.

Whatever their treatment at the hands of others, the army's doctors did little to improve their status by indulging in periodic bouts of infighting. There was particular rivalry between the physicians and surgeons. In general, periods of peace promoted the status of physicians whereas it was the surgeons who, in relative terms, thrived in war. The pre-eminence of physicians in civilian life is evident from the salaries in the Emperor's court. The senior physician received an annual wage of 30,000 francs and the senior surgeon only 15,000 francs. Similarly, a middle ranking physician received 15,000 francs compared to 12,000 francs for the equivalent surgical post. However, in war all was different. At the headquarters of the *Grande Armée* the pay scales for physicians and surgeons were the same. As early as the Revolutionary Wars it was clear that the inability of the military physicians to understand and cope with disease was leading to disenchantment with their services and an erosion of their stature. Conversely, the surgeons were prominent on the battlefield and escaped blame for the epidemics decimating the army. In 1793 the assistant minister of war wrote to all hospital personnel suggesting that rather than attempting to replace physicians lost through illness or death, their duties should be taken over by senior surgeons. The gap between the traditionally academic and aristocratic physicians and the humble surgeons was beginning to close.

This trend continued under the Empire. The ascendancy of surgery was symbolised by the award of the *Légion d'honneur* to *officiers de santé*. In 1804 in the camp of Boulogne, the first granting of the honour to army doctors, thirty-eight received the award; twenty-seven surgeons, five physicians, five pharmacists and a single *officier de santé*. Two years later, there was a further round of awards with twenty-three surgeons honoured and no physicians included. The senior physician Coste was moved to write to Lacépède, grand chancellor of the order, pleading the case for his fellow physicians, stressing that many had lost their lives in the recent campaign.[45]

Such a fundamental shift in status and influence from one medical speciality to another was bound to lead to tension and recrimination. The army's senior physician and surgeon, Coste and Percy, appealed for understanding between the two parties, but with limited success. In a pamphlet written in 1808, Principal Physician Gilbert argued that the dominance of army surgeons over physicians was detrimental for soldiers. He fully understood why the soldiers favoured the surgeons.

> Surgery assaults all the senses. For those of limited understanding it makes a completely different impression to the delayed action of medicines. The brutal savage will presume that a man who bleeds and handles him with dexterity has much more talent than the man who knows how to prevent the need for bleeding. Thus, the soldiers in the camps will have a lot more affection for the surgeon who bandages him and shares his sufferings and way of life than for the physician who he sees only in the odious hospitals, who gives him only disgusting things, and who appears only to impose privations upon him.[46]

On the other side, Percy was never slow to extol his surgeons at the expense of the physicians. When the occasion permitted, he ensured that the Emperor was given an account biased in favour of his own speciality. A case in point was the affair at the hospital at Kustrin in November 1806 where, for reasons that are obscure, there was a complete lack of medical staff. Napoleon was appalled and took issue with his senior doctors. Percy had the first audience and was quick to extract the absent surgeons from blame. It was the feeble ageing Coste – unfairly held responsible for both the absent physicians and pharmacists – who took the full force of the Emperor's wrath.[47] Although this ill will between surgeons and physicians can hardly have improved the image of the army's doctors there is no evidence that sick or wounded soldiers were poorly treated because of these rivalries.

It may be argued that the most important relationship of the *officiers de santé* was not with their fellow doctors, military officers or ordinary soldiers, but with the army's administrators. We have seen that the authority of the *service de santé* and the autonomy of its doctors were increasingly subjugated to the administrative department. The administration receives a poor press in most accounts of the medical services of the *Grande Armée*, being seen as incompetent, lazy and grasping and ultimately responsible for many of the failings of the *service de santé* and the difficulties of its officers.

In the two most recent English biographies of Larrey, the French Army's most famous doctor is seen to fight a long and frustrating battle as much with his own administration as with the enemy.[48] *Officiers de santé* are portrayed as the whipping boys of the self-seeking and heartless *commissaires des guerres*.

Whilst there is undoubtedly some truth in this portrayal, the reality is certainly more complex. It is unfair to suggest that all administrators were cowardly, incompetent and corrupt and too simplistic to attribute all the woes of the army and its medical service to the administration. There is evidence that at least a few *commissaires des guerres* were honest and competent and performed a thankless role with dignity and dedication. The journal of Commissaire des Guerres Alexandre Bellot de Kergorre gives valuable insights into the role of an administrator in the *Grande Armée*. Bellot de Kergorre appears to take his duties seriously and, indeed, he was commended for his actions at Mojaisk in 1812, where, in the course of a month, he succeeded in bringing together and feeding 3,000 wounded under the most difficult circumstances. The army's senior administrator, Intendant-General Pierre Daru, was generally well regarded. Bellot de Kergorre describes Daru's considerable efforts to organise hospitals in Poland in 1807. In Warsaw:

> He worked so hard that in just three days, to the great astonishment of the locals, twenty-eight hospitals were opened in a town where most of the inhabitants were sleeping on straw. M.Daru had written to the Polish governor that he would not tolerate one French soldier being thrown onto a pallet when one Count was resting on a mattress.

The personal relationship of the army's *officiers de santé* with the *commissaires des guerres* was likely to be strained. Even the honest administrators frequently had little understanding of medicine. Conversely, army doctors may have underestimated the difficulty of supplying their needs. The increasing subservience of the *service de santé* to the army's administration often placed the doctors at the mercy of the *commissaires*. Mutual antagonism and misunderstanding were the norm. The degree of authority which the *commissaires des guerres* came to have over the *officiers de santé* is evident from the following excerpts from Bellot de Kergorre's account of his role at the Battle of Leipzig in 1813. The italics are mine.

> When the general had placed his troops in battle order I asked him where he wished me to place *my ambulances* … Our troops were advancing and I followed my ambulance, keeping always at the same distance; *my officiers de santé* wanted to set up in the open but I did not want this and I ordered *my first wounded* to be carried to my colleagues … My *officiers de santé* were so busy, that when I arrived *to give orders*, I held the legs of the unfortunates when they were amputating; I drew on all my courage

to overcome the most dreadful repugnance ... I concluded that we were retreating and I loaded all my wounded not leaving one behind.[49]

Bellot de Kergorre seems to have fulfilled his duties admirably but the tone of this account leaves no doubt as to who was in charge.

We do not know how Bellot de Kergorre was viewed by his medical colleagues. Undoubtedly, some *commissaires des guerres* lacked tact and openly treated the *officiers de santé* as inferiors. Physician Salomon-Louis Laurillard-Fallot recalls an incident before the Battle of Wagram in 1809 where, in the company of several senior military officers, he was treated with disdain by a young man of roughly his own age who had only recently been promoted to assistant *commissaire des guerres*. Laurillard-Fallot was provoked into an argument as he admitted, at that time, 'I did not know the amount of power and influence that the *commissaires* exerted over the *service de santé*'. The young doctor managed to extract himself without any serious damage. Not all altercations between the two services were so simply settled. In 1807 in Berlin, Percy had to personally intervene after a quarrel between a *commissaire des guerres* and Surgeon Jean-Pierre Gama had led to the latter being placed under arrest. The army's senior doctor understood that this incident highlighted a wider malaise.

> Since the departure of His Majesty, several *commissaires des guerres* have come out of their shells and taken a tone towards the surgeons which general opinion, the reality of the service, and the goodwill of the Emperor all dictate to be misplaced. I have complained to the *Intendant General* and pointed out that a *commissaire* might be chief of a hospital but never a chief of *officiers de santé*: there is still much to be said and done relating to this subject.

Percy was correct but the tide was flowing against him. By 1812 the power of the *commissaires* was such that even Larrey struggled to combat them. As Chief Surgeon of the Imperial Guard he had often used Napoleon's favour to bypass the administration but when he was promoted to Surgeon-in-Chief of the *Grande Armée* the administrators were quick to take revenge, keen to exploit his lack of military rank or real authority.[50]

Although Larrey and Percy were senior enough to be immune to serious personal harm from the administration, this was not the case for their more junior colleagues. Often a convenient excuse would be found to sideline a doctor who was prepared to criticise the unseemly aspects of the administration. Physician Joseph Tyrbas de Chamberet tells of a divisional inspector of hospitals in Spain who risked fighting the administrative corruption around him. Tyrbas de Chamberet notes that such an enemy of the administration was rarely allowed to remain with the army for long and when the doctor developed a trivial leg ulcer this was promptly used as an excuse to get rid of him back to France.[51] All such anecdotes must be interpreted in the context of the enmity between the two services. Tyrbas de Chamberet attributed his lack of promotion in Italy in 1810 entirely to the scheming of the *commissaires des guerres*. This may have been true but, equally, it is likely that the administrators, whether good or bad, were a convenient scapegoat for a multitude of evils and failings.

The most overt recognition of the status and worth of any group of army personnel was the awarding of official honours. Napoleon constructed an intricate and hierarchical system of military honours and took great interest in its application. It was not unusual for the Emperor to personally bestow awards on an ordinary soldier, often with a few words displaying a surprising knowledge of his bravery and the battle record of his regiment. This was an integral part of the creation of the Napoleonic legend, the potential for the lowliest ranked soldier to ultimately receive his marshal's baton. The *officiers de santé* took their place in this system and the relative number of *Légions d'honneur* awarded to surgeons and physicians has been alluded to. But how were Napoleon's doctors rewarded with honours compared to military officers or the other specialist services of the *Grande Armée*?

For the army's most senior doctors, men such as Percy, Larrey, Coste and Desgenettes, there were many prestigious honours – we will further discuss these eminent men in the next chapter. However, for the ordinary *officiers de santé* Napoleon's official recognition was more elusive. The *Légion d'honneur* was an essentially military award and *officiers de santé* who received it, men like Urbain Fardeau, were often distinguished by their bravery in action rather than by exceptional professional service. Honours for purely medical services were relatively rare. Some eminent army doctors were made barons of the Empire – Boyer, Desgenettes, Girardot, Heurteloup, Larrey, Percy, Yvan – but this was out of over a thousand barons created between 1808 and 1814. When the Emperor did honour ordinary medical officers, this was often only after intense lobbying by Percy or other senior army doctors. At times, these honours appeared to be randomly distributed with men with little exposure to danger receiving inexplicable awards. For example, Marie François Vergez, at his death in 1831, was the most decorated officer in the *service de santé* despite not having appeared on a battlefield since 1792.[52]

These inconsistencies can only have increased the frustration of the many *officiers de santé* whose services received little official recognition. Ultimately, the only reward for most diligent army doctors was the gratitude of their patients. Not that this was any small recompense. Physician Tyrbas de Chamberet recalls that when he entered a Spanish town in 1812, a cavalry officer came over to him and thanked him profusely for the care he had received from him in the hospital in Madrid. He gave the doctor a large quantity of sugared almonds and pralines which had been pillaged from a confectioner's shop. Percy notes that nothing distressed the wounded more than being removed from the hands of their own surgeons whom they knew and trusted. The cumulative effect of these thousands of small services gratefully received was an increase in the status of doctors not just within the *Grande Armée* but within French society. This change was subtle but almost certainly real. Many Frenchmen owed their lives to the army's doctors. This is reflected in popular literature where the pompous ineffectual doctors portrayed by Molière were now replaced by the competent and concerned *officiers de santé* of Flaubert and Balzac. The wars of the French Revolution and Empire had been a catalyst for change and this was particularly the case for Napoleon's doctors.[53]

Notes

1. Heller, R, *Officiers de Santé: the second-class doctors of nineteenth-century France*.
2. Lemaire, J-F, *Napoléon et la Médecine*, p. 141; Percy, Baron, *Journal des Campagnes de Baron Percy*, p. 106.
3. Lagneau, L-V, *Journal d'un Chirurgien de la Grande Armée 1803–1815*, pp. 19–33.
4. Poumiès de la Siboutie, Doctor, *Recollections of a Parisian (1789–1863)*, pp. 76–108.
5. Tyrbas de Chamberet, J, *Mémoires d'un Médecin Militaire*, pp.37, 39, 53.
6. Fardeau, U, *Urbain Fardeau. Mémoires d'un Saumurois chirurgien-sabreur*, pp. 42–4.
7. Pigeard, A, *Dictionnaire de la Grande Armée*, p. 180; d'Héralde, J-B, *Mémoires d'un Chirurgien de la Grande Armée*, p. 12.
8. Lagneau, pp. 32–3.
9. Pigeard, A, *L'Armée de Napoléon*, p. 182; Percy, p. xxiii; Roos, H de, *Avec Napoléon en Russie*, p. 5.
10. Roos, p. 7; Tyrbas de Chamberet, p. 131; Pigeard, *L'Armée de Napoléon*, p. 182.
11. Lemaire, p. 202.
12. ibid., p. 200.
13. ibid., p. 204.
14. Vess, D M, *Medical Revolution in France 1789–1796*, p. 66.
15. Percy, p.xxxiii; Lagneau, p. 21.
16. Fenech, E, *Mémoires d'un Officier de Santé Maltais dans l'Armée Française (1809–1813)*, p. 22.
17. Brice, Docteur and Bottet, Capitaine, *Le Corps de Santé Militaire en France*, p. 210.
18. Percy, pp. 478, 403, 463.
19. Lagneau, pp. 37, 65, 159.

20. Jacob, P-I, *Le Journal Inédit d'un pharmacien de la Grande Armée*, p. 197; Fenech, p. 94.
21. d'Héralde, p. 111.
22. Roos, p. 168; Guilmot, A N J, *Journal de Voyage d'un officier de santé à Saint-Domingue (1802)*, p. 94.
23. Pigeard, A, *Le Service de Santé de la Révolution au 1er Empire 1792–1815*, p. 46; Laurillard-Fallot, S-L, *Souvenirs d'un Médecin Hollandais sous les Aigles Françaises 1807–1833*, p. 15; Tyrbas de Chamberet, p. 148.
24. Percy, p. 302.
25. Lemaire, J-F, *Coste: Premier Médecin des Armées de Napoléon*, pp. 328–9; Tyrbas de Chamberet, p. 147.
26. Vess, p. 156; Dible, J H, *Napoleon's Surgeon*, p. 211.
27. Percy, p. 208; Milleliri, J-M, *Médecins et Soldats pendant l'expédition d'Égypte (1798–1799)*, p. 180.
28. Lagneau, p.40; d'Héralde, pp. 75–6.
29. Fardeau, pp. 59, 173.
30. Vess, p.156; Percy, pp. 403, 188, 353, 351.
31. Morvan, J, *Le Soldat Impérial*, Vol. II, p. 368; Gonneville, *Recollections of Colonel de Gonneville*, Vol. I, p.156; Vossler, H, *With Napoleon in Russia 1812*, p.30; Tyrbas de Chamberet, p. 57.
32. Milleliri, pp. 210, 221; Guilmot, p. 88; Brice, Bottet, p. 147.
33. Morvan, Vol. II, p. 329; Jacob, p. 257; Roos, p. 116.
34. Percy, p. 245; Larrey, D J, *Mémoires de Chirurgie Militaire et Campagnes 1787–1840*, p. 132; Brice, Bottet, p. 232; Fardeau, p. 133.
35. Percy, pp. 200, 472, 492; Dible, p. 218.
36. Lemaire, *Napoléon et la Médecine*, p. 229; Lejeune, Baron, *Memoirs of Baron Lejeune Aide-de-Camp to Marshals Berthier, Davout and Oudinot*, Vol. I, pp. 172, 331; Pelet, J J, *The French Campaign in Portugal 1810–1811*, p. 203.
37. Lemaire, J-F, *Les blessés dans les Armées Napoléoniennes*, p. 195.
38. Fenech, p. 77; Jacob, p. 85; Percy, pp. 17, 198.
39. Tyrbas de Chamberet, pp. 108–9, 119.
40. ibid., p. 110
41. Fenech, p. 62.
42. Lagneau, p. 53; Laurillard-Fallot, p. 98.
43. Percy, pp. 222, 438–40, 206, 260.
44. Brice, Bottet, p. 183.
45. Lemaire, *Napoléon et la Médecine*, pp. 128–9; Vess, p. 140; Lemaire, *Coste*, p. 271.
46. Lemaire, *Napoléon et la Médecine*, p. 131.
47. Lemaire, *Coste*, pp. 284–5.
48. Dible; Richardson, R, *Larrey. Surgeon to Napoleon's Imperial Guard.*
49. Bellot de Kergorre, A, *Journal d'un Commissaire des Guerres pendant le Premier Empire (1806–1821)*, pp. 20, 142, 114–5.

50. Laurillard-Fallot, p. 32; Percy, pp. 392–3; Richardson, p. 155.
51. Tyrbas de Chamberet, p. 95.
52. Percy, p. 190; Lemaire, *Napoléon et la Médecine*, p. 102.
53. Tyrbas de Chamberet, p. 128; Percy, p. 371; Weiner, D B, *French Doctors Face War 1792–1815*, p. 73.

CHAPTER III

Percy, Larrey and Napoleon

In the higher echelons of the *service de santé* there was a small group of doctors who attempted to shape the medical services of the *Grande Armée*. They achieved some notable successes despite the perfidious influence of the despised administration. Four of the men – Percy, Larrey, Desgenettes and Coste – deserve special consideration. One of them, Larrey, has become immortalised, an integral part of the Napoleonic legend. He is the only one of the four to have had biographies published in English. The others, unfairly, are less remembered today. We will start with Pierre-François Percy as he had arguably the greatest impact on the French army's medical services. The only men with claims to greater influence than Percy were Larrey and Napoleon himself.

Pierre-François Percy

Percy was born in 1794 in the small French town of Montagney-les-Pesmes, the son of a local surgeon.[1] At 21 years old he qualified as a doctor at the faculty of Besançon where he was a pupil and friend of the great surgeon Louis. He joined the army as *aide-major* to the Scots company of *la petite gendarmerie* at Lunéville in 1776. By 1782 he had progressed to become *chirurgien-major* to the regiment of *Berry-Cavalerie* in garrison at Béthune. Unlike many other army surgeons of the era, he dedicated all his spare time to study and was brilliantly rewarded. After winning the most prestigious award of the Academy of Surgeons four times, he was named *associé libre* both as a mark of respect and as a way of debarring him from further entry to give his competitors a chance.

His great military reputation was built upon his role as *chirurgien en chef* in Flanders and Artois in 1789 and then as *chirurgien en chef* to the Army of the Rhine. During the Revolutionary Wars, he pioneered a mobile ambulance termed a '*wurst*' which was to be overshadowed by Larrey's flying ambulance. In 1800 he was one of the first army doctors to seriously explore the concept of inviolability of hospitals during war, an action that was much later supported by the Red Cross and the Geneva Convention. Under the Empire, Percy continued to press for change, drawing up detailed plans for a proper surgical service in battle (*chirurgie de bataille*) and promoting the use of specially trained orderlies for the management of wounded and sick in the field and in the hospitals, the so-called *infirmiers* and *brancardiers*. He was amply recognised for his efforts, becoming an inspector general in 1803, member of the Institute in 1807, commander of the *Légion d'honneur* after Eylau, and baron of the Empire after Wagram in 1809. Serious ophthalmia kept him away from the *Grande Armée* during the later campaigns of Russia and Saxony and he only returned to active military service during the Waterloo campaign in 1815, although even then he was debilitated by heart problems. He spent much of the later years of the wars teaching in Paris, dividing his time between the Academy of Sciences and the Faculty of Medicine. After the Restoration, he became a prolific writer on mainly medical matters. He died of a heart disorder in 1825. Percy is one of only three of Napoleon's doctors (with Larrey and Desgenettes) to have his name engraved on the Arc de Triomphe.

Percy was not a great technical surgeon in the mould of Larrey. He did have strong views on surgical procedures which carried some influence, notably his relative reluctance to amputate and his support of local resection. He also pioneered some novel pieces of surgical equipment. However, his great contribution was not in the sphere of medical or surgical treatment, but as a leader, reformer and, above all, as an advocate for the *service de santé* and its doctors. We can say with some confidence that he was compassionate, charming, brave, dedicated, scholarly, principled, determined and highly independent. On occasions, the last quality amounted to a streak of anti-authoritarianism. His opponents, and there were many, especially in the administration, may have regarded him as stubborn and overly sensitive to criticism. We have evidence for all the above character traits from his journal and the contemporary descriptions of his peers.

That Percy was willing to serve at the front and not shirk danger was apparent from the earliest years of his army career. In 1793, when he was *chirurgien en chef* of the Army of the Moselle, he carried a wounded officer on his back across a bridge which was under fire from a dozen enemy cannons. He also showed a disregard for his own safety away from the battlefield. In 1800 he and a fellow surgeon arranged the escape of thirty-one French émigrés, among them women and children, who had been condemned to death by a military commission. Only three days earlier, ten people had been shot for giving similar help to other émigrés. This action reveals his deeply compassionate nature. In his own words:

> It is necessary that a surgeon sympathise with the sufferings of the wounded and show them respect; he is their only friend, the only one to give consolation on the battlefield or in the hospitals … He must be careful not to add to the great distress of an unfortunate soldier who is

going to lose a limb or undergo another major operation by the hastiness of his manners.[2]

Percy was always the first to reprimand *officiers de santé* who adopted a flippant attitude towards the wounded. Two junior surgeons who referred to the limbs they had just amputated as *gigots* (legs of lamb) felt the full force of his anger.

Percy was idealistic. He did not accept honours indiscriminately. He was content to accept the gold medal from the Prussian Academy and the Order of Saint Ann from Russia but he firmly refused any gifts or awards from Britain, France's greatest and most constant enemy. He could also be pragmatic when the need arose. He openly supported Napoleon, littering his journal with admiring references to the Emperor's actions. When Napoleon returned to France from Elba in 1815, Percy responded to the call and served in the campaign of the Hundred Days. However, following Napoleon's further fall at Waterloo, he pledged himself to the new regime.

There is no doubt about Percy's academic ability. He was a prolific writer of scholarly works, notably a study on the surgery of the army published in 1792 and a treatise on the health of the troops of the *Grande Armée*, co-authored with Coste, which appeared in 1806. After his retirement from the army, he continued to submit papers to learned journals such as *Le Dictionnaire des Sciences Médicales* and the *Biographie Universelle*. His scholarship extended beyond medicine as he was an enthusiastic amateur archaeologist. In the campaigns of 1806 and 1807 he gathered information for a later treatise on the 'Altars and Tombs of the Ancient Peoples of the North'. He avidly collected armour and there are several references to this in his journal – we are not informed how he transported it back to France.

Percy was charismatic and a fine conversationalist. Pharmacist Jacob met him in Paris in 1812 and noted that he could tell an anecdote with 'grace and dignity' and that his 'charming voice captured the attention of the listeners'[3]. Jacob was not universally complimentary regarding his senior colleagues so his comments are probably not mere sycophancy. Most biographers of Larrey refer to the great surgeon's friendship with Sir James McGrigor, the most eminent British army doctor of the period. However, when McGrigor visited Paris in 1815, he unequivocally favoured Percy.

Among the professional gentlemen to whom I was introduced at Paris by my friends Barons Desgenettes and Larrey was Baron Percy, likewise a medical officer of the army. The appearance and manner of this gentleman was more pleasing than those of his confreres and, in giving information, he had a singular appearance of openness and candour.

Napoleon also genuinely liked his senior surgeon. Whereas, at Tilsit in 1807, he was only 'Monsieur Percy' to the Emperor, a year later in the Spanish campaign it had become 'My dear Percy'.[4]

If these accounts give an impression of a 'benign' personality, this would be to ignore Percy's iron will and his willingness to take on authority, whatever the risks. In the Revolutionary Era, all those who resisted the official agencies of *La Patrie* were in danger of at least peremptory dismissal and, at most, of the guillotine. When Percy perceived that the *service de santé* was not being well used or that he was being personally maligned he did not hesitate to correspond directly with the Minister of War. The following was written at Basle in June 1799.

> I have only received this morning the letter that you wrote on 21st [May]. You admit to it? – it neither surprises or affects me. I am not used to, indeed I do not aspire to, praise from Paris. Paris is too far from the army. It is here, it is on the battlefield and in the hospitals that I obtain worthy recognition; if you had made one military campaign you would then understand that in my situation there is no time for the pointless letter writing that appears so popular and which is so productive for so many in Paris. I believe you fair and they say that you are wise, but you have been circumvented. Disappointments and cowardly flattery will not make me resign. I remain firm and resolute at my post; I want to stay there and brave new disgusting actions and improprieties with which the envious and mediocre will no doubt continue to pursue me. They will call me back perhaps; I expect it without desire or fear. But then it will not be me who has removed from the unfortunate victims of war their friend, sustainer and sympathiser.

This was not an isolated episode as Percy was quick to use his pen as a weapon. He went so far as to argue with the members of the *conseil de santé* over the cost of his correspondence with them. Such insubordination was not widely tolerated and Percy's superiors must have understood his value to the army. When he did threaten to resign following a further round of unhelpful regulations in October 1800, the Minister of War was quick to placate him with a flattering letter.[5]

A senior figure with such strong opinions was likely to have his enemies and detractors. Percy is criticised in a number of medical memoirs of the wars including those of his junior colleagues d'Héralde, Fardeau and Tyrbas de Chamberet.[6] Much of this antagonism arose from a perceived lack of support for their promotion or even a bias for his own favourites. This appears inevitable in view of Percy's considerable powers of patronage – he could hardly promote every *officier de santé*. Louis-Vivant Lagneau's journal shows him to have been helpful and considerate to a well deserving junior surgeon. Tyrbas de Chamberet's accusation that

Percy hypocritically transferred his support from the Emperor on the entry of the allies into Paris in 1814 is more serious. He says that on the eve of the allied takeover Percy praised Napoleon, who still had the veneer of power, but that, only two days later, he was eulogising the Bourbons and Tsar Alexander. Perhaps so, but it would be harsh to decry Percy for this. To have continued to overtly support Napoleon would have been an act of gratuitous self-destruction both for the senior doctor himself and the institutions with which he was associated.

With the hindsight of two hundred years, it is clear that one of Percy's greatest achievements was his campaign journal. This was kept on a daily basis giving it a truth and immediacy lacking in many retrospective memoirs. It was tracked down in Egypt after the wars and, unfortunately, is incomplete as several of the notebooks have disappeared. The remaining thirteen small notebooks, each easily fitting into a pocket, cover the campaigns of 1799–1800 and 1805–9. The entries have an intimate tone and there is no indication that Percy ever intended them to be published. The eminent Napoleonic historian Alain Pigeard describes the journal as one of the ten best contemporary texts of the Napoleonic Wars because of its 'rigour, honesty, and the quality of detail'. Another French historian acknowledges Percy's brilliant reportage in a journal which 'will be long esteemed'.[7] Despite this high praise for his writings, it is indicative of the relative lack of interest in Percy that his journal has never been translated into English and that he has been the subject of only two French biographies published almost 180 years apart.

Dominique Jean Larrey

In marked contrast to Percy, Dominique Larrey has become the most lauded and famous military doctor of the Napoleonic era. Larrey was born in 1766 in a small village in the French Pyrenees, the son of a master shoemaker.[8] He initially served as a naval surgeon and voyaged to Newfoundland before transferring to the army as an *aide-major* in the army of the Rhine in 1792. After the capture of Mayence he was named *aide-major principal* and was then successively *chirurgien-en-chef* to the armies of Corsica, Spain and Italy. He followed Bonaparte to Egypt and, on his return, was promoted to *chirurgien-en-chef* to the Consular Guard and made Officer of the *Légion d'honneur* at its inception. He accompanied Napoleon in all his campaigns, being with him as surgeon-in-chief to the Imperial Guard at Ulm, Vienna, Austerlitz, Berlin, Eylau, Friedland, Madrid, Aspern-Essling and at Wagram. In the Russian Campaign he was *chirurgien-en-chef* of the *Grande Armée* and was again at the Emperor's side at Lützen, Bautzen, Dresden and Leipzig, the battles in France in 1814, and finally at Waterloo where he was captured by the Prussians. He was widely recognised for his services being, in addition to a Commander of the *Légion d'honneur*, a baron of the Empire, an inspector general of the *service de santé*, and, in civilian life, a member of the Institute, the Academy of Medicine, and a number of scholarly societies. After the wars, he was ultimately restored in his duties by the Government of Juillet. He died aged 61 years after returning from a medical inspection in Algeria.

Larrey's greatest achievements were as an innovator of the ambulance system of casualty evacuation and as a brilliant military surgeon. His unprecedented contribution in these areas is discussed in later chapters. Larrey was a complex personality who was rarely treated with indifference by his peers, apparently attracting either adulation or disdain. That he had enormous determination and stamina is unquestionable. His memoirs are replete with instances of his prodigious capacity for work; for instance, in a letter to his wife during the 1809 campaign, 'More than 10,000 wounded have passed through our ambulances … I have operated for five days and nights and have performed all the urgent dressings'. No doctor could perform such feats on the battlefield without some disregard for his own safety. Larrey demonstrated his bravery as early as the campaign in Egypt where, at St Jean D'Acre in 1799, he continued to calmly dress a soldier's wound despite his own hat lying at his side being riddled with shot.

Such episodes show not only Larrey's heroism and professional commitment but also his devotion to the ordinary soldiers of the *Grande Armée*. The following is from his 1813 campaign journal.

> I confess I have never had any desire other than that of helping the wounded, no intention other than that of doing right, and in all actions – most of which I did unobtrusively – I have had no end other than the well-being of these unfortunate men … to perform a task as difficult as that which is imposed on a military surgeon, I am convinced that one must often sacrifice oneself, perhaps entirely, to others, must scorn fortune and maintain an absolute integrity, and must inure oneself to flattery.[9]

Larrey's preoccupation with the well-being of the ordinary soldiers was not always to his own benefit. When Bonaparte decided to abandon his army in Egypt in 1799 he took Larrey to one side, fully expecting his senior surgeon to accompany him back to France. But Larrey, although undoubtedly anxious to return home, resisted: 'I can be ready in two hours if that is your wish General; but if my presence is not indispensable, it is more important that I stay with my wounded.' The astounded and disappointed Bonaparte concurred with this but it was a major political mistake by Larrey – Napoleon never forgot what he regarded to be a betrayal. Larrey, on the other hand, was always loyal to the memory of the Emperor. In later times, old imperialists were inclined to gather in selected Paris salons to ruminate over the war years. Larrey had little truck for those he regarded as having been traitors under the Empire. In one reputed incident, he was addressed by an officer who had deserted to the Prussians on the eve of Waterloo. Stopping before Larrey, the officer held out his hand. The old surgeon regarded him coldly. 'What, don't you remember me? I'm d'Y......' 'The officer of that name I once knew died at Waterloo.' And he turned away. Conversely, Larrey could be loyal and gracious to those of his medical peers whom he respected. In his memoir of the campaign of 1793 he applauded the physician of the army, Laurenz, and also Percy and Lombard, for 'their great understanding and constant solicitude' for the soldiers.[10]

Larrey was amply rewarded for his services to the *Grande Armée*'s soldiers by their adoration and profound respect. Few men held such a high status with the grumbling veterans. When a rumour that Larrey had been killed spread through the Army of Spain in 1808, men of the Imperial Guard broke down and wept and vowed terrible vengeance. The surgeon's sudden reappearance in the town of Aranda was greeted with cheers of joy. He was rarely short of a helping hand. At the chaotic re-crossing of the Berezina in 1812, he was rescued from the crush on the river banks by soldiers who carried him on their shoulders. Anecdotes of Larrey's selflessness and goodwill to the common soldier appear in several memoirs. François-Frédéric Billon of the Imperial Guard recalls that, after the Battle of Eylau, Larrey emptied the floor of a house to convert it into an ambulance. A colonel arrived from headquarters with an order from Napoleon to Larrey directing that he return to Mohrungen to undertake the embalmment of General Dahlmann, commander of the *chasseurs à cheval* of the Guard. Larrey replied to the officer, who towered over him.

> Return, Monsieur. Tell his Majesty that I will not abandon seven to eight hundred wounded, of whom I might save half, to occupy myself with one dead man, however glorious his memory.

Billon was much impressed by 'l'admirable Dr Larrey'.[11]

Although he may, at times, have been frustrated by Larrey's stubborn independence, Napoleon was not stinting in his praise. In the Egyptian campaign, the surgeon was applauded for 'performing miracles', after Eylau he was gifted the Emperor's own sword, and most famously of all, Napoleon's will referred to him as 'the most virtuous man that I have known'. In his *Memorial de Sainte-Hélène*, Las Cases quotes Napoleon as saying that: 'If the army were to raise a memorial to the memory of one man, it should be that of Larrey. All the wounded are his family.'[12] The greatest possible praise from the highest possible source.

Larrey deserves to be remembered as one of the greatest of all military surgeons. However, there was a less savoury side to his character. Larrey himself refers to his 'extreme self-assurance' in a letter to his wife. He was immodest and vain. In his memoirs he was not averse to stressing his own vital role and, worse still, denigrating the contribution of others. This poisoned his relationship with other senior army doctors. Even his more junior colleagues noticed the shortcomings in Larrey's personality. Pierre-Irénée Jacob, who was so generous to Percy, is damning in his description of Larrey.

> He is as boastful on his own as three young men put together. He speaks loudly and with a singular assurance of things of which he is entirely ignorant. His audacity in this exceeds all description … In the army, in the eyes of the officers and even the generals of Empire who for the most part were upstart soldiers, this assured effrontery passed for merit … Out of this grew the enormous disproportion that we now see between the man and his reputation. His writings inspire little confidence; his boasting removes all credibility from them.

André Cosse, a medical student in Paris, agreed with Jacob, noting that Larrey 'was full of pretension' and that his vanity led him to elaborate the truth. Although there is considerable evidence of Larrey's dedication to the wounded, there are also anecdotes suggesting that the surgeon's pride could impair his better judgement. For instance, at Benavente in Spain in 1809 he was irritated by a Chirurgien-Major Baudry who was in charge of the local hospital and rather peevishly refused him use of the Guard's surgical instruments. Baudry, who seems to have been motivated only by a desire to operate on his own wounded men, was forced to borrow instruments from another regimental surgeon. The incident was in some ways trivial but it did lead to at least one wounded man having a delayed operation.[13]

Although Larrey may have received some bad press during the wars, events in later years ensured that his name would be woven into the Napoleonic legend, that mixture of fact and fiction that was to glorify the memory of Napoleon and an elite group that surrounded him. If there was some disproportion between the man and his reputation – and this is contentious – then it was in the post-war years that this chasm developed. Jean-François Lemaire argues that Larrey's subsequent popularisation was largely politically motivated. Whilst closely allied to Napoleon, he remained a republican at heart. The Second Republic, instituted shortly after Larrey's death, was badly in need of heroes and the dedicated surgeon was as good a candidate as any. His name was already symbolic of the military surgery of the era and the laudatory comments of Napoleon and others were the ideal substance with which to create the legend from the man. The following widely quoted Waterloo anecdote, very likely apocryphal, is typical. On seeing a French surgeon near the farm of Belle Alliance, Wellington reputedly asked his entourage:

'Who is that bold fellow over there?'
'That is Larrey,' said someone.
'Tell them not to fire at him. Give the brave fellow time to pick up his wounded.' And so saying he raised his hat.
'Whom are you saluting?' asked the Duke of Cambridge.
'The honour and loyalty you see yonder,' Wellington answered, pointing to the surgeon with his sword.[14]

The wording of the anecdote varies but the identity of the surgeon is constant. Of all the surgeons in the French army present at Waterloo, the legend demanded that only Larrey could be the recipient of such praise.

Larrey's memoirs are one of the great works of military surgery. These consist of four volumes of *Mémoires de Chirurgie Militaire et Campagnes, 1812–1817* and *Relation Médicale de Campagnes et Voyages de 1815 à 1840*, effectively a fifth volume of memoirs. An unparalleled account of the army surgery of the period, the memoirs are not such a valuable record of the reality of life in the *Grande Armée* and in the *service de santé*. Larrey's was not an unpremeditated daily account in the style of Percy's journal. He was unequivocally writing for posterity. Whilst it may be unfair to concur with Jacob's view that Larrey's account of events is worthless, there are discrepancies between Larrey's oft favourable view of the wars and the difficulties and suffering described by his contemporaries. Historian Jean Morvan, who consulted innumerable memoirs, is frequently dismissive of Larrey's observations. Where Larrey sees no sickness and the wounded well cared for, others see only death and starvation.[15] This may have been deliberate obfuscation by Larrey. Perhaps he was trying to portray himself and the *service de santé* in the most favourable light, unwilling to acknowledge the failings so apparent in Percy's journal. More prosaically, it may be that, as surgeon to the Imperial Guard, Larrey was simply protected from the worst of the miseries of the line regiments and their doctors. The Guard was a privileged organisation and this applied equally to its medical staff.

What was the relationship between Larrey and Percy? We know that Larrey was not universally popular among his medical peers. This is apparent from his difficulty in gaining election to the Academy of Sciences and to the Institute. It appears that Larrey and Percy were on friendly terms in the earlier years of the wars. Larrey praises Percy in his memoirs for his actions at Jena in 1806 whereas Percy makes a number of complimentary references to Larrey in his journal of 1805. Indeed, when Larrey fell ill in 1807 it was Percy who cared for him. In the same year, before the Battle of Friedland, we find the two men happily dining together with Alexandre Yvan, Napoleon's personal surgeon, and the administrator of the corps. It was in the following year in Madrid that a rift developed which was never completely resolved. The quarrel arose over the men's relative roles in the functioning of the *service de santé* and in the development, such as it was, of the army's ambulance system. Larrey perceived that Percy had 'borrowed' his idea of the flying ambulance. He may also have felt that he had to work overtime to compensate for the shortcomings of the *service de santé* of the rest of the army, which was Percy's responsibility. Certainly, he had recently been asked to act as inspector general of the hospitals of the line, a post that appears well outside his remit as chief surgeon to the Imperial Guard. Percy's views are well represented by the following extract from his journal dated September 1808.

> Monsieur le grand-maréchal [Duroc] returned to the hospital [in Madrid] to distribute gifts; I found him there and, following my invitation, he saw the confusion the service was in and stopped the distribution; tomorrow he will have a list of wounded who are worthy of it; I have asked him for some *infirmiers* and have begged him to tell His Majesty that it is necessary to have these immediately and that bringing them from Paris is putting the service in danger. Monsieur Larrey, who pokes his nose in everywhere in his own boisterous way, interrupted me and dared to say to His Excellency with me present, that there was nothing good or useful in my suggestion, unlike the project which he had had the honour to submit to His Majesty the Emperor of Russia, which had been greatly welcomed and which it was necessary to bring to the attention of His Majesty Napoleon, who ... The grand-maréchal, accustomed to these boastings, smiled at me and, none-the-less, invited me to detail my ideas. The same presumptuousness [of Larrey] is directed at the service of the Line which does not concern him; he speaks to me of pharmacy, pharmacists, etc ...

Percy describes Larrey as becoming 'mad with pride' and even implies that he was a little deluded, 'he proposes the formation of ambulances of Africa, Asia etc.'[16]

After this time, it seems that the two men, despite their mutual commitment to the *service de santé*, were in frequent conflict with each other. In 1813 Larrey instituted some changes to the medical equipment of the *Grande Armée* without consulting the inspector generals – Percy, Coste and Gallée. Although this was not as personal as their earlier disagreement, Percy and Larrey were again on the opposite sides of an argument, Percy, unusually for him, being on the side of authority. The Inspectors were disgruntled at Larrey's unilateral actions and rejected most of his suggestions, at least for the Army of Spain. Percy's brusque response was followed by a more ponderous and diplomatic letter from Coste. Larrey was also to feel aggrieved at the arrangements made for the Campaign of One Hundred Days in 1815, when Percy was appointed surgeon-in-chief to the *Grande Armée*. It is probable that Napoleon favoured Percy because of his greater administrative skills. Larrey had previously been criticised for his preoccupation with the details of surgery at the expense of the wider service. However, due to poor health, Percy had not seen active service since 1811 and Larrey's irritation was understandable. Furthermore, he held Percy personally responsible for his demotion. He withdrew, leaving the ambulances to the Guard's more junior surgeons, and was only persuaded to march on the eve of the campaign. 'I must have Larrey for the Guard and the General Headquarters,' the Emperor snapped. 'He sulks because he has been replaced by Percy. Go and tell him that he is indispensable and that I count on him.'[17]

Posterity has been kinder to the memory of Larrey than to Percy's. This modern perspective of the two men has been honed by a number of eulogistic biographies of Larrey appearing during the later 19th and then 20th centuries. The evolution of a symbolic picture of the Battle of Eylau suggests a different contemporary view. In April 1807 Larrey learned that such a painting had been commissioned and that Napoleon wished to include a surgeon in the picture to honour the contribution of the *service de santé*. Among the artists likely to win the commission, Girardet was a particular favourite. Larrey lost no time in writing to him to demand that it should be him who featured.

> My request is very well founded as I was the only senior doctor who directed, without intervention, the dressing of all the wounded. It was me who did all the major operations … My colleague, Monsieur Percy, made only an appearance on this terrible day and did not perform a single operation.

Concerned that Napoleon might not have specified him by name, Larrey was quick to add that, if this was the case, it was simply an oversight. In the event, the work was eventually undertaken by Antoine-Jean Gros and the surgeon in the foreground of one of the most famous of all Napoleonic paintings is Pierre-François Percy.

René-Nicolas Desgenettes

René-Nicolas Desgenettes was arguably the greatest physician in the French army. He was born in Alençon in 1762 of an old family of the town and went to Paris to pursue medical studies. He interrupted these in the 1780s to travel to England and Italy. After passing his thesis for a doctorate in medicine at Montpellier, he spent a further period studying in the capital before being attached to the Army of Italy as a physician in 1793. He was soon elevated to physician-in-chief and commenced a long friendship with Napoleon. He was an obvious choice to direct the medical services for the Army of the Orient and it was in the Egyptian Campaign that Desgenettes reached the peak of his career. He combated the plague with enormous devotion and bravery, even inoculating himself to try and convince the soldiers of its non-contagious nature and therefore restore their morale. Of course this was a delusion but Desgenettes' action had the desired impact and he survived the experiment with few ill effects. On his return from the Orient he was named chief physician of the military hospital in Paris. Officer of the *Légion d'honneur* in 1804 and baron of the Empire in 1809, he followed the *Grande Armée* from Vienna to Berlin and from Madrid to Moscow. In the 1812 campaign he fell into the hands of the Russians and was ultimately freed by Tsar Alexander with the words, 'Men like you have the right to be recognised by all nations.' After the Battle of Leipzig in the following year, he spent a miserable period in the town of Torgau struggling against typhus. In the decades after the wars, he was elected to the Academies of Medicine and Sciences and taught hygiene to the faculties. He died in 1851.[18]

Desgenettes was an aristocrat and, by all accounts, he had the assurance, grace and charm associated with his class. He was also intelligent and eloquent. Pharmacist Jacob met Desgenettes when the latter visited his bivouac during the 1813 campaign in Germany. Jacob describes him as distinguished, honest and principled. He was also great company, telling numerous amusing anecdotes with a gift for impersonation. 'I do not know if he was a good physician but he might have been an excellent comedian.' The events of the Egyptian Campaign and its aftermath show a different side to Desgenettes' character. He was one of the very few men who were prepared to argue against the highest authority in favour of the sick and the medical services of the army. He first clashed with Napoleon, at that time General Bonaparte, when the latter notoriously ordered poisoning of a number of plague victims at Jaffa. In fairness to Bonaparte, his request that the debilitated men should be given high doses of laudanum to prevent them falling into the hands of the ruthless Turks can easily be seen as a humanitarian gesture rather than as the evil act portrayed by his detractors. Whatever the motivation, Desgenettes refused to play any part in poisoning the patients, and the laudanum, probably in insufficient doses, was given by the pharmacist Royer. At least some survived and were subsequently protected by the British admiral, Sir Sydney Smith.[19]

Simmering resentment from this affair may still have been in the air when Bonaparte later convened a sitting of the Institute of Egypt at Cairo. He requested that the Institute appoint a commissary to draw up a report on the plague at Jaffa and Acre. It was widely suspected that Bonaparte was preparing to place the blame for his failed campaign in Syria either on the plague itself or on the medical services' inability to recognise the danger quickly enough. Desgenettes, surprisingly, was not nominated to serve on the commission but he was at the initial meeting. When Bonaparte allowed himself a few cheap and disparaging comments at the expense of the medical profession, Desgenettes leapt to his feet and 'with a vehemence that astounded the numerous audience', he proceeded to speak his mind. He made transparent allusions to a 'certain criminal action' which he had resisted and also made telling comments regarding moral principles. Bonaparte tried to silence him in a friendly manner, as did the president. By now, the meeting was in uproar with shouts of 'mercenary adulation', 'oriental despotism', and 'armed guards up to the very doors of a peaceful literary society', referring to the general-in-chief's guides who had come with him to the meeting. This was all reminiscent of the recriminatory days of the Revolutionary Era. Desgenettes kept his calm but lacked any discretion. He was not intending to mix words and reproached Bonaparte for 'being something other than a member of the institute when here', and for 'wanting to be top dog everywhere'. He refused to retract any of this, almost taking pride in saying things which he acknowledged would 'have their recriminations far from here'. He ended by quoting a triumphant reply given by the physician Philippos to Alexander the Great, 'I take refuge in the gratitude of the army.' Immediately after this astonishing scene, Desgenettes requested authorisation to return to France because of health and family reasons. Bonaparte refused to replace him, one presumes out of recognition for his merits.[20]

Napoleon took no further steps against Desgenettes and, indeed, it appears that the physician had no serious enemies. There was one possible exception. Falling out with Dominique Larrey was an occupational hazard for other senior doctors in the *Grande Armée*. In Desgenettes' case the rift occurred following his imprisonment by the Russians in 1812. Larrey made considerable efforts to get his colleague freed, writing personally to the Tsar. Desgenettes was duly released; an outcome that he attributed, possibly correctly, entirely to his own reputation but which Larrey believed was due to his lobbying. Desgenettes' lack of gratitude to Larrey was extremely irritating to the latter who wrote to his wife of the army's senior physician, 'Without me he would be no more than a memory in people's minds.' The situation was exacerbated by Desgenettes making a claim for the loss of his own equipment in Russia but not, as Larrey alleged he had promised, speaking up for his surgical colleague. In Larrey's words to his wife, 'That's that then.' Once again, a chasm had developed between two of the army's greatest doctors.[21]

Jean-François Coste
Arguably the fourth great doctor of the *Grande Armée*, unlucky not to have his name also inscribed on the Arc de Triomphe, was the physician Jean-François Coste. Less well known than Larrey, Percy and Desgenettes, his modern reputation has been enhanced by a recent comprehensive biography.[22] Coste was considerably older than his three illustrious peers and made significant contributions to the *service de santé* prior to the Wars of Revolution and Empire. Born into a medical family in 1741, he mixed in elevated circles from an early age, being an acquaintance of Voltaire. After studying medicine he took a particular interest in military hospitals and,

in 1780, he was appointed chief physician to Rochambeau's expeditionary force to America. Here, Coste laid the foundations of his later work in the *Grande Armée*, dealing effectively with outbreaks of smallpox and dysentery and writing an academic work on hospitals. Coste's reputation as an army physician and eminent citizen was on the rise and this was reflected by his election as the first mayor of Versailles. He survived the Revolutionary Period unscathed and, probably in part due to his close friendship with Berthier, Bonaparte's ablest lieutenant, in 1803 he found himself as chief physician to the camp of Boulogne and then to the *Grande Armée* itself. This was the culmination of Coste's career as his lot under the Empire was not an entirely happy one. Despite retaining senior positions in the army hierarchy, notably in the *conseil de santé*, he was gradually brought down to earth by a combination of age, ill health and Napoleon's prejudice against the physicians of the army. In 1806 an increasingly enfeebled Coste unfairly bore the brunt of the Emperor's anger at the lack of physicians in the hospitals around Warsaw and he was sent back to Paris to be replaced by Desgenettes. After the Restoration, in the few years before his death in 1819, he dedicated himself to re-establishing the military hospitals. Never one of Napoleon's favourites, he was not made a baron of the Empire despite representations from Daru and Berthier. He deserves recognition for his patient administrative work in the highest levels of the *service de santé* and for his contributions to the health of the army including the promotion of improved hygiene and the introduction of vaccination.

Beyond these four giants there are a number of other surgeons, physicians and pharmacists of the *Grande Armée* who merit a brief mention either because of their contribution to the *service de santé* or their closeness to Napoleon. Alexandre Yvan was of doubtful calibre but he gained fame as the Emperor's personal surgeon.[23] He had modest success as a surgeon in the Army of Italy in the closing years of the 18th century and he was picked from relative obscurity to fill this elevated position. Percy had difficulty in hiding his irritation, writing to Berthier: 'The most prestigious post in military surgery has been given to a young man ... one who was in a crowd of pupils when I occupied already, not without distinction, the premier place in the army'. Despite the perceived injustice, Yvan carried out his role until late in the wars, always just behind the Emperor, 'his shadow'. He was not a great technical surgeon and generally took a conservative view, opposing the vigorous approach to amputation advocated by Larrey. It was Yvan who made the dressing when Napoleon was slightly wounded in the ankle by a spent ball at the Battle of Ratisbonne in 1809. His relationship with his master ended dramatically and unhappily at Fontainebleau in April 1814 when Napoleon made a bungled suicide attempt. Yvan's precise role remains obscure, he may have prepared the poison, but he did himself little credit by then panicking and deserting the Emperor, never to see him again.

Perhaps more deserving of memory is Nicolas Heurteloup, who was an inspector general of the *service de santé* and a baron of the Empire. He received many of the same distinctions as his more famous surgical colleagues, Percy and Larrey, but he was more of an administrator and man of action than a practising doctor and man of science. Rising through the ranks in the Army of Revolution he was chief surgeon to the army in 1800. His greatest moment was his superb organisation of the surgical services during the Austrian campaign of 1809 where his direction of the hospitals at Vienna and Ebersdorf was commended by Napoleon in the official bulletin. He was still working towards the improvement of the *service de santé* when he died in Paris in 1812.

The final surgeon worth of introduction is François Girardot, *chirurgien-major* of the Polish *chevau-léger* of the Imperial Guard. He was wounded for the first time at the Battle of Montereau in France in 1814 and was promoted to Officer of the *Légion d'honneur*. Two months later, at the Battle of Craonne, he got off his horse in a hail of fire to tend the wounded. Struck by a ball, he still rallied the cavalry around him. Finally, pulling himself to his feet, covered with blood and his leg only attached to his body by a few fibres, he collected his strength and shouted a vibrant *'Vive L'Empereur!'* Napoleon witnessed the whole episode and made the gallant surgeon baron of the Empire at the same time that his leg was being amputated on the field. He was one of only seven army doctors to receive this honour.[24]

We will only briefly consider the most famous physician of the Napoleonic Era as he had little impact on army medicine. Jean-Nicolas Corvissart was Napoleon's personal physician and was responsible for the *service de santé* of the imperial household. The Emperor had great faith in him, once commenting, 'I do not believe in medicine but I believe in Corvissart.' After accompanying the Emperor in the campaigns of 1805 to 1809 he increasingly distanced himself in the later years of the Empire. Criticised for being a fawning courtesan in Napoleon's entourage, Corvissart is more fairly remembered as a pioneer of the new more rational approach to clinical diagnosis and an early authority on diseases of the heart. The greatest army pharmacist of the period was undoubtedly Antoine-Augustus Parmentier, born at Montdidier in 1737. He was pharmacist in chief at the *Invalides* as early as 1776. A proponent of the potato, he personally cultivated the plant and managed to interest King Louis XVI in its more widespread consumption. For a long period he was a member of the *conseil de santé* although he had little direct contact with the *Grande Armée*. Modest and hardworking, he championed practical advances such as the use of vaccination and the provision of better bread for the soldiers. In 1802 he wrote and published his *Code Pharmaceutique*, a guide for the pharmacy services in military hospitals.[25]

The cumulative influence of all these senior doctors on the *service de santé* of the *Grande Armée* was probably less that that of a man who held no medical qualifications. Napoleon moulded the army in his own image. It was a familiar tool in his hands. This has been conclusively shown in countless books on the Napoleonic Wars and does not require detailed reiteration here. Just as the infantry were 'Napoleon's infantry', the cavalry 'Napoleon's cavalry', and the artillery, 'Napoleon's artillery', the *service de santé* also functioned according to his tastes and dictates. Its *officiers de santé* were unequivocally 'Napoleon's doctors'. If we accept that this is true, then it is clear that to fully understand why the *service de santé* worked as it did, we need to understand something of Napoleon's attitude to it. How did he regard medicine? What was his opinion of doctors? Above all, what did he believe to be the role of the *Grande Armée*'s medical services? It is possible to address these key questions using a combination of Napoleon's own correspondence and the accounts of those around him.

Jean-François Lemaire has argued coherently that Napoleon's rule was the catalyst for the emergence of modern medicine in early 19th-century France.[26] This is ironic as the Emperor is frequently portrayed as a man who disliked doctors and was contemptuous of medicine. On reviewing the evidence, it may be more accurate to state that he was distrustful of doctors and sceptical of their vocation. We have to acknowledge the frequent inconsistencies in his statements and behaviour pertaining to medicine in general and the *service de santé* of his army. Where we try to analyse Napoleon's interaction with doctors we are all too often confronted with non sequiturs.

Napoleon's antagonism to medication was well known. He took pride in the fact that he rarely had to resort to it. His favourite physician, Corvissart, was famed for his therapeutic nihilism. In one outburst directed at Desgenettes, Napoleon claimed that 'Chemistry is the cookery of medicine and medicine is the science of assassins!' Desgenettes rather obtusely replied, 'And you, how would you define the science of conquerors?' Napoleon did not reply but he obviously enjoyed his sally against medicine and therapeutics as he confronted Corvissart with identical statements. The court physician, a more polished diplomat than Desgenettes, refrained from replying. But Napoleon was not uninterested in medicine and drugs. Marchand, the Emperor's valet, noted that, 'though he did not have a high opinion of medicine he liked to discuss it with his doctor'. On one occasion, after viewing some anatomical charts, Napoleon observed that he had wanted to study anatomy but had been put off by the odour of the cadavers which he found repulsive. Percy records that, during the campaign of 1806 in Poland, the Emperor was 'much preoccupied' with the supply of medicines and talked in detail of kina, emetics and camphor. He was disturbed at the lack of medical supplies with the army. Two years later, in Spain, when the French army came across a large amount of quinine, one of the few effective drugs of the period, Napoleon took elaborate measures to allocate it to forty 'good towns' of the Empire. Although there was a public relations element to this exercise, it appears unlikely that he would have gone to such trouble unless he believed that the drug would be beneficial.[27]

Napoleon preferred prevention over treatment. He agreed with Lord Nelson's tenet, 'It is easier for an officer to keep a man healthy than for a physician to cure him.' His favourite medicines were good hygiene, fresh air, rest, nutritious food and high morale. He went to great lengths to preserve his own health. Las Cases describes his regimen which was based on establishing 'equilibrium'. If he had spent some time resting he would then deliberately undertake a period of exercise. Conversely, after a period of intensive activity he would studiously take some absolute rest. With respect to the troops, he was particularly preoccupied with the concept of 'unhealthy air', and always took great care in their placement. Two hundred years later, it is difficult to argue with Napoleon's views. Much of his cynicism regarding the efficacy of contemporary medical treatments was entirely justified. Where he did support specific medical interventions, for instance vaccination and quinine, he more often than not got it right. He certainly had more understanding of disease than most of his enemies. When the British invaded the Island of Walcheren off the Dutch coast in 1809, Napoleon ordered his generals not to intervene. 'Walcheren has for its defence fever and poor air ... in this season the island is one of the unhealthiest places on earth.' The Emperor was soon proved entirely correct in his prediction, the British army being decimated by 'Walcheren fever', a mixture of malaria, typhus, dysentery and other infectious diseases.[28]

Although Napoleon had some real understanding of medicine and perhaps was intellectually fascinated by it, this interest was not convincingly translated into genuine and concerted support for the medical services of the army and the care of sick and wounded soldiers. The evidence is conflicting but the bulk of it weighs against him. We are left with the impression that he was a master of the timely gesture but that he was not prepared to invest the effort required to give the *Grande Armée* the *service de santé* it surely deserved. There are endless anecdotes of the Emperor revisiting the battlefield strewn with wounded men. For instance, the following written by Vélite Billon.

> I was sitting on a bank of stones, leaning against a wall, when he [Napoleon] passed close to me. The Emperor was making every effort to avoid the hooves of his horse treading on the human remains. Not being able to cross the field, he abandoned the attempt and it was then that I saw him cry.[29]

It was commonplace for him to give orders relating to the collection and dressing of men left on the field. This included the enemy. On the day after the Battle of Bautzen in 1813, Eugene Fenech met the Emperor as he was dressing a Prussian officer. 'He stopped to advise me to have the same regard for the foreign wounded as for our own. Twenty five paces further on he saw several of them and sent me an aide-de-camp to tell me not to forget them.' Such excursions were often followed by gifts to the wounded men in the nearby hospitals and generous payments to the widows and orphans of the dead.[30] He was careful to enquire as to the health of individual wounded officers. Napoleon's supporters see these actions as characteristic of a man who took a sincere concern in the wellbeing of the ordinary wounded soldier, be he friend or foe. His detractors see only a superficial ritual, an act which was habitual and cost the Emperor little in real time or effort. Some have gone so far as to suggest that Napoleon derived a vicarious pleasure in viewing the mangled remains of those slaughtered in his own name, a true consummation of his megalomania.

Napoleon was capable of short periods of interest in the *service de santé* during which he involved himself in the most mundane details of its functioning. This is apparent from his correspondence and his conversations with his senior doctors. As early as 1796, in the Army of Italy, General Bonaparte was giving detailed orders regarding the evacuation of the wounded and particularly the separation of the amputees from those men who were more likely to recover. Three years later, in Egypt, he addressed the minutiae of the evacuation of the wounded and again he showed great concern that the wounded be divided up according to the severity of their injuries. The full extent to which Napoleon was prepared to dictate the finer details of the *service de santé* is well illustrated by his correspondence with Daru and Berthier regarding hospitals in the 1806 campaign. In December, he wrote to the *intendant general* from Paris.

> The *infirmiers* will be paid daily at a rate of 20 *sous* and will additionally receive one ration of food which will be distributed to them. The Intendant General, out of the funding put at his disposition by the Minister of War, will take the necessary measures so that each hospital director always has in his accounts, and in advance, a fund of 12 francs for each sick man in the hospital. These funds will pay the salaries of the *infirmiers* and will meet the cost of minor requirements such as eggs, milk, etc.

It is odd that Napoleon should have felt the need to address the means of purchase of eggs. There is much more correspondence of the same ilk concerning the supervision, inspection and security of hospitals. The Emperor ordered that each hospital was to have a Catholic priest as chaplain who would contribute to the administrative duties. He ensured that the pharmacy of the *service de santé* had supplies adequate for two months. Other detailed correspondence of the period pertains to the organisation of ambulances and the lack of surgeons. 'The number of surgeons in the

French hospitals is ridiculous. It is not in proportion with the number of employees of the army.'[31]

In his conversations with his senior doctors, Napoleon often requested information about the number and state of sick and wounded men. In Spain in 1809, he quizzes Percy as to the precise nature of the prevailing diseases and their management prior to a more wide-ranging discussion of the relative merits of French and English surgery and the pay of army doctors. In Russia in 1812, it is the Emperor who personally directs the medical services at headquarters at Vilna, telling Berthier to make the ambulances and surgeons ready for departure. A year later, in Germany, his letters once again return to the evacuation of wounded and to the organisation of the hospitals and, belatedly, he makes some suggestions for a proper ambulance service. This all demonstrates that Napoleon was interested in the well-being of the sick and wounded of the *Grande Armée*. That this interest was sustained and more than opportunistic is less clear. Much of the Emperor's preoccupation with his medical services occurred at the outset of a campaign or even on the eve of a major battle. There is an almost desperate air to his enquiries regarding surgeons, ambulances and hospitals, giving the impression that he was reacting to events rather than dictating them.[32]

Napoleon's public pronouncements regarding the *service de santé* are inconsistent. After the Egyptian campaign in 1801, he wrote to Larrey via Berthier acknowledging, 'the unbounded devotion and great success that you and your colleagues have displayed in the preservation of this most valuable army'. Similarly, in 1807, the Emperor corresponded with Percy, praising the surgeons who had shown, 'courage, zeal, devotion and, above all, patience and resignation'. The bulletin of the *Grande Armée* after Wagram emphasises the satisfaction of the Emperor with the *service de santé* and especially the surgical services and the surgeon-in-chief Heurteloup. On the other hand, the Emperor was quick to publicly criticise the army's doctors whenever he believed they were not serving him well. His best known outburst is contained in a letter of January 1812 to Jean-Gérard Lacuée. 'The inexperience of the surgeons does more harm to the army than the guns of the enemy. The *comité de santé* is entirely guilty of sending surgeons so ignorant.'[33]

On occasions, the Emperor used perceived shortcomings in the *service de santé* to conceal problems of his own making. In the town of Vitebsk in 1812 he held regular reviews of his troops to try and maintain morale. He was well aware of the grumbling about the supply situation and he used one of the parades to vent his anger publicly at the *commissaires* and those in charge of the medical services. Shouting loudly enough for the soldiers to overhear, he derided them for failing to honour the 'sanctity of their mission'. He sacked a senior pharmacist and threatened the hapless doctors that he would send them back to treat the whores of the Palais Royal. There is little doubt that if they had known what was in store for them in

Russia many of the *officiers de santé* would have jumped at this offer. This unsavoury spectacle had the desired effect on the watching soldiers who cheered the Emperor who appeared to care for them so deeply.[34]

By failing to support the autonomy of the *service de santé* Napoleon allowed it to be subjugated to the administration. He could easily have reversed this situation but he chose not to. He later claimed that this was to allow the *officiers de santé* to appear as advocates of the soldier and so that they were not tainted with the problems of actually managing the hospitals, 'they could still complain of the poor medicines and the soldiers saw them as men who protected them'. Whatever his reasons, it is obvious that he did not have high regard for most of the administrative officers. His admonitions against the *service de santé* hardly compare with his attacks on his own administration. In Warsaw in 1806, Percy describes Napoleon's tirade against the administration's management of the hospitals. 'He went so far as to say that, with respect to the hospitals, the Nation had become the most barbarous in Europe, below that of our neighbours, and that even the Cossacks treated the wounded better than us.' In the face of ongoing short-ages of hospital equipment and the lack of hospital employees the Emperor later accused the administration of ruining the medical services: 'They have lost my surgery by worrying it and delivering it over to their foolish proj-ects.'[35] It was convenient for him to displace the blame for the inadequacy of the hospitals onto the administrators who were often struggling to maintain the service in an inhospitable country against overwhelming odds.

Napoleon failed his doctors. His sporadic bursts of intensive involvement in the workings of the medical services cannot disguise the reality that, over the whole course of the wars, he was not prepared to invest the time or effort required to provide a first class *service de santé* for the *Grande Armée*. Neither was he prepared to delegate adequately to allow others to achieve this. His correspondence confirms these assertions. French medical historian Jean-François Lemaire has combed the Emperor's 22,000 letters and found fewer than five hundred pertaining to health. Many of these relate to rather peripheral subjects and are not strictly military in nature. Of the latter, many contain warnings against the dangers of 'unhealthy air', a near obsession of the Emperor. There are fewer than a hundred (less than 0.5% of the total) directly addressing the management of the wounded.[36] Napoleon may have revolutionised the art of war but he was reluctant to support any new inno-vations in the medical care of his troops. He paid little more than lip service to the well intentioned suggestions and plans of men such as Larrey and Percy and the status quo remained. As will be seen in the following chapters on the battlefield medicine of the wars, the projects that would have made a real difference – a formal ambulance system, Percy's *chirurgie de bataille*, *brancardiers* – all failed to materialise. He complained of the quality of his surgeons but it was he who had closed the *hôpitaux d'instruction* in 1803 and he who had failed to motivate them by depriving them of permanent commissions and a proper infrastructure in which to work. When he did try to address some of these issues in the later years of the wars, for instance his own tentative suggestions for an ambulance service directed by surgeons made in 1813, it was largely irrelevant because, by this stage, his star was waning and he no longer had the necessary resources. For too long the Emperor had agonised over the health of the Empire but had been too little concerned about the health of his troops. He had taken both them and their doctors for granted. Not for nothing did Kléber refer to him as a '*général à 6,000 hommes par jour!*'[37]

What did Napoleon's doctors think of their Emperor? Napoleon had a gift for drawing people towards him, particularly those whose skills and influence he required. Senior doctors who had close contact with him often expressed their admiration. Percy's journal is replete with complimentary references emphasising the Emperor's humanity, vision, bravery and tirelessness. Before Eylau, in the miserable depths of Poland, the roads were littered with French dead. 'His Majesty's heart must be torn by these sights, but he moves on to fulfil the great destiny that he has prepared for Europe.' At the subsequent battle, Percy describes Napoleon standing on a small hill in the midst of the fighting, ignoring the numerous shells falling about him. In Spain, it is his stamina which impresses Percy:

> What a man! What a body! Yesterday he astonishingly rode from Burgos to Aranda, always at the gallop, and was only relieved three times. Today he has been in the saddle nine hours, seeing everything, giving all the orders, giving departures for the march etc.

Percy's journal was a contemporary account and it may have been risky to record the Emperor's actions in less reverential terms. The surgeon did permit himself the occasional criticism of his master and we can therefore interpret his admiring comments as sincere. Conversely, when Percy wrote for public consumption, his account of the Emperor and his circle was so immoderate as to be considered simple propaganda. In a piece written for a French newspaper in 1810 he describes the visit of Napoleon's brother, Joseph, the King of Spain, to the Madrid hospitals. The prose is adulatory. The local inhabitants are portrayed as being astonished by the philanthropy of their new ruler. We are reminded that he has inherited this characteristic as a family trait.[38]

Larrey also admired Napoleon and showed him great loyalty but as much of his memoirs were written retrospectively he is more circumspect in his comments. Indeed, it is noticeable that whereas in the early memoirs Larrey refers to Napoleon as the 'Emperor' or the 'Commander in Chief', from 1813 onwards he is simply the 'Head of the Army'. This probably reflects nothing more than Larrey's fastidious correctness and not any lesser regard for Napoleon. The army's more junior doctors had mixed views. They acknowledge the Emperor's charisma and his unparalleled ability to inspire those around him in the most calamitous of circumstances. In Russia, Physician Heinrich Roos says that 'all the faces of the troops were directed towards him with a mixture of admiration, trust and hope. At this time, as later, I heard the officers of different nations say, "Whilst Napoleon is in our midst we will not lack courage".' Even those who were politically opposed to Napoleon, for instance, Chirurgien-Major René Bourgeois, were infected by these sentiments.

> Although this man was, rightly, regarded as the author of all our misfortunes and the unique cause of our disaster, his presence still elicited enthusiasm and there was nobody who would not, if the need arose, have covered him with their body and sacrificed their lives for him.

Such mixed feelings towards the Emperor were common among doctors and medical students both in the army and in civilian life. Medical student Poumiès de la Siboutie describes the lack of support for Napoleon among the students of the *École de Médecine* when Paris was under attack by the allies in 1814. Few were prepared to join the makeshift local companies of artillery. Poumiès de la Siboutie claims that Napoleon's name was 'reviled everywhere'. In contrast, when Napoleon returned from Elba the following year the students 'offered him their devotion and service', eagerly joining the newly formed artillery companies and attending drill in the gardens of the Luxembourg Palace.

> We were filled with a fervent desire to blot out the recollection of our pusillanimous conduct in 1814. It was not merely blind passion for Napoleon that animated us. Our susceptibilities had been hurt in every conceivable way under the Restoration and we really looked upon him as our avenger. How he deceived us history has since made clear!

Not all were so easily won over by the Emperor's dramatic return. Chirurgien-Major Jean-Baptiste d'Héralde was angry at the news: 'I understood well that Bonaparte did not come for the good of my country.' Physician Joseph Tyrbas de Chamberet is relentlessly antagonistic to Napoleon. Bonaparte's rise to absolute authority is achieved through 'the power of charlatanism, intrigues and ruses'. His subsequent empire is founded upon 'hypocrisy, imposture, the violation of laws, brutal force, blood and tears'.[39]

Napoleon's attitudes and actions with respect to his doctors and the *service de santé* all too often appear paradoxical. He was friendly and helpful to army doctors he knew and trusted but he failed to support their profession. He was capable of intensive involvement in the workings of the *Grande Armée*'s medical services but he failed to take the necessary steps to consolidate the service and improve it. He took a close interest in the well-being of wounded and sick soldiers but was capable of callously sacrificing enormous numbers of men in ill-prepared schemes of dubious military merit. Any discussion of Napoleon is an 'argument without end'. This applies equally to an analysis of his role in the *service de santé* of the *Grande Armée*. Peter Geyl, in his brilliant resume of French historical interpretations of Napoleon, writes: 'History can reach no unchallengeable conclusions on so many sided a character, on a life so dominated, so profoundly agitated, by the circumstances of the time.'[40]

Notes

1. For biographical details of Percy see Ducoulombier, H, *Le Baron P-F Percy. Un chirurgien de la Grande Armée*; Brice, Docteur and Bottet, Capitaine, *Le Corps de Santé Militaire en France*, p. 244; Tulard, J, *Dictionnaire Napoléon*, Vol. II, p. 488; Pigeard, A, *Dictionnaire de la Grande Armée*, p. 455; Lemaire, J-F, *Les blessés dans les Armées Napoléoniennes*, p. 206; Percy, Baron, *Journal des Campagnes de Baron Percy*, p. xxi.
2. Percy, p. lxxxviii.
3. Jacob, P-I, *Le Journal Inédit d'un pharmacien de la Grande Armée*, p. 198.
4. McGrigor, J, *The Autobiography and Services of James McGrigor Bt. Late Director of the Army Medical Department*, p. 353; Percy, p.lxxxi.
5. Damamme, J-C, *Les Soldats de la Grande Armée*, p. 240; Percy, pp. 43, xlviii.
6. D'Héralde, J-B, *Mémoires d'un Chirurgien de la Grande Armée*, p. 29; Fardeau, U, *Urbain Fardeau. Mémoires d'un Saumurois chirurgien-sabreur*, p. 59; Tyrbas de Chamberet, J, *Mémoires d'un Médecin Militaire*, p.146.
7. Pigeard, p.455; Blond, G, *La Grande Armée*, p. 102.
8. For biographical details of Larrey see Richardson, R, *Larrey. Surgeon to Napoleon's Imperial Guard*; Dible, J H, *Napoleon's Surgeon*; Soubiran, A, *Le Baron Larrey chirurgien de Napoléon*; Triaire, P, *Dominique Larrey et les campagnes de la Révolution et de l'Empire*; Pigeard, p. 366; Tulard, Vol. II, p. 154; Lemaire, p. 210.
9. Richardson, p. 203.
10. Dible, p. 332; Larrey, D J, *Mémoires de Chirurgie Militaire et Campagnes 1787–1840*, p. 53.
11. Damamme, p. 251.
12. Richardson, pp. 228–9.
13. Jacob, p. 206; Lemaire, p. 215; Percy, p. 455.
14. Dible, p. 238.
15. Morvan, J, *Le Soldat Impérial*, Vol. II, pp. 338, 354.
16. Lemaire, p. 215; Larrey, p. 463; Percy, pp. 69, 287, 436–7; Richardson, pp. 131–2.
17. Lemaire, pp. 197–203; Dible, p. 236.
18. Brice, Bottet, p. 239.
19. Jacob, p.261; Herold, J C, *Bonaparte in Egypt*, p. 358.

20. Charles-Roux, F, *Bonaparte: Governor of Egypt*, p. 327; Herold, p. 317.
21. Richardson, p. 188.
22. Lemaire, J-F, *Coste: Premier Médecin des Armées de Napoléon.*
23. Lemaire, *Les blessés dans les Armées Napoléoniennes*, p.218.
24. Brice, Bottet, p. 247; Lemaire, *Les blessés dans les Armées Napoléoniennes* , p. 221.
25. Tulard, Vol. I, p.564; Brice, Bottet, p. 240.
26. Lemaire, J-F, *Napoléon et la Médecine.*
27. Milleliri, J-M, *Médecins et Soldats pendant l'expédition d'Égypte (1798–1799)*, p. 37; Marchand, L-J, *In Napoleon's Shadow*, p. 92; Percy, p.115; Lemaire, *Napoléon et la Médecine*, p. 244.
28. Howard, M, *Wellington's Doctors. The British Army Medical Services in the Napoleonic Wars*, p. 187; Lemaire, *Napoléon et la Médecine*, pp. 63, 52; Howard, M, *Walcheren 1809: A medical catastrophe.*
29. Lemaire, *Les blessés dans les Armées Napoléoniennes*, p. 116.
30. Fenech, E, *Mémoires d'un Officier de Santé Maltais dans l'Armée Française (1786–1839)*, p. 79; Percy, p. 475.
31. Lemaire, *Les blessés dans les Armées Napoléoniennes*, pp. 119, 126; Brice, Bottet, p. 176; Lemaire, *Coste*, pp. 287–8.
32. Percy, p. 469; Lemaire, *Les blessés dans les Armées Napoléoniennes*, pp. 155, 168.
33. Percy, p. 183; Lemaire, *Napoléon et la Médecine*, p. 91; Brice, Bottet, p. 179.
34. Zamoyski, A, *Napoleon's fatal march on Moscow*, p. 193.
35. Percy, pp. 124–5.
36. Lemaire, *Les blessés dans les Armées Napoléoniennes*, p. 119.
37. Morvan, Vol. II, p. 369.
38. Percy, pp. 137, 420, 497.
39. Roos, H de, *Avec Napoléon en Russie*, p. 163; Zamoyski, p. 455; Poumiès de la Siboutie, *Recollections of a Parisian (1789–1863)*, pp. 130, 153; d'Héralde, p. 213; Tyrbas de Chamberet, p. 128.
40. Geyl, P, *Napoleon for and against*, p. 15.

CHAPTER IV

The Battlefield 1792–1802:
Birth of the Ambulance

The French Revolutionary Wars were fought between the years 1792 and 1802. They were more than simply the last conflict of a century already disrupted by continual warfare. They marked the sudden and brutal end of the era of 'limited warfare' which had begun in the period of Enlightenment. Previously, the affairs of Europe had been settled by surprisingly small professional armies, often with minimal involvement and disruption of the local population. The Revolutionary Wars ushered in the era of 'modern war' not so much because of new technology but because of the birth of the 'citizen army'. Universal conscription enabled France to field massive forces which initially turned back the tides of counter-revolution but ultimately flowed over France's natural boundaries crushing all before them. The soldiers were men with little military training but motivated by patriotic fervour for *La Patrie*. As Marshal Foch declared a century later, 'The wars of kings were at an end. The wars of the people were beginning'. Despite the cataclysmic nature and historical importance of the Revolutionary conflicts, they have received relatively little attention compared to the later Napoleonic Wars. There are several reasons. The Revolutionary Wars were fragmented with no obvious single form or theme. Often there were as many as ten separate campaigns being fought simultaneously with two or three battles per week worldwide. There is a dauntingly complex political aspect and no single unifying personality, such as Napoleon, to provide continuity and a simplistic explanation for the evolution of the struggle.[1]

As Revolutionary battles tended to be frequent but small, the number of casualties was relatively few compared with the later blood baths of the Empire. For the major battles between 1792 and 1796, the normal number of casualties was around ten percent, approximately 15% for the French and 7% for the allies. In the battles of the Empire after 1804 the average French loss was 21% and the allies 23%. Thus, not only were the later battles larger in absolute terms but they resulted in double the proportion of casualties.

This increase was relatively greater for the allies (from 7% to 23%) than for the French (from 15% to 21%).[2] We can conclude that although the French casualties increased under the Empire, it was the allies who had to absorb the greater increase in attrition from battle.

This new philosophy and type of warfare was not accompanied by any great step forward in weaponry. The muskets used by the Revolutionary and Napoleonic armies had heavy spherical bullets, large windage and low muzzle velocity, a combination of factors that led to poor ballistic performance. Although there must have been some improvement in the musket between 1650 and 1850 this was probably entirely in the rate of fire. The musket bullet or ball followed a trajectory that was extremely curved and erratic at all but the shortest distances. At the outset of the Revolutionary Wars it was estimated that only between 0.2 and 0.5% of the bullets fired hit their targets and it was commonly stated that a soldier had to fire seven times his own weight in lead to kill a man at whom he was aiming. Some contemporary texts suggest that this may have been an exaggeration. Picard in *La Campagne de 1800 en Allemagne* gives some interesting figures relating to the use of the French musket by soldiers under battle conditions. Against a target measuring 1.75 by 3 metres, the number of shots hitting at 75 metres was 60%, but this fell to 20% at 300 metres. The rifle was carried by specialist units in the British, Austrian and Prussian armies but did not find favour in France. The rifling of the barrel made it a far more accurate weapon than the musket and trained marksmen could reliably hit a target up to 300 metres away, albeit at a slower rate of fire.[3]

Cannon were described according to the weight of their projectile. The lightest three and four pounders were mobile field weapons whereas the larger six and twelve pounders supported armies in static positions. The range and destructive power depended on the precise type of cannon and the nature and weight of ammunition. The commonest projectile, used in 70 to 80% of cases, was round shot, solid cast iron spheres or 'cannon balls'. Round shot was designed to break the walls of fortresses in siege operations and to destroy men, horses and equipment. It could have horribly damaging effects in the field as the close formations adopted by troops made them particularly vulnerable to this type of fire. There are records of a single shot at around 700 metres killing up to forty men standing in line. Other artillery projectiles included common shells, often fired from howitzers, spherical case (shrapnel), and case or canister shot. The latter consisted of a tin case containing a number of loose bullets. The term 'grapeshot' was used imprecisely and was probably case shot.

There were innumerable different models of swords but, in simple terms, they were either straight and used mainly for thrusting or curved and designed for slashing. In the French army, heavy cavalry such as the *cuirassiers* or *carabiniers* carried a large straight broadsword whilst light cavalry such as the hussars and *chasseurs-à-cheval* carried curved sabres.

In view of the inaccuracy of the musket, many French experts advocated shock action with the bayonet but, in practice, this seems to have been rarely employed. Larrey studied the wounds of two hand-to-hand melees between French and Austrian troops and concluded that whereas the bullet wounds exceeded one hundred, there were only five wounds definitely attributable to the bayonet. The impact of the bayonet appears to have been psychological rather than material.[4]

Knowledge of the nature of the weaponry facilitates understanding of the types of wounds suffered by soldiers in the Revolutionary and Napoleonic Wars. The destructive power of lead musket balls depended much on the range of firing. At short ranges, for instance less than fifty metres, the ball could shatter major limb bones and joints. At medium range, the soft balls tended to flatten on impact and cause large conical wounds. These injuries were often complicated by the presence of clothing fragments and other foreign bodies. At ranges exceeding 200 metres, the ball might only cause a flesh wound or even be deflected by pieces of equipment or objects in packs or pockets. Superficial bullet wounds could cause little immediate pain and some soldiers even dug the ball out themselves. Pierre Lafargue, a volunteer of the second battalion of Lot-et-Garonne, was wounded by a musket ball in the hip in late 1792. He reputedly had sufficient courage to extract the ball, load it into his musket, and return it to the enemy shouting, 'Look! This is how republicans fight!' This nonchalance was not unique. Pierre-François Briot, an army surgeon of the period, recollects revolutionary soldiers with gunshot wounds walking into the ambulances and having the bullet quickly removed with a minimum of fuss, the ball being finally presented to the soldier as a memento. Others tolerated musket ball wounding less well having immediate violent reactions such as convulsions or vomiting, or screaming with pain. There was no close correlation between these reactions and the true severity of the injury.[5]

Any soldier unfortunate to find himself in the path of a round shot was likely to be killed outright or suffer a major limb injury. The awesomely destructive cannon ball caused extensive damage to bones and soft tissues and amputation of the remnant of arm or leg was usually needed. There are many anecdotes of soldiers stopping an apparently harmless ricochet ball with a foot and suffering severe bone injuries. Artillery shell fragments caused jagged wounds with compound (open to the air) fractures of the bones and torn flesh. The type of sword wound depended on the shape of the sword, straight or curved, and whether it was wielded in a thrusting or slashing action. Thrusting led to penetrating injuries, frequently of the chest and abdomen, whereas slashing with a sabre caused lacerations, often to the head and arms. The formidable broadswords of the heavy cavalry were capable of breaking bones and severing limbs. Lances were less common causes of injury but where used they predictably caused penetrating wounds. The vulnerable soldier also ran the risk of crushing injuries from falling masonry and horses and burns from exploding shells and fires in undergrowth and buildings.

Anecdotal information relating to the wounds of soldiers in the Revolutionary and early Napoleonic Wars can be gleaned from the memoirs of active campaign surgeons such as Percy and Larrey. Understandably, they emphasise the more severe injuries. Thus, in 1799 at Engen, we find Percy in an ambulance in an inn attending to the only three men who cannot be moved; one with a grapeshot wound to the spine and paralysis of the legs, the second with a musket ball wound to the bladder and the third with a ball in the chest. At Wadeleux the following year the wounded arrived in large numbers in the village, many men having severe sabre cuts and fractured leg bones. Although less often fatal than musket ball wounds, injuries from cold steel were frequently disfiguring and distressing. Percy describes the dressing of wounded at Ostrach in 1799 where a number of hussars had received sabre slashes to the face. One had a sabre cut extending from the left temporal region (forehead) to the mouth leaving a considerable flap of skin and a hole in the face which Percy repaired with three large sutures. Of the 4,360 wounded men admitted to the French military hospitals at Landau and Metz between June and October 1793, only ninety-five died, a surprisingly low mortality rate of 2%.[6] Of course, much severe trauma would not have resulted in admission to hospital with an earlier demise on or around the field. Equally, some of the wounded men may in fact have succumbed to disease, a much more common cause of death in the Revolutionary armies.

The types of wounds suffered by French soldiers depended on the weapons of their adversaries and in the more exotic theatres of war, such as Egypt, the army's surgeons were faced with new challenges. Larrey remarks that the musket balls of the Turks and Arabs were cast with a pedicle of iron or copper. Because of this the ball tended to cause more destruction and was more difficult to extract than the European version. 'This metallic fibre tears the soft parts, breaks the vessels, punctures the nerves and fixes the ball firmly in the bones, more especially when it strikes a joint.' The enormous curved swords of the Mamelukes also caused fearful wounds, on occasion completely removing a limb. The Egyptian Campaign was unusual for the period in that the number of deaths from wounds in the French army exceeded that from disease; 4,468 compared with 4,157.[7] This can be attributed more to the heroic efforts of the senior physician Desgenettes and his colleagues in the prevention and control of disease rather than to an exceptionally high mortality from wounding.

The collection of the wounded from the battlefields of the Revolutionary Wars was generally haphazard and opportunistic. It was normal 18th-century practice to leave wounded men on the field until the end of the battle.

Only then would a variable number of hastily selected litter bearers carry those still alive to the field hospitals a mile or more away. This improvised casualty evacuation system was deeply flawed. Many of the men designated to carry the wounded were distracted by looting whilst other soldiers gave unwanted help simply to preserve themselves from the dangers of battle. Surgeon Briot describes the scene.

> Three or four soldiers carried the wounded soldier in their arms or on their guns, on branches, on cloaks, on coats, sometimes by means of his own clothes; a fifth carried his bag; a sixth his gun; another his shako; until six or eight soldiers left the front for every one who was struck; and a regiment which had twenty or thirty wounded was soon reduced to one third of its strength.

This encouraged the early evacuation of lightly wounded men whilst the more seriously injured were likely to remain on the field for up to twenty-four or thirty-six hours. Any subsequent medical treatment had to also combat the resultant effects of exposure, dehydration and shock caused by bleeding. At the Battle of Fontenoy in 1745 nine tenths of the amputees died and nothing had changed significantly by the start of the Revolutionary Wars.[8]

There is evidence that not all the *officiers de santé* of the Revolutionary armies were motivated by a great desire to treat their fellow citizens on the battlefield. At least some favoured the traditional system where the army's doctors remained safely behind the battle lines until a lull in the fighting permitted their intervention. The Revolutionary authorities saw it differently and, after the Battle of Wattignies in 1793, their representatives on mission pursued the reluctant army doctors, ordering that they 'remain with the men in battle instead of withdrawing safely to the rear'. Those not complying risked a charge of desertion. Similar demands were made of the stretcher-bearers and wagon-drivers that had shown 'slackness and indifference'. Severe punishments, up to six months in prison, were promised for those who did not play their full part in the evacuation and treatment of wounded soldiers.[9]

Percy's accounts of battlefield medicine towards the end of the Revolutionary period suggest that many army surgeons were fully committed to their work but there is still an impression of an ad hoc service. For instance, during the Rhine Campaign of 1799 after fighting near the town of Engen.

> Our poor surgeons are exhausted; since half past five this morning they have not stopped working or running behind the lines to collect together the wounded; they have had twenty complicated fractures to dress which has taken them ten hours; the major operations are ongoing and then

there are endless dressings to be done; those of a grenadier with thirty sabre cuts took five and a half hours. We have evacuated on Geisingen where the headquarters of the administration is situated; there are there at present, one surgeon of the first class, four of the second class and several of the third class including the surgeons of the hospital previously established in the town to take the wounded. It has been necessary to fill the barns with wounded where they are cold. The miserable state of the wounded after the fighting is a major obstacle to their cure; if they could be kept warm in winter and kept out of the burning sun in summer the wounds would be less problematic. Several compound fractures of the thigh and leg have been reduced after deep incisions and removal of bony splinters; we evacuated them during the night. One should never have to evacuate men with such wounds but what could be done to care for them once the army has left? They would be better left in a hospital but a handful of sick men can hardly be left alone.[10]

In the following year at Marengo, the last great battle of the Revolutionary Wars, the fate of the wounded was little better. Because of the lack of wagons to transport them off the field, up to a third of the infantry deserted the ranks to 'help' their injured comrades. Many were still left on the field as night fell. Joseph Petit, *grenadier à cheval* in the Consular Guard, witnessed the dreadful scenes at the field hospital at headquarters.

We all lay down among the dead and dying, the violence of sleep shutting out the cries and moans. The next day, hunger got the better of me and when I entered into the courtyard of headquarters to procure some food for myself and my horse a most awful spectacle made me shudder. More than three thousand French and Austrian wounded were piled one upon the other in the yard, in barns, in the cowsheds, on the stairs, even in the cellars and the lofts, all letting out lamentable cries and cursing the surgeons who could not do so many dressings at once.[11]

There was thus a considerable gulf between the well intentioned proclamations of the revolutionary authorities and the reality of the battlefield. One would have expected that the revolutionary emphasis on the rights of the wounded soldier, a valued citizen of *La Patrie*, would have catalysed real improvements in battlefield medicine. Perhaps an innovation to match the unprecedented change in the nature of warfare itself. In one specific way this did actually happen. The well meaning initiatives of the authorities and the unstinting efforts of a few army doctors, notably Larrey, led to the creation of one of the greatest inventions of military medicine, the 'ambulance'.

The term ambulance was frequently used at the time to describe a field hospital close to the action. The ambulance pioneered by Larrey and others was much closer to our perception of the term today, a means of rapidly bringing initial medical care to wounded men and then promptly removing them from the field for more sophisticated treatment elsewhere. Although the ambulance was truly born in the Revolutionary Era it is a common mistake to regard it as an entirely new concept, unknown before the wars. In fact, Larrey adopted and perfected an idea that was in circulation and even being actively advocated by the National Convention. A crude ambulance service was in place as early as 1772 with heavy wagons drawn by as many as fifty horses. These were effectively mobile hospitals, each attending to an army of 20,000 men and able to cater for 2,000 wounded, one tenth of the effective force. These 'ambulance hospitals' were staffed by 134 men; a mixture of surgeons, physicians and employees such as cooks, bakers, priests, drivers and assorted workers.[12]

Despite this initiative there was a perception that there remained fundamental problems with the French army's methods of casualty evacuation and transportation. In 1788 a royal ordinance was issued requiring the creation of a better system and in the early years of the Revolutionary Wars the National Convention made significant efforts to improve the situation. This was undoubtedly in part politically motivated as the authorities were keen to suppress the damaging eye-witness accounts of the battles fought in their name, tales of 'wagons where wounded men are piled up, jolted, and painfully transported'. In November 1792 the Convention went as far as to organise a competition to design a carriage suitable for the transportation of the wounded and sick of the armies. The competition was advertised on the walls of Paris. Coste, president of the jury, captured the spirit of the event.

> The French nation was the first in Europe to routinely establish hospitals following the armies. It will be the first to give the example of all that must be done for the brave warriors who are wounded fighting for *La Patrie*. It will reduce as much as possible the sufferings of the wounded in the transports. You will be impressed, citizens, to see what has not been seen before, scholars and artists coming together to compete on equal terms for the good of humanity.[13]

Among the specifications was the requirement for the carriage to be 'light, solid, suspended and comfortable'. It had to carry four or six casualties lying down, eight at most. It had to be simply constructed and easy to repair but also insulated, waterproof and well ventilated. However, after eight months of consideration of twenty-nine designs, the commission realised that its stringent specifications were unrealistic. Ultimately, this contest led only to delay and compromised the introduction of more feasible ambulance designs which, as we will see, were under development in the field. Whilst the judges deliberated in Paris the war continued. At the Battle of

Wattignies in 1793, the wounded were crammed into clumsy four-wheeled wagons which were likely to exacerbate their wounds. Many wounded soldiers preferred to walk. The War Ministry did eventually produce two designs for evacuation vehicles but these were soon scrapped. In a final attempt at a central politically motivated solution, the Committee of Public Safety ordered the construction of vehicles based on a compromise of several designs but the result was another heavy hospital on wheels far removed from the original specifications and destined to fail.[14]

In the event, the real progress in ambulance design and introduction was made not in the political corridors and workshops of Paris but in the army itself. Some of the earliest initiatives were taken by Percy whilst he was serving with the Army of the Rhine. In 1792 he pressed a number of old soldiers and slightly disabled men into action as a corps of stretcher bearers. Provided with a uniform, a knapsack of first aid materials, a pike and a knife, the men worked in pairs to remove the wounded from the battlefield and take them to the nearest mobile hospital. Once the wounded were cleared from the field, the stretcher-bearers doubled up as orderlies in the hospitals helping the physicians and surgeons. Percy's second innovation was to design a mobile hospital or ambulance to bring the surgeons and their instruments closer to the fighting. Following the example of the French army's flying artillery, Percy mounted his battle surgeons astride a *'wurst'* ('sausage' in German), an elongated carriage which contained the dressings and surgical instruments. The body of the wagon was suspended and the top covered with leather and rounded to serve as seating for up to ten surgeons and assistants. A shelf running along each side of the vehicle served as a stirrup.[15] In his journal, Percy proudly describes his new creation and also acknowledges the problems in its introduction.

In 1799 the French army under the orders of General Jourdan crossed the Rhine. Towards midday, the corps of ambulance departed, marching with the advance guard. It was made up of only six wagons instead of the twelve or fifteen that it should have been, but in view of the usual shortage of supplies and the carelessness of most of those involved in the administration of our hospitals, we felt ourselves fortunate, by dint of our own perseverance, to have procured these feeble means. The six wagons contained in all one hundred *demi-fournitures* [units of bedding] and tools in proportion. Following the ambulance of the advance guard, marching on foot in accordance with custom, were the surgeons of all grades attached to the service. Attached to them was a *wurst* of horse artillery to carry them everywhere where they rendered help to the army and especially to enable them to arrive more quickly and freshly on the battlefield. The proposition which I had made to our generals, to give to my colleagues in all divisions of the advance guard this type of light vehicle on which ten men could sit astride with ease, and the explanation that I had made to them of the particular advantages which might result, pleased them so much that it was arranged that several of these unhitched *wursts* were put at my disposal on the battlefield, something done with pleasure and eagerness by the senior artillery officers. But it was necessary that the ambulances be supplied with horses and this was the stumbling block of our plan. The horses were not refused but they [the administration] multiplied the hindrances, the problems, the excuses, and the *wursts* drawn from the arsenal for the relief of the surgeons and the well-being of the wounded had to return there because, perhaps, *officiers de santé* on a vehicle would have been a dangerous spectacle … These men had been long condemned by a system of malevolence, oppression and humiliation to be covered in dust and mud; the administrators wanted them to go on foot and to be unhappy; otherwise, they said, the *officiers de santé* would become too insolent.[16]

Percy had a vested interest in proclaiming the utility of his new invention but his fellow surgeons supported him. Pierre-François Briot was attached to a *wurst* and was impressed.

I prepared in advance everything which my colleagues and I would need for dressing two, three, or four thousand wounded, sometimes an even greater number, according to estimated needs. Supplies of rags, strips of all sizes, elastic sticking plasters, compresses of all types, bandages of all sorts; all was prepared, stacked, labelled, numbered in the boxes which never left the ambulance; everything was at our fingertips when we needed it. With one eye we saw the nature of the wound and with the other the most appropriate treatment.

The *wurst* was also fulsomely praised by military officers. In his report on the Battle of Memmingen in 1800, General Lecourbe noted that the soldiers were greatly reassured by Percy's ambulances on the field as they knew that if they were wounded they would receive first aid with 'an unprecedented rapidity'. Later in the year, at the Battle of Oberhausen, Lecourbe again applauded the performance of the ambulances and stressed that none of the French wounded had fallen into the hands of the enemy. Percy himself enjoyed seeing the astonishment on the faces of the soldiers as the *wursts* passed by with the surgeons sitting on top.[17]

Whilst highlighting the advantages of the *wursts*, Percy did not try to disguise the difficulties he encountered in bringing the ambulance service to full fruition. He hoped to staff his ambulances with companies of 120 *infirmiers* taken not from state employees but from willing volunteers among the soldiers. These men would give vital assistance to the surgeons. However, he was continually frustrated by the lack of resources. Apart

from the shortage of horses, or at least the administration's unwilling-
ness to release them, he was frequently denied wagons and basic medical
supplies. Carts that might easily have been adapted for use as ambulances
were instead used to carry the women and children who followed the
army. The *wursts* were soon devoid of dressings and the surgeons relied on
stripping the curtains from the windows of the local houses. At Engen in
1800, a *wurst* was in attendance manned by three surgeons and an *infirmier*
but it was soon overwhelmed by the number of wounded. It still required
considerable ingenuity to reach the surgeons, wounded soldiers being carried by their comrades on their shoulders or on stretchers improvised from
branches and muskets.[18] The full implementation of Percy's innovation was
thus impeded by a lack of logistical support and it seems that, apart from a
few notable examples, the *wursts* never saw widespread battlefield use.

In his efforts to solve the army's evacuation problems Percy was to be
overshadowed by Dominique Larrey whose concepts for an ambulance
system better stood the test of time. Larrey first had his idea for a 'flying
ambulance' or *ambulance volante* in 1792 when he was serving with the
Army of the Rhine commanded by General Lucker. At the first operation
of the campaign, the capture of Spire and the passage of the Rhine, the
surgeon was struck by the deficiencies of the ambulances. He particularly
noted that they were kept off-limits until after the fighting and it was then
difficult to bring the ambulance wagons to the crowds of wounded with
the result that many were only treated after twenty-four to thirty-six hours
or died without any help. Larrey personally saw many wounded soldiers
perish because of these clumsy arrangements and he vowed to create a
better ambulance system which would be able to bring succour to the field
itself. Larrey's early opportunity came after a number of French wounded
fell into the hands of the enemy at Limbourg.

> This unfortunate contretemps determined me to propose to the senior
> general [Houchard] and the commissaire général Villemanzy the setting
> up of an ambulance capable of following all the movements of the army
> in the manner of the flying artillery. My proposal was accepted and I was
> authorised to construct a carriage which I called an *ambulance volante*.[19]

Larrey had at first envisaged carrying the wounded on horses fitted with
pack-saddles and suitable panniers. He soon realised that this was insufficient and he instead conceived 'a system of carriages which combined
sturdiness with speed and lightness'. A number of these light ambulances
were built and apparently performed well. Briot was attached to a flying
ambulance when the Army of the Moselle was united with the Army of
the Rhine and he describes 'twenty five suspended carriages, covered, and
with well lined interiors; in each one two patients could lie down comfort-
ably'. He says that each carriage took the wounded to the nearest hospital

making up to six trips per day.[20] However, it was not until May 1797 that Larrey, who at this time was with the Army of Italy in Milan, received official approval to organise the fully fledged flying ambulance system. This went far beyond his original conception of 1792, consisting not only of the novel ambulance wagons but also of a legion of 340 men subdivided into divisions. Every man in the ambulance had a specific role to play. The best description of this historic development in battlefield medicine is contained in Larrey's own memoirs and is worth quoting in full.

FLYING AMBULANCE

This ambulance which may be given the name of 'legion' was made up of three divisions or 'centuries'. The first was at Udino, the second at Padua and the third at Milan.

Each of these was arranged in the following manner.

One *chirurgien-major* of the first class commanding;

Two *chirurgiens aides-majors* of the second class, 12 *chirurgiens sous-aides* of the third class [two of which will serve as pharmacists]

One *lieutenant-économe* [lieutenant serving as commissary officer] of the ambulance division;

One *sous-lieutenant inspector de police* as *sous-économe* [a second lieutenant from the military police also acting as assistant commissary officer]

One *maréchal de logis chef commis* of first class ambulance [mounted company sergeant major as chief clerk in charge of records]

Two *brigadiers commis* [two medical corporals as assistant clerks] of third class ambulance

One trumpeter carrying the surgical instruments

12 *soldats infirmiers à cheval* [mounted medical orderlies] including a farrier, a boot maker and a saddler

One sergeant-major clerk of first class

Two *fourniers commis* [supply sergeants as assistant clerks] of second class

Three *caporaux sous-commis* [corporals as assistant clerks] or heads of other services;

One drummer in charge of surgical dressings;

25 *soldats infirmiers à pied* [foot medical orderlies]

There will be twelve light carriages and four heavy vehicles per division.

This number of carriages requires

One *maréchal de logis en chef conducteur* [company sergeant major in command]

One *maréchal de logis sous-chef* [a sergeant second in command]

Two *brigadiers* [corporals] one of which is a farrier

One trumpeter

20 supply train drivers

The total number of staff attached to each legion is 340, 113 for each of the divisions and the senior surgeon commanding. Each division of the ambulance had twelve lightly sprung carriages for the transport of the wounded; they were of two types with two and four wheels. The former, of which there were eight, were designed for flat country; the others with four wheels were intended to carry the wounded in the mountains. The carriage of the first type was an elongated tube curved on the top; two small windows opened out of each side; two double doors were at the front and rear; the floors of the carriage were a movable frame with a horsehair mattress and bolster covered in leather. The frame slid easily on the two side beams of the carriage by means of four small rollers and it was provided with four iron handles set into the wood; these handles were intended to receive the straps or the belts of the soldiers so that they could carry the wounded on the frame like a stretcher; they could dress the wounded on these frames when the season did not allow them to be dressed on the ground. When the army was engaged in steep mountains it was necessary to have mules or horses with panniers with compartments for the carriage of dressing materials, surgical instruments, medicines and other items necessary for first aid.

The small carriages were drawn by two horses, one of which was ridden. Inside they were 32 *pouces* [about 1.1 metres] wide. Two wounded could be conveniently accommodated lying full length. There were pockets inside to hold bottles and other items necessary for the sick. These carriages combined solidity with lightness. The second type of lightly sprung carriage was a wagon with four wheels. The body was a little longer and wider than that of the carriage with two wheels but was otherwise similar. It was also suspended on four springs. Its floor was covered with a fixed mattress and the panels were padded up to a foot like the small carriages. The left side of the carriages opened for almost the whole of its length by means of two sliding doors so that the wounded could be placed on the carriage in a horizontal position. Small windows, suitably placed, renewed the air by encouraging its movement. To fix the centre of gravity these carriages had to have a stretcher which could be put to other uses. The large carriages were drawn by four horses and had two drivers; they were light, solid and well suspended. We carried in these carriages four wounded lying full length with their legs crossed a little. The equipment wagons were four wheeled and not different from other wagons in military service.

There was an administrative committee for the three divisions which was made up of *officiers de santé* and administrative officers.

A regulation specifically determined the order of march of the ambulance, its interior policing and the duty of each individual. These ambulances were intended to remove the wounded from the battlefield after having given first aid and then to transport them to the hospitals of the first line.

The ambulance legion was under the immediate orders of the senior surgeon of the army and each division under the orders of a *chirurgien-major* of the first class.

It was also intended to remove the dead for burial. The unmounted medical orderlies were specifically charged with this duty under the orders and supervision of the inspector of police who was authorised to requisition the working men who were necessary from among the local inhabitants.[21]

Only by reading this comprehensive account can we fully appreciate the scope and sophistication of the flying ambulance. In the interests of space, Larrey's careful description of the uniforms and equipment of his medical staff has been omitted. Here there was also considerable attention to detail. For example, the surgeons each carried 'a small cartouche box ... divided into several compartments, containing a case of portable surgical instruments, some medicines and articles necessary to afford immediate assistance to the wounded on the field of battle'. The military officers were supplied with courier bags on their saddles which contained field dressings instead of pistol holsters.

The concept of the flying ambulance complemented Larrey's views on the importance of early surgery for seriously wounded men.

When a limb is carried away by a ball, by the burst of a grenade or a bomb, the most prompt amputation is necessary. The least delay endangers the life of the wounded ... I may even assert that without the assistance of the flying ambulance ... a great number would have died from this cause alone.[22]

It is natural to make comparisons between Percy's *wurst* and Larrey's flying ambulance. The two ambulance systems had fundamentally different objectives. Percy's ambulance was primarily a means of transporting surgeons and their instruments as close to the fighting troops as possible. Stretcher bearers could then fan out from the parked *wurst* to collect the wounded. Larrey's ambulance, in contrast, was quicker and lighter and was designed to keep up with the advanced sections of the army most likely to be involved in fighting. Although first aid was administered on the field, a central objective was the quick transfer of the more seriously wounded men away from the battlefield to receive potentially life-saving surgery in hospitals in the rear. The two systems were similar in that they created a specialist ambulance corps and removed the chore of caring for the wounded from their fellow soldiers. Both greatly increased the mobility of the army's surgeons and allowed them to take vital equipment with them. In Percy's *wurst* instruments were contained in the ambulance vehicle itself whereas in the flying ambulance the tools were carried both in the carriages and in the saddlebags of the medical officers. Both systems were welcome sights to troops in battle where morale was bound to be improved by the appearance of such high profile surgical help at the hour of greatest need.

Larrey's ambulance had the edge. It was less vulnerable to the dangers of battle. Because it was composed of a large number of smaller carriages, the loss of an ambulance vehicle was not a crushing blow to the flying ambulance whereas the loss of a single *wurst* and its surgeons would have been a major setback. Larrey's ambulance was quicker both on and off the field than the *wurst* and the wounded men could be removed more rapidly from danger than by Percy's stretcher bearers. The surgeons of the flying ambulance, either on foot or horseback, brought only vital surgical instruments to the field. They were not encumbered by the major surgical instruments of the *wurst*, their objective being only to perform immediate minor surgery to stabilise the patient.[23]

Larrey was not a modest individual (see previous chapter) and he was very keen to take every plaudit for the 'invention' of the ambulance. He does make a fleeting reference to Percy's ambulance in his memoirs but otherwise he acknowledges it little. He was always quick to take offence if he perceived that the role of the flying ambulance had been underestimated or if his own contribution had not been fully appreciated. When he received the *Légion d'honneur* in 1807, he took aside the grand chancellor and asked him to add the flying ambulance to the list of achievements for which he was being honoured. The bemused official acceded to Larrey's demand. His colleagues recognised Larrey's role in the development of the flying ambulance but they stopped short of giving him all the credit. When, in 1804, Coste wrote to Larrey following a minor falling out between the two men, he reminded him that he had supported him in acknowledging the 'great part' he had played in creating the *ambulance volante*. The army's senior physician well understood that this was a subject close to Larrey's heart. His words were carefully chosen and remind us that, although Larrey was the chief architect of the flying ambulance, he did not create it in splendid isolation. Percy and Coste deserve at least some of the fulsome praise that has all too often been given to Larrey alone.

Larrey had a further opportunity to test the new ambulances in the campaigns in Egypt and Syria. The army embarked at Alexandria in July 1798 and the French suffered around 250 casualties in fighting around the city. Larrey attached two divisions of ambulance to each wing of the army and he remained in the centre with a third division where he could receive Bonaparte's orders and watch the ambulances in action. All the wounded were taken to a hospital in the convent of the Capuchins. In preparation for the advance on Cairo, he added a light ambulance to each of the five divisions of the army and retained a sixth reserve ambulance at headquarters. Larrey does not specify the size of these ambulances but it is very likely that they were considerably smaller in scale than his prototype ambulance divisions of the Army of Italy.

The light ambulances performed creditably in the subsequent conflicts of the campaign although the number of French casualties was modest compared with the later battles of Empire. At the Battle of the Pyramids, Larrey took the precaution of visiting the ambulances of the divisions prior to the fighting to check that all necessary preparations had been made. The wounded were taken to the castle of Giza which Larrey had converted into a 'superb hospital'. A year later, at the Battle of Aboukir fought against the Turks, the ambulances were again in the midst of the action. Larrey writes:

> During the engagement, the ambulances were placed at the principal points on the line and gave immediate assistance to the wounded. I then united them to that of the centre which I had placed as near as possible to the fort. The most severe wounds were all brought to this ambulance. I dressed them myself and performed the necessary operations. More than forty amputations were immediately performed and with astonishing success. Among them were more remarkable cases than I have seen elsewhere. After this affair, the wounded received the most prompt and effectual assistance from the surgeons of the ambulances and of the line; none were left more than a quarter of an hour without being dressed. They were then carried in litters to the boats which were conveniently moored in a creek out of the view of the enemy's squadron and transported to Alexandria without accident.

In 1801 the French hold on Egypt was loosening but in fighting with the British around Alexandria the ambulances proved their worth to the 1,300 French wounded. The light ambulance wagons were again attached to the divisions whilst Larrey directed the ambulance of the centre.[24]

The mobile ambulances were just the first step in casualty evacuation. Larrey set up small hospitals in close proximity to the fighting (*hôpitaux ambulants*) to which the wounded could be carried by the mobile ambulances once first aid had been administered. These small hospitals, often of only twenty to fifty beds in improvised local accommodation, were also generally referred to as ambulances. It is unfortunate that, in much of the French literature, the word 'ambulance' is used interchangeably to mean a system of casualty evacuation such as Larrey's, a small mobile hospital or a carriage for the wounded. In English parlance the *hôpitaux ambulants* would be termed 'field hospitals'. From these smaller makeshift hospitals, the more seriously wounded and sick men were then transferred to the larger fixed hospitals which will be discussed in a later chapter.

Larrey was a great improviser and his talents were fully tested in the inhospitable terrain of Egypt and Syria. There was a severe shortage of draught animals to transport the wounded and the surgeon turned to the only animals available in abundance, camels. He devised light panniers in the form of cradles slung over the camel's hump and suspended by elastic straps. Each pannier was long enough to carry a man lying full length. Unfortunately, the quartermasters later commandeered the camels and Larrey, unusually, acknowledges that 'we were much embarrassed in carrying our wounded'. He was reluctant to admit such difficulties and it is fair to say that his memoirs must often be taken with a small pinch of salt. He had a vested interest in portraying the light ambulances as a success. Whereas there is no reason to doubt that the ambulance did make a significant contribution in the battles of the Orient, it is clear from Bonaparte's correspondence that even the relatively modest number of battle casualties was putting considerable strain on the army's medical services. In May 1799 we find letters desperately commandeering any available horses and donkeys for the carriage of wounded. In another letter, Bonaparte demands that the artillery's gunners are sent to the ambulances to help carry the wounded men. Larrey, on at least one occasion, at the fort of el-A'rych in 1799, had to request the regimental surgeons to assist the surgeons of the ambulances in the management of casualties. These necessities do not belittle the role of the light ambulances but they do suggest that these were not the self-sufficient units that Larrey had originally envisaged.[25]

As Larrey's writings dominate most accounts of the *service de santé* there is a tendency to portray his *ambulance volante* as a dominant theme of the service. This is far from the reality. During the wars of Empire there were many types of ambulance in service on and around the battlefield. The role of ambulances in particular battles will be described in the next two chapters but it is appropriate to give an overview here. From a quick perusal of regulations, correspondence and memoirs for the period 1803–15 we can list the following types: ambulance of headquarters, ambulance of the corps, ambulance of the division, ambulance of the depot, sections of ambulance, *ambulance volante* and regimental ambulances. This excludes the Guard's ambulance which was entirely separate from the dispositions for the line and the Emperor's own personal ambulance.[26]

The largest single unit was the ambulance of the corps which was composed of administrators, *officiers de santé* and equipment. The army corps was a major innovation of the *Grande Armée*, a body of 20,000 to 30,000 men capable of giving battle unsupported. It was composed of two or more infantry divisions of 8,000–12,000 men and a brigade of light cavalry of 2,000–3,000 men in addition to six to eight companies of artillery and the supporting staff including administration, engineers, transport and doctors.

Percy describes the ambulance of the Fourth Corps in action at the Battle of Heilsberg in 1807. Manned by a large number of surgeons working under the orders of a senior surgeon, it was established in a hut near the field. It was common practice for the ambulance of the corps to be divided up before the action into the smaller ambulance types of division, section, depot and *volante*. The divisional ambulances played a key role in battle.

Each followed a column of the corps. They were organised such that they had enough staff, equipment and infrastructure available to immediately set up small temporary hospitals around the battlefield where first aid could be given. Their supervision was the responsibility of the *commissaires des guerres* who in turn were accountable to the *ordonnateur* who was in overall administrative charge of the ambulances.

In April 1809 the ambulance of a division of infantry contained the following personnel: one physician, six surgeons (one *chirurgien-major*, one *aide-major* and four *sous-aides*), four pharmacists (one *major*, one *aide* and two *sous-aides*), four employees (one clerk (*econome*) and one employee each of the first, second and third classes). They might also be supplemented by a company of *infirmiers* attached to the army (see Chapter V). The ambulance vehicles usually consisted of two ambulance caissons and some light carts. On the day of battle the divisional ambulances were well placed to support the wings of the army and bring immediate surgical help and improvised field hospitals to the wounded. Percy describes divisional ambulances working in combination with the smaller regimental ambulances in skirmishing before the Battle of Friedland in 1807. As the bloodiness of battles increased so did the demands on the ambulances. In March 1813 Napoleon wrote to Marshal Ney asking him to attach ambulances of six caissons to each of his four divisions. He expected these to cater for the dressing of 40,000 wounded. In 1799, in Egypt, Napoleon had made detailed arrangements for the evacuation of fifteen wounded men. In the final years of Empire, he was planning for tens of thousands.[27]

Where a limited and flexible ambulance was required to provide a service to the outposts or smaller groups of men detached from the divisions, then 'sections of ambulance' were formed. Like the divisional ambulances, these were drawn from the ambulance of the corps. Their size varied with the task in hand. The number of surgeons and *infirmiers* was decided by the *officier de santé en chef* and, in general, there would be one or two ambulance caissons containing surgical instruments, dressings and supplies, the latter entrusted to employees. The *ambulance volante*, another fragment of the corps ambulance, carried the name of Larrey's invention but it was a much more modest affair manned by one or two mounted surgeons and perhaps four *infirmiers* with an ambulance caisson hitched to four horses. As was the case for its illustrious predecessor, it was designed to gallop onto the field at short notice to give first aid. Two stretchers in the caisson gave some limited capacity for casualty evacuation. Once the ambulance of the corps had been split into the above subdivisions, the ambulance left behind was termed the 'ambulance of the depot'.

In battle, the depot ambulance would usually be placed in the centre rear of the army, as close as possible without compromising its safety. Apart from the surgeons, ready to give urgent treatment, the depot contained a number of stretchers and covered wagons intended to take the more seriously wounded to the nearest hospital. Marshal Ney, in his *Instructions for the Troops Comprising the Left Corps*, describes the normal procedure for the ambulances in battle. They were divided between the right, left and centre and, if they were overwhelmed at any point by the number of casualties, then the commander of the reserve was to give the authority and resources to the *directeur général de l'ambulance* to promptly requisition the local carts of the country to plug the gap.[28]

The headquarters ambulance, sometimes referred to as that of the reserve, generally contained around fifty surgeons, some mounted and others in carts. This leaves just the regimental ambulances, which Napoleon believed to be the most important, 'because the esprit de corps means that the *officiers de santé* are attached to the men and are rewarded by the esteem of the officers of the regiment'. These regimental facilities were under the orders of the colonel and always followed the regiment on campaign. The legislation of late 1803 had specified one ambulance caisson (*fourgon*) per battalion (four per regiment) but in the legislation of September 1805, on the eve of the campaign of Austerlitz, this was unaccountably watered down to one per regiment.

> His Majesty decrees that a *fourgon d'ambulance* will be attached to each regiment entering on campaign to provide first aid. This will be hitched to four horses and designed to transport at least six wounded men. To permit this, each caisson must contain complete sets of surgical instruments and drugs, 50 kg. of lint, two mattresses and six stretchers. The *fourgons* will be made in one of the workshops of Sampigny according to a standard design.[29]

The caissons often also contained 100 kg of linen for dressings. This was not a generous provision when one considers that the standard size of a four-battalion infantry regiment was 3,360 men. The regimental ambulances were staffed by the regimental surgeons and operated separately from the ambulances of division and section, playing a role more similar to that of the *ambulance volante*.

In the early years of the 19th century, the horses and wagons for the various ambulances were supplied by private companies, Breidt for the *Grande Armée* and Gayde for the Army of Italy. Because of the frequent problems and exorbitant cost of this arrangement, Napoleon decided to militarise the system as the *équipages des transport militaires*, specific battalions of which were reserved for ambulance use. As the *Grande Armée*'s casualties escalated in the later years of the wars, the ambulances required increased supplies. A document of March 1813 issued by the *conseil de santé*, probably mainly the work of Percy, makes detailed recommendations for the staffing and supplying of the divisional ambulances which were intended to treat around 5,000 wounded in the course of a campaign. It was noted that the traditional

French surgical instruments were too heavy and that there was a need for an employee with the ambulance to clean and organise them. Other articles relate to splints and stretchers, the latter to be carried by the 'soldiers' of the ambulance, the number of which is not specified. This illustrates that the demands on the ambulances were increasing and that the *conseil de santé* was acutely aware of the need for well resourced ambulances. It was easier to write documents than to make change on the ground and it is unlikely that many of the suggestions were instituted in the subsequent campaign.[30]

The documentation detailing the arrangement of the army's ambulances for the early years of Empire makes no mention of Larrey's flying ambulance. There is the allusion to the *ambulance volante* but this small offshoot of the corps ambulance was far removed from the impressive legion of 340 men. This leads to an obvious question; how much was Larrey's famous flying ambulance actually used in the Napoleonic Wars? We must remember that, for the majority of the wars, Larrey was the senior surgeon of the Imperial Guard's medical service and had relatively little authority or influence over the service provided for the remainder of the army. Within the Guard, there is good evidence that Larrey's ambulance was well organised and had all the attributes of a 'flying ambulance'. It was adequately staffed. In 1806 an Imperial decree attached five companies of medical workers or *infirmiers*. By the time of the Battle of Eylau in 1807, each of the three of Larrey's *ambulances volantes* contained a *chirurgien-major* of the first class, two *aides-majors*, ten *sous-aides* and two pharmacists. There were twelve mounted *infirmiers* and twenty-five on foot. This meant 113 men in each ambulance, a total close to 350.[31] The medical staff of the active ambulance transferred to the Guard's hospital at Gros-Caillou in Paris during peace-time. On campaign, the ambulance was in a constant state of readiness. Physician Salomon-Louis Laurillard-Fallot served with the Guard's ambulance in 1813 and has left a brief description.

> The ambulance of the Guard was properly organised; it was a corps in which the ranks were clear and the duties well understood; in a word, the position of each man was well defined. It was kept up to date with all the movements of the part of the army to which it was attached. The billets of the staff of the ambulance were as well organised as they were for the other officers. It was much different in the line where each individual usually had to arrange their own billet with the local authorities when they arrived in a town in the evening. I have seen Monsieur Larrey himself do this chore for the Guard's ambulance.[32]

The far more numerous regiments of the line benefited little from Larrey's ideas. His well organised ambulance system was meant to serve only the precious Guard. In practice, the Guard's ambulance did sometimes tend to the wounded of the line regiments simply because no other provision was available. The ambulance service for the rest of the army, with its numerous subdivisions and specific duties, may have appeared well enough on paper but, in reality, it was hopelessly inadequate. This became obvious as early as 1805 as the newly formed *Grande Armée* marched towards its first great victory at Austerlitz. According to Marshal Davout, always the most reliable of witnesses, the ambulance service was in a state of 'complete destitution' and there was effectively no resource to give first aid.[33] The *Grande Armée* was on the brink of glorious conquest. With the exception of a few elite units, its wounded soldiers lying on the field were unlikely to be cared for by the famed flying ambulance. Indeed, it was all too likely that they would see no ambulance at all.

Notes

1. Griffith, P, *The Art of War in Revolutionary France 1789–1802*, pp.7–8.
2. ibid., pp.230–3.
3. Hughes, Major-General B P, *Firepower. Weapons effectiveness on the battlefield 1630–1850*, pp. 26–9.
4. Chandler, D, *The Campaigns of Napoleon*, p. 343.
5. Howard, M, *Wellington's Doctors. The British Army Medical Services in the Napoleonic Wars*, p. 126; Vess, D M, *Medical Revolution in France 1789–1796*, p. 118; Briot, P-F, *Histoire de l'état et de progrès de la chirurgie militaire en France pendant les guerres de la Révolution*, p. 381.
6. Percy, Baron, *Journal des Campagnes de Baron Percy*, pp. 18, 25, 63; Vess, p. 143.
7. Larrey, D J, *Mémoires de Chirurgie Militaire et Campagnes 1787–1840*, p. 302; Desgenettes, R, *Histoire Médicale de l'Armée d'Orient*, Vol. I, pp. 177–8.
8. Vess, p. 78; Briot, p. 400; Morvan, J, *Le Soldat Impérial*, Vol. II, p. 297.
9. Vess, p. 100.
10. Percy, pp. 28–9.
11. Masson, F, *Aventures de Guerre 1792–1809*, pp. 137–8.
12. Vess, pp. 26–7.
13. Lemaire, J-F, *Les blessés dans les Armées Napoléoniennes*, pp. 235–6.
14. Oritz, J M, *The Revolutionary flying ambulance of Napoleon's surgeon*, p. 3; Vess, pp. 81–2.
15. Brice, Docteur and Bottet, Capitaine, *Le Corps de Santé Militaire en France*, pp. 72–3.
16. Percy, pp. 2–3.
17. Briot, pp. 380–1; Laurent, C, *Histoire de la vie et des ouvrages de P.-F. Percy*, p. 178; Percy, p. 13.
18. Percy, pp. 19, 26–7.
19. Larrey, p. 47.
20. Briot, p. 404.

21. Larrey, pp. 91–5; Richardson, R, *Larrey. Surgeon to Napoleon's Imperial Guard*, pp. 34–8; Brice, Bottet, pp. 70–1.
22. Oritz, p. 5.
23. Oritz, p. 6; Longmore, T A, *A treatise on the transport of sick and wounded troops*, p. 31.
24. Larrey, p. 208; Dible, J H, *Napoleon's Surgeon*, p. 46.
25. Larrey, pp. 155–6; Lemaire, p. 128.
26. Brice, Bottet, p. 177.
27. Pigeard, A, *Le Service de Santé de la Révolution au 1er Empire 1792–1815*, p. 23; Percy, p. 289; Lemaire, p. 166.
28. Pigeard, A, *Dictionnaire de la Grande Armée*, pp. 25–7; Ney, Marshal, *Memoirs of Marshal Ney published by his family*, Vol. II, p. 355.
29. Brice, Bottet, pp. 178, 130.
30. Pigeard, *Dictionnaire de la Grande Armée*, p.568; Lemaire, pp. 137, 181.
31. Lemaire, p. 242.
32. Laurillard-Fallot, S-L, *Souvenirs d'un Médecin Hollandais sous les Aigles Françaises 1807–1833*, p. 93.
33. Morvan, Vol. II, p. 306.

CHAPTER V

The Battlefield 1803–1809:
Chirurgie de Bataille

When, in August 1805, the *Armée des Côtes de l'Océan* turned its back on the English Channel and marched towards Austria, it was renamed the *Grande Armée*. There were seven corps, a cavalry reserve and the Imperial Guard. The army corps were commanded by Marshals Bernadotte (I), Marmont (II), Davout (III), Soult (IV), Ney (V), Lannes (VI) and Augereau (VII). As has been described, each of these corps was divided into divisions. In turn, each division was usually split into two brigades of one or more regiments. After some experimentation, the regiments were now composed of four battalions of six companies, a total of around 3,500 men. Each corps had its own artillery support of forty-eight to sixty-four guns, two companies of which were under direct corps control and the rest attached to divisions or brigades. The *Grande Armée* of 1805 was the most French army that Napoleon ever commanded. Even so, about a quarter of its 200,000 troops were foreign. The number of foreign soldiers increased every year and by 1812 the army was hardly more than half French with more than fifty percent of the infantry and one third of the cavalry being Austrian, Prussian, German, Spanish, Italian, Portuguese, Dutch, Polish and Croatian. Many of these 'allies' were reluctant or, at best, indifferent.[1]

The losses of the *Grande Armée* during the wars are not clear-cut, the frequently quoted figures being derived from a mixture of intelligent research into original sources and wild guesswork. Among the former efforts, the conclusions of French historian Jacques Houdaille may be closest to the truth. Acknowledging the difficulties of interpreting the sources, Houdaille estimates that, between 1803 and 1815, the French army recruited 2,015,000 Frenchman and 645,000 foreigners. For the French, 1,190,000 were lost, either killed in combat, perished in hospital, made prisoner, struck off the registers due to 'long absences', or disappeared without explanation. Perhaps, up to 300,000 returned surreptitiously to their villages in France, some after a period of captivity. For the foreign troops, the losses up to 1814 amounted to 450,000 men, of which an indeterminate number may simply have returned to their homeland. If the losses for French and foreign troops are merged, we are left with the following revealing statistics: 4.5% of lost troops died in combat or as a direct result of wounds, 15% died of disease in hospitals, 22% were made prisoner of which a quarter ultimately returned, 13% were struck off the register after a long absence, one half returning to their villages, and 11% deserted. The rate of desertion was greater among the foreign contingents.[2]

Napoleon introduced a new form of war based on speed and mobility, unsettling the majority of his opponents who were steeped in a tradition of more leisurely warfare. However, the weaponry of war changed little from the Revolutionary Period and, accordingly, the *Grande Armée*'s soldiers suffered the same types of wounds as their predecessors fighting for *La Patrie*. Jean-François Lemaire, in his superb study of the wounded of Napoleon's army, cogently argues that the best source that we have for the nature of these wounds, the 3,000 officers' files in the *Service Historique de l'Armée de Terre*, must be interpreted with caution. There are multiple examples of inconsistencies, probable exaggerations of the severity of wounds, and unlikely sequences of injuries. Nevertheless, Lemaire's study does give a unique view of the wounds received by the army's officers – unfortunately, the files of the ordinary soldiers are not detailed enough to allow a similar analysis. One truth which emerges is the greater lethality of fire compared with steel. Officers survive multiple sabre slashes but later die of a single musket ball wound. The second striking observation is the frequency of multiple wounding. Of the 2,200 officers studied, more than half had been wounded at least once. There were over 4,000 wounds in total meaning that, among the wounded, the average number of woundings was greater than three.

In the records there are some celebrated examples of multiple injuries. For example, Marshal Oudinot, Duc de Reggio, received as many as twenty-seven wounds between 1793 and 1814 but still died in his bed at 80 years of age. General Rapp, one of Napoleon's most trusted personal aides, began fighting at the start of the Revolutionary Wars and commanded the small attachment at the Rhine that continued resistance until almost two weeks after Waterloo. He was wounded on eight occasions between 1793 and 1812, including at least three gunshot wounds. Less well known than Oudinot and Rapp is Colonel Nicolas Thurot who gave twenty-three years of uninterrupted service despite being wounded most years. The list of his wounds is both a testament to his durability and an insight into the typical wounds of the wars.

Wounded by gunshot in the hip between Maubeuge and Mons in 1792.
Wounded by gunshot in the right shoulder at Vannel (Holland) in 1792.
Wounded by two sabre cuts to the head at Grave (Holland).
Wounded by gunshot in the right leg at the camp of the Lune.

Wounded by a gunshot wound in the left knee.
Wounded by two sabre cuts and a bayonet cut at Kempten (Germany).
Wounded by a gunshot wound in the left leg at Munich.
Wounded by a gunshot wound through the body at Zurich.
Wounded by a musket ball in the right hip at Austerlitz (1805).
Wounded by three sabre cuts at Jena (1806).
Wounded by gunshot in the right leg at Elsberg.
Wounded by gunshot in the head at Eylau (1807).
Wounded by sabre cuts to the left hand and forehand at Kenisberg.
Wounded by gunshot to the right leg at Santarem (Portugal).
Wounded by a bullet wound in the right thigh at Leipzig (1813).

Thurot was retired at the Restoration not because of his wounds but because he had served at Waterloo. Nineteen of the twenty-one of Napoleon's marshals who saw active service were wounded. Oudinot suffered the most but Ney was hit six times, Lannes four times, and both Grouchy and Poniatowski on three occasions. The remainder were wounded once or twice.[3]

As the official files detailing officers' injuries are inconsistent we can conclude that there is no ideal written source for the wounds of the era. The closest we get to an objective account are the surgical treatises of the period by Larrey, Briot and others. In recent years, these have been supplemented by archaeological evidence from a number of grave excavations around the sites of Napoleonic battles and hospitals. The excavated bones give incontestable evidence of the injuries inflicted by musket ball and cold steel. In Spain, bone collections from the Peninsular War have been unearthed at Léon, Valladolid, Tolosa and Zaragoza. Among the 115 complete skeletons found in the cemetery of the French hospital at Tolosa in the Basque country are a number showing signs of trauma to the legs. Lead bullets are embedded in bones and pieces of shell located around the centre of injuries. There are signs of remodelling of bony fractures indicating survival after the wound.[4] Even this evidence is not always unequivocal – is the hole in the pelvis (coccyx) of a soldier due to a musket ball or a bayonet? In 1994, in the course of construction of a McDonald's restaurant on the outskirts of the village of Jiríkovice in the Czech Republic, a grave pit containing twenty-two skeletons was discovered. The dating of the bones and other objects in the find such as French and Russian uniform buttons established that it was a trench dug as a grave for soldiers who died of their wounds at the Battle of Austerlitz. Predictably, most of the skeletons were of young men but there were also two women and two children. The most common findings were of severe fractures caused by musket balls but there was also evidence of stabbing wounds.[5]

The *Grande Armée* of 1805, thundering across Europe from the Channel coast, sweeping up the Austrian army of the hapless General Mach at

Ulm, relied upon the surgeons of its regiments and ambulances to manage its battle injuries. As fighting unfolded, there would be deployment of the general ambulances whilst the regimental surgeons would set up their ambulance caisson as a dressing station as close as possible to the action to give urgent first aid to their own soldiers. The colonel of the regiment would detail a few of his men, rarely the best or brightest, to collect the wounded for them. It was to be hoped that this two-tier approach, local provision at regimental level and the divisions of the corps ambulance on the wider battlefield, would be able to deal with the inevitable flood of casualties.

As the great battles of the Napoleonic Wars loomed it was clear that not all was well with the *service de santé*. The ambulances were in short supply. There was also a lack of surgical instruments. Percy says that the ambulance of the division of the advance guard had none at all. This situation is confirmed by Jean-Baptiste d'Héralde, *chirurgien-major* of the divisional ambulance: 'In these great campaigns, nothing was provided to give help to the sick and wounded. At Ulm, on the day before and after the battle, we had not a single case of amputation instruments.' Surgeons were also thin on the ground. After early fighting around Elchingen, the 600 wounded were gathered in the local abbey although many had already died of cold on the field. Part of the service was performed by Larrey and his surgeons of the Guard but Percy had to improvise, removing his own surgeons from the hospital at Donauworth. Some of the wounded were then actually evacuated to Donauworth where, Percy acknowledged, they must have been 'miserable'. In their quest to minimise deaths from wounds, the army's doctors were not helped by Napoleon. According to d'Héralde:

> Before we started the campaign, they gave us a lecture, on the authority of the Emperor, ordering that the wounded should only be removed after the battle. An order which one might regard as either heroic or barbaric, but which was not reassuring.[6]

This was the state of the army's medical services at the Battle of Austerlitz on 2 December 1805 where the 71,000 troops of the *Grande Armée* faced a combined Austro–Russian force of 93,000 men commanded by Kutusov in the presence of the Tsar. The allies attempted to turn the French right but they were frustrated by the stubborn resistance of Davout's 3rd corps. This manoeuvre fatally weakened the allied centre around the plateau of Pratzen and whilst Lannes' and Murat's cavalry held the enemy right in check, Soult cut through splitting the Austro–Russian army in half. There followed a rout in which many of the Austrians and Russians drowned in the frozen marshes and lakes of the battlefield. An intense French artillery attack added to the panic. The allies lost 4,000 dead and 15,000 wounded and the French 1,290 killed and 6,943 wounded.

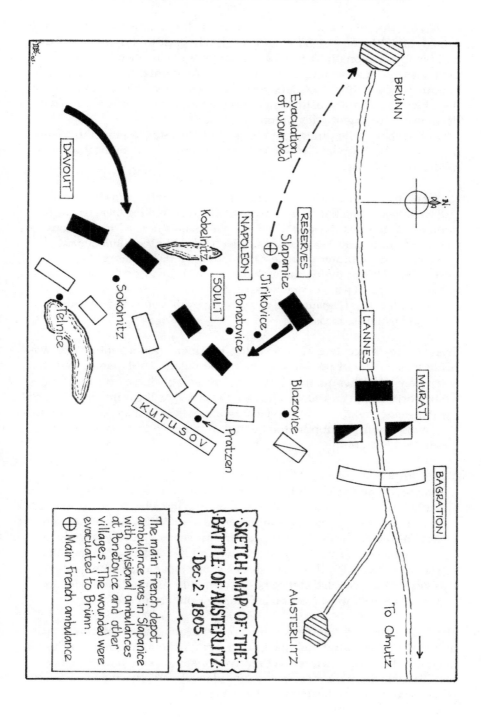

BRÜNN

Evacuation of wounded

DAVOUT

Kobelnitz

RESERVES
Slapanice

NAPOLEON

Jirikovice

SOULT

Ponetovice

Sokolnitz

Telnice

KUTUSOV

Pratzen

Blazovice

LANNES

MURAT

BAGRATION

AUSTERLITZ

To Olmutz

SKETCH · MAP · OF · THE ·
·BATTLE · OF · AUSTERLITZ·
· Dec · 2 · 1805 ·

The main French depot
ambulance was in Slapanice
with divisional ambulances
at Ponetovice and other
villages. The wounded were
evacuated to Brünn.

⊕ Main French ambulance

101

D'Héralde describes a large column of French walking wounded of the 1st, 4th and 5th corps making its way slowly back to the town of Brünn and being occasionally struck by the enemy's shells.[7] It was, however, a great victory. That evening, in the château of Austerlitz, Napoleon read his famous proclamation: 'Soldiers. I am happy with you; you have on this day at Austerlitz, fully justified my expectations of your bravery. You have decorated your eagles with an immortal glory.'

Because Percy, the director of the medical services, was still in Vienna organising the hospitals, it fell to Larrey to make the medical arrangements for the battle.

> After I had visited all the ambulances, I was at great pains to instruct their surgeons and the chief surgeons of the corps and regiments on their duties for the next day and to site the ambulances near to the divisions. In conformity with His Majesty's order, I wrote to the commandant of the hospitals at Brünn to request him to furnish the means of transport, stretchers etc. for the central ambulance which I had previously established at a mill. I was admirably assisted in every way by the commissary of war, Monsieur Dagiaut, who was charged by the commandant with the execution of these measures.

From Larrey's account, it seems that the main depot ambulance was behind the centre of the French line in the village of Slapanice and that there were two other main ambulances, presumably large divisional units, to support the first and second lines of the army. As the number of French casualties increased, the divisional ambulance in the village of Ponetovice was withdrawn to support the central ambulance at Slapanice. Larrey continues his account:

> The Inspector General, Monsieur Percy, having rejoined the army, I returned to my post with the Imperial Guard during the course of the battle. The first wounded received were from the terrible charge made by this unit against the Russian Imperial Guard. All were operated on and dressed on the field and carried back as soon as they were ready in the wagons of our light ambulances which I had organised at the mill. The speed with which these vehicles could move enabled us also to transport the wounded of the line. I myself followed the Guard with my ambulance halting wherever our presence would be of use.[8]

The battle probably ended around 5 o'clock in the afternoon. Larrey returned to the central ambulance at 4 o'clock the following morning to attend to those who had not yet received first aid. The following day, he says that all the wounded in the ambulance were evacuated to Brünn where a convent had been opened as a hospital.

This description of the medical arrangements at Austerlitz is broadly in keeping with what we would expect. As the best organised and resourced ambulance, Larrey's *ambulance volante* of the Guard had to work overtime. The divisional ambulances of the line, at least those that were available, fanned out across the field and set up local temporary hospitals in any suitable buildings or even in tents. These gave the initial surgical help to the wounded. In English terminology, the smaller temporary facilities were dressing stations and the larger were field hospitals. Surgeon La Flize has left an account of his work in a typical field hospital of the era.

> We erected a long tent made of tarred canvas and attached to some trees; we covered the ground with stubble containing tufts of horse hair which we had picked up from a neighbouring field. Near to this tent another smaller one was set up in which we placed the operating table … we started by operating on those most gravely affected. In the small tent we had driven four metal chandeliers with candles into the ground around the operating table. Their light allowed the most delicate operations to be performed … As soon as an operation was finished, we transported the wounded man to the large tent of the ambulance and he was given some soup and wine. We had slaughtered some cattle and the cooks of the ambulance were charged with the preparation of the food.

Apart from the inevitable favourable treatment of the Guard, it was intended that the more severely wounded men should be operated on first, a process known as 'triage'. Larrey supported this prioritisation of surgery, stating that 'those who are dangerously wounded should receive the first attention without regard to rank and distinction'.[9] This made sound medical sense as it was apparent that many of the more lightly wounded men were not at great immediate risk of complications and could safely afford to wait and even retire to the hospitals of the rear as the more severely injured men received first aid and surgery on or near the field.

In practice, it is obvious that such lofty principles were rarely applied and the speed of treatment was more often than not determined by status and nationality. Whilst an ordinary wounded soldier was likely to lie unattended on the field, a senior officer with a similar injury would attract one or more surgeons. At Austerlitz, d'Héralde was ordered by his colonel to leave his allotted post to attend to General Valhubert who had had his leg fractured by a burst shell. D'Héralde picked his way across the dangerous field, narrowly avoiding volleys of grapeshot, and found the wounded Valhubert lying on the ground in front of the 88th line regiment. To his credit, the general warned back men of the regiment who had left the ranks to help him, reminding them of the Emperor's orders not to remove wounded until after the battle. Later in the day, d'Héralde had Valhubert taken to a nearby village from where he organised Russian and Austrian prisoners to carry him on a stretcher to Brünn. The surgeon makes little mention of his other work during the battle and we can presume that the care of this one wounded man took up much of his time.[10]

The degree of medical attention that might be lavished on a senior officer is well illustrated by the case of General Thiébault who received a severe wound at Austerlitz in leading a charge on a Russian battery. Thiébault's account of his wounding and subsequent treatment is one of the most detailed of the era. A musket ball had passed through his left shoulder breaking the clavicle and part of the scapula.

> At my lodgings [in Brünn] on the following day, there gathered, to assess my state and prepare my first major dressing, Monsieur Percy, *chirurgien en chef* of the French army; Monsieur Yvan, the Emperor's personal surgeon; Monsieur Larrey, *chirurgien en chef* of the Imperial Guard; the *chirurgien-major* of the 8th regiment of Hussars and, finally, the surgeon who was lodged with me.

Despite this astounding assembly of surgical expertise, the outlook for Thiébault appeared poor with death likely within thirty-six hours from secondary haemorrhage. When he survived this initial period of danger the prognosis improved although his arm swelled up enormously and, if it had been feasible, it is likely that the limb would have been amputated. One of the chief characteristics of Thiébault's narrative is his obvious preference for Percy over Larrey.

> Having two openings, one in the chest and the other in the arm, I had decided that I had been struck by two musket balls and that, consequently, I had two separate wounds, not imagining that a single wound could extend over such a distance. They had not disillusioned me; but Monsieur Larrey, who was better at cutting off limbs than looking after a sick man, proved me wrong when he was doing the dressing on his own one morning. To the great annoyance of Monsieur Percy, he stuck a sound in my shoulder and I was disagreeably surprised to see it appear under my chin.

Thiébault cannot praise Percy highly enough. When he finally overcame episodes of infection and a chronic shortage of dressings and was recovered enough to be able to leave his lodgings, he parted company with the army's senior surgeon with regret, describing him as 'the greatest man in the world both as a surgeon and friend'.

In a recent imprint of Percy's journal, Thiébault's account is quoted verbatim, serving as a eulogy to the surgeon.[11] However, the general's denigration of Larrey is almost certainly unfair. Larrey asserts in his memoirs that Thiébault had appropriated a surgeon entirely for his own use, a fact supported by the patient's own version of events. When Larrey suggested that the surgeon should be freed for other duties and be replaced by an orderly, Thiébault was indignant and refused. This appropriation of surgeons by senior officers was well established and Larrey had tried to get the practice stopped. Only a week earlier, he had written to the chief-of-staff in Brünn,

> I have to report with reluctance that the generals, believing the best surgeons to be entirely at their disposal, sometimes attach them to their persons so as to have immediate attention when wounded. This seems to me to be a waste when the surgeons could be more profitably occupied.[12]

From this point on, Thiébault took a dislike to Larrey and this is well reflected in his account of his wound treatment. Larrey's passage of a sound through the path of the wound, decried by the patient, was standard surgical practice. In his version of the episode, Larrey takes his retribution against the general, claiming that he would not give up his personal surgeon to the hospitals at Munich despite the dire staffing situation and Berthier's orders to do so. Larrey also implies that Thiébault over-emphasised the severity of his wound. This is quite possible as Thiébault's memoirs are well known for a degree of exaggeration. Percy makes no mention of this unsavoury episode in his journal.

Larrey's description of the evacuation and management of the wounded at Austerlitz implies that this was successful. 'The French wounded were almost all treated on the field of battle because the weather was favourable.' French historians have asserted that the wounded from the battle received prompter attention than after any other conflict of Empire and this may well be correct. There are, however, some discordant voices. Larrey makes few references to specific difficulties or shortages, yet d'Héralde paints an entirely different picture.

> On the day before Austerlitz, at 9 o'clock in the evening, Monsieur Larrey did not have a single compress available to him; he requested what I had, which was some linen, enough lint to dress four or five hundred wounded and a double case of amputating instruments. He asked me to tell the *directeur* to send him our caisson and requested that my surgeons and I stayed close to him during the night. He put some sentries of the Guard in the only house reserved for the care of the wounded. The supplies for the Guard's ambulances only arrived in the night after the battle at 11 or 12 o'clock!

Larrey complimented the local *commissaire de guerre* on the scene but the administrators at Brünn were less helpful and the requested supplies, including carriages, food and stretchers, were either not sent immediately or held up on the roads. His claim that nearly all the wounded were dressed quickly is also challenged by other accounts. Aide-de-Camp Lejeune recalls spending the night on the snow under a tree in the garden of the village post-house. 'It was intensely cold though the day had been so fine, but I counted myself lucky and I was indeed a thousand times more fortunate than the 20,000 wretches lying out on the ground not far from me, all wounded, many dying, without fires and quite unattended.' Of course, it is not possible to know how many of these neglected men were French and how many from the allied army.[13]

It seems that the Guard did receive high quality medical care at Austerlitz. Quickly collected from the field, they were evacuated on the following day to Brünn where a hospital specially prepared by Larrey was waiting for them. These almshouses were well away from the other hospitals and the populated parts of the town and were clean and well ventilated. The hospital service was assiduously carried out by the medical officers and orderlies from the mobile ambulances. The more numerous troops of the Line were much less well served. The shortage of ambulances left them largely dependent on their own regimental surgeons and, after the battle, many were piled up in houses around the field or left on the ground. One witness states that, on the day after the battle, 'One could tell the houses occupied by the French by the cries, The Russians remained silent.' They were only slowly evacuated to Brünn, often on local carts mixed with the Russian wounded. D'Héralde claims that everything was lacking for such a large number of wounded and that every house was a hospital. Disease was inevitable and typhus was soon cutting swathes through both wounded soldiers and the local population. As d'Héralde bitterly recalled: 'The three months back pay in Austrian notes which the Emperor gave to each wounded man gave them no protection from this.' Similar scenes were to follow other battles of Empire. There was also a recurrent shortage of medical officers. Most moved with the army, either manning the ambulances or serving with their regiments and when the wounded finally arrived in the rear it was likely that they would fall into the hands of local doctors who could be incompetent or hostile or both. To be fair, there is anecdotal evidence that after Austerlitz at least some of the French wounded were well looked after by the local medical fraternity. The young General Kellerman was wounded in the leg by a musket ball while charging at the head of his hussars and was left behind in Brünn after the French army retreated. He received competent, if expensive, care from his German physician and apothecary. Two and a half months later his wound was much improved and he was evacuated to Paris in a carriage.[14]

Following the Battle of Austerlitz, the bulk of the *Grande Armée* did not return to France but remained billeted in Germany. Napoleon imposed a tough peace on Austria which licked its wounds and started to rebuild its army. The Austrians would not be in a fit state to re-enter the conflict until 1809 but it was now Prussia which was spoiling for a fight. In July 1806 Frederic William III, allied with Alexander I of Russia, mobilised his field army of 145,000 men. Napoleon, anticipating Prussian intent, left Paris in September and rejoined the *Grande Armée*. The two armies came together in mid October in the dual battles of Jena and Auerstädt. The Emperor was quick to take full credit for his own victory at Jena over the forces of the Prussian Generals Hohenlöhe and Rüchel, but in fact the greater victory was to the north at Auerstädt where the outnumbered single corps of Marshal Davout defeated the larger part of the Prussian army under the command of the Duke of Brunswick. Davout got little recognition for this at the time. Two years later, when the French population was distracted by other campaigns, Napoleon belatedly gave him the title of Duke of Auerstädt.[15] French losses at Jena were between 4,000 and 7,500 killed and wounded whilst, at Auerstädt, Davout had 8,000 casualties, almost one third of his corps.

The Jena campaign highlighted the deficiencies of the *service de santé* in the field. There was administrative disorder in the hospitals and a lack of proper organisation and resources on the battlefield. The few ambulances available at Jena were placed too far away from the fighting and thus only arrived very late in the day to dress the wounded. There was little attempt at triage and the ambulances soon filled up with the walking wounded leaving the more seriously injured on the ground. Larrey was not at Jena as he had to remain with the Guard at the nearby town of Gera. The Guard had no wounded and the flying ambulances dressed a number of wounded of the Line who arrived in the town. Percy was on the field and personally performed several operations. It is clear that the surgeons were overwhelmed. They were hardly helped by a shortage of staff and equipment. Only a week before the battle, at Bamberg, neither lint nor dressings or instruments had yet arrived. In the few days prior to the fighting, Percy wrote to the administration requesting an extra ten *chirurgiens-majors*, twenty *aides* and twenty *sous-aides*. In the event, at the church of Naumburg fifteen surgeons had to dress over a thousand wounded. In Jena, the large church, local asylum, town hall and college had all been converted into temporary hospitals. Percy says that he and his colleagues operated on and dressed more than 2,000 wounded, 'These unfortunates had been lying on the floor without straw, food or water; we scarcely had enough dressings.' A young officer was shocked by the sight of blood running through the street next to the church at Jena. 'I did not believe that one could see anything more horrible ... The dying were piled on top of the dead, pell-mell on the stone floor; bits of arms and legs were lying next to the surgeon's chair. What a sight for those awaiting their turn!'[16]

Hospitals were hastily arranged at Wurzburg, Schweinfurt, Bamberg, Anspach, Nuremberg and Frankfurt with *gîtes d'évacuation* at Offenheim,

Closter-Oberbach, Langfeld and Seligenstadt. The French relied heavily on local hospitals and were short of all supplies which were still stranded in the rear. Despite all this, the medical arrangements at Jena-Auerstädt retained some semblance of organisation and many men did receive vital surgery from the over pressed *officiers de santé*. The provision compared favourably with later battles of the wars. Indeed, d'Héralde, working with his comrades in the 5e corps at Jena, comments that the care of the wounded on the field was the best that he had seen. Many of the operations were successful. He also notes that 'several' surgeons were killed or wounded, implying that at least some were close to the action.[17]

At the end of 1806 France invaded Poland and called upon the Polish people to rise up against their Prussian rulers. The *Grande Armée* was not in the best of spirits. There was no respite in the fighting and the troops could only expect to be sent home if they were seriously wounded or if their units were judged a liability. Poland was an infertile and primitive country and ill equipped to maintain an army on the march. The cries of *'Vive l'Empereur!'* still rang out but more weakly than in previous campaigns. To the north, the Russian army was mobilising under the command of General Bennigsen. Napoleon's forces marched to meet them and the two armies clashed at Eylau, currently the town of Bagrationovsk on the Russian–Polish border, in one of the most murderous of Napoleonic battles. Fought in glacial conditions, the two exhausted armies stubbornly slugged it out without any decisive result. Napoleon was able to claim victory as he remained in possession of the field but the cost was considerable. The quoted French losses vary widely: a note from Berthier suggests that these were as great as 237 officers and 4,193 men killed and 784 officers and 23,589 men wounded. On the Russian side, Bennigsen admitted 9,000 killed and 7,000 wounded but this was almost certainly an underestimate.[18]

From a medical viewpoint, the Battle of Eylau is possibly the best documented of all Napoleon's battles. Both Larrey and Percy were in attendance and have left detailed descriptions of their work on the day. Predictably, Larrey's account emphasises his own achievements whilst Percy provides a more objective description of the proceedings. Larrey had to deal with some wounded caused by skirmishing on 7 February, the eve of Eylau. He commandeered the largest house in the village of Preuss-Eylau as a temporary hospital, scratching the word 'hospital' in large letters on the door. When General Louis Caulaincourt later arrived to reserve the house for Napoleon, Larrey sent the indignant officer away, saying that he could not move his wounded. Caulaincourt reported back to his master who sided with his favourite surgeon. 'Larrey has done well to keep a large house for the wounded ... It is up to you to find another lodging.'[19]

At the outset of the battle on the 8th, Larrey established the main ambulance for the Guard in some barns at the entrance to Preuss-Eylau near to the church where Napoleon had his headquarters. This was just to the left of

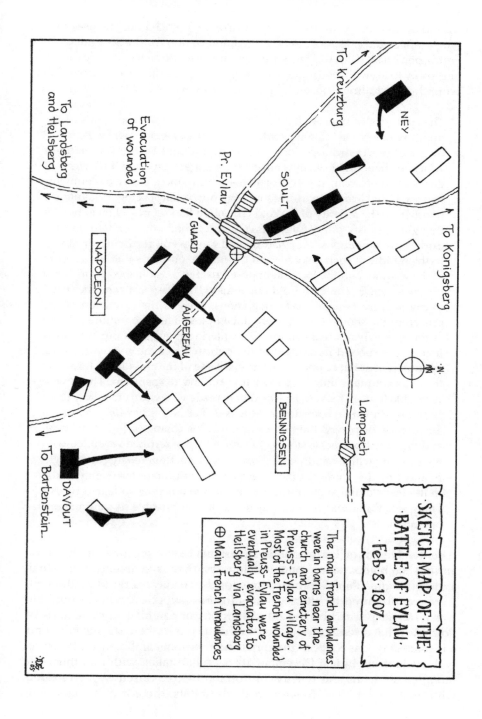

SKETCH MAP OF THE
BATTLE OF EYLAU
Feb 8 1807

The main French ambulances
were in barns near the
church and cemetery of
Preuss-Eylau village.
Most of the French wounded
in Preuss-Eylau were
eventually evacuated to
Heilsberg via Landsberg
⊕ Main French Ambulances

the Guard infantry, roughly in the centre of the French line. The use of these barns reflected the lack of suitable accommodation for the wounded. They were open on all sides with no straw and holes in the roof allowing the wind and snow to blow through them. Although large, the barns were soon full of wounded, including troops of the Line. Larrey was equal to the challenge.

> The cold was so intense that the instruments fell from the hands of the pupils who were helping me with the operations. As for me, I was driven by a really extraordinary force, inspired no doubt by the keen interest which the honourable victims must have inspired in me and by the fervent desire I had of saving the lives of all these brave men. The two sentiments had separated in some way my soul from my physical being. I was almost numb from the severity of the cold. The night had set in and I had not yet thought to satisfy powerful needs of nature; I had not even noticed that, during my operations, they had offered me several fortifying drinks …
> In the middle of such disorder and the infinite obstacles that the severity of the weather and the location opposed us, I was astonished by my own perseverance, by the sang-froid I maintained, and especially by the speed of my surgery. Several major operations, such as the extraction of the arm from the shoulder joint, were done in less than two minutes. It was at the time when a real comfort was entering the soul of our wounded that an unexpected movement of the right wing of the enemy designed to outflank our left happened at the exact site of the ambulance throwing these unfortunates into a state of turmoil and desperation. Those who were able to walk took flight. The others made vain efforts to follow them … In this difficult circumstance, Monsieur Pelchet, *officier-directeur* of the ambulance, displayed the full resources of his character, his ardent zeal, and rare intelligence. He stopped a large group of terrified wounded who were fleeing with a handful of *infirmiers*. An impetuous charge at the right moment by the cavalry of the Guard on this column of the enemy, made in the middle of a snowstorm, prevented the outcome so feared by our wounded. Calm was re-established and it was possible to continue our operations.[20]

After twelve hours, Larrey and his assistants took a short rest in the snow around the bivouac fire. The following day, they recommenced dressings and operations. Percy's preparations for the medical services of the Line were compromised by shortages of surgeons, supplies and transport. He was also exasperated by the difficulties of campaigning in the depths of Poland, 'What a season! What cold! What a country!' He struggled to find adequate surgeons for both the corps and divisional ambulances. When he had left Warsaw in late December 1806, he had taken with him thirty-six mounted surgeons and twenty-four on foot with a dozen wagons loaded with medical supplies. To support the hospitals in the rear, he left a few

French surgeons but relied largely on the local Polish doctors. This short-age of surgeons was sorely felt at Eylau where Percy acknowledges, 'the massacre was dreadful and our surgeons were not sufficient to cope with the flow of wounded.' Arriving on the field later than Larrey, Percy was forced to share the miserable barns already used by the Guard's ambulance. The quality of the surgery was not universally of the standard practised by Larrey. 'Whilst nineteen-year old surgeons hacked and butchered, the orderlies stood and shouted "Arms to the left. Legs to the right".'[21]

Like Larrey, Percy was deeply affected by what he witnessed. 'The noise of the artillery, the smoke of the fires, the smell of the powder, the cries of the wounded on which we operated, all that I saw and heard will never be forgotten.' The remainder of Percy's account is more matter of fact than Larrey's. He acted in an operational capacity, not personally performing any surgery, which was quite appropriate for the army's senior doctor.

> I returned to our barns where Chirurgien-Major Laurenchet and his divi-sion were busy dressing the wounded. We had not been able to give this help earlier because the ambulance wagons had not then arrived; once they did come we opened one and there was no lack of dressings, lint and instruments. We made a large fire close to one of the barns to pass the night around because the cold became more and more intense and the snow continued to fall.

Percy now took a little time out to go to the neighbouring cemetery to obtain a better view of the battle. Perhaps it was this absence, at the height of the action, that made Larrey so indignant that it was not he who was later featured in Gros's painting of the battle. Percy then returned to the barns, passing close to Napoleon who was observing proceedings from a small hill.

> I found the surgical service in the barns in full activity, but what a service! Some amputated legs and arms thrown together with the dead bodies in front of the door; some surgeons covered with blood; some unfortunates with scarcely any straw and shivering with cold! Not a glass of water to give them; nothing to cover them; the wind blowing from all parts through the sheds from which the soldiers had removed the doors to make their bivouac close by. I ordered some armfuls of crushed straw to be brought to cover a few of these brave men; the doors of the barn were put back on the side where the north wind blew the most strongly and, having exhorted my colleagues all around me to work as long and hard as they could, I returned to the equipment wagons a quarter of a league away. Passing by some ambulance wagons, I made sure that they were giving some soup to the wounded; I arranged for some candles, a new supply of dressings and more instrument cases to be taken to the surgeons.[22]

After the battle, Percy used Russian prisoners to remove the dead from the roads, houses and ambulances. A number of seriously wounded were not collected from the field until the next day. Larrey states that all the seriously wounded of the Guard and most of the Line had been dressed by the following morning but he later acknowledges that it took eight days to attend to all those who had not received help in the first twenty-four hours. Inevitably, large numbers of wounded ended up in Eylau where the troops had caused extensive destruction and many buildings had been wrecked by fires and Russian shells. Percy's surgeons moved from house to house as 'there was no single building where it was possible to place more than fifty wounded'. Efforts were made to provide some basic protection from the elements and by the day after the battle most of the wounded had received a little soup and bread. Water remained in short supply. The dreadful conditions in Eylau raised the spectre of epidemic disease, 'Everywhere, there was excrement, manure, entrails of animals, crushed horses and rotting and infected refuse; the smell of gangrene came from every house and one smelt the hospitals in every street'.[23]

Just when Percy's surgeons were starting to come to terms with the enormity of their task, the foot regiments of the Imperial Guard seized houses from surgeons and wounded for their own billets. They even took the food. The Guard's most severely wounded had been taken to a single large house in Eylau reserved by Larrey. The Emperor had directed that the Russian wounded be given the same care as the French. Three hundred Russians were in the church at Eylau where the conditions were especially horrific. They were crammed together 'like herrings in a tin'. It was almost impossible for the French doctors to access them, in part due to the extreme overcrowding and also because of the suffocating smoke as the less disabled soldiers were burning the contents of the church to keep warm. Retrieving the dead was difficult as the living preferred to lie on the bodies rather than on the hard stone floor. Percy tried to force Russian surgeons to enter the building but they absconded at the earliest opportunity.

On 13 February Napoleon ordered that all the wounded in Eylau be evacuated to Heilsberg, twenty miles to the south, where there was a château in preparation to receive 1,500 patients. Wagons and sledges were hastily commandeered and Russian prisoners loaded the wounded onto them. Napoleon had also directed that ten men be put in each wagon but this was not feasible. Percy watched the evacuation with horror. 'My heart bled when I saw these unfortunates lifted on a ladder over the sides of the wagons to be deposited near naked on the bare planks; this was nearly as bad as torture on the wheel.' Eight *officiers de santé* accompanied the column of wagons and sledges. 'The pain of these sad victims of the war was reflected on the faces of our surgeons; they are pale, haggard, depressed and exhausted.'[24]

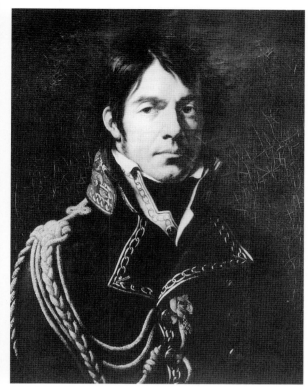

1. Dominique Larrey.

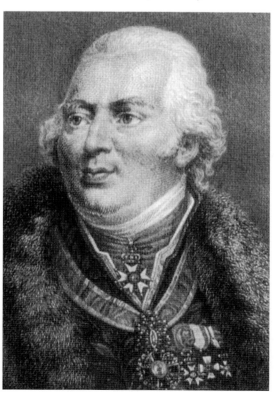

2. Pierre-François Percy.

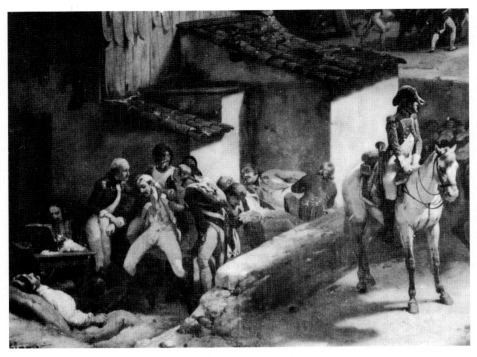

3. An improvised field hospital at the Battle of Valmy.

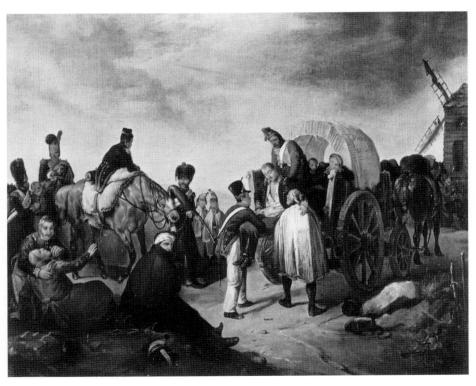

4. Wounded evacuated in local wagons.

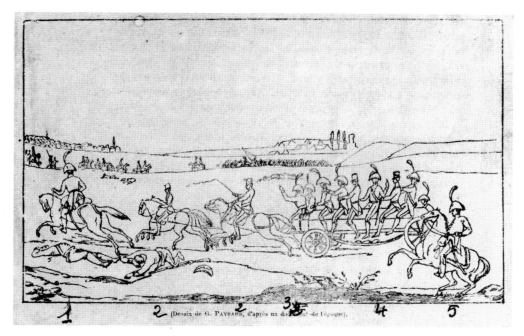

5. Percy's ambulance (*wurst*) in action.

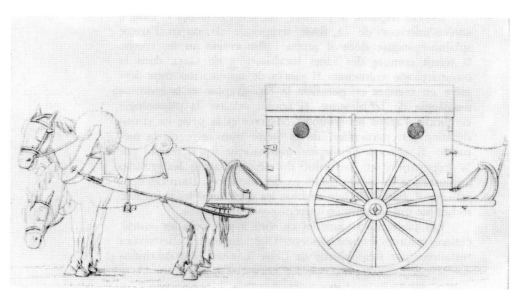

6. Larrey's flying ambulance.

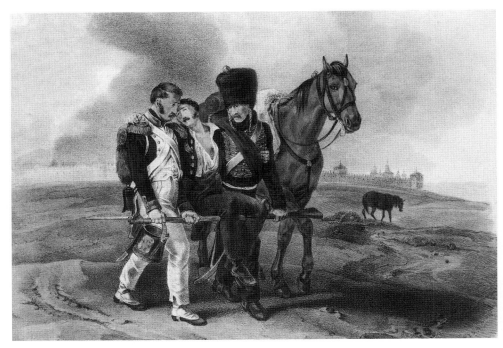

7. Wounded soldier carried from the field at Smolensk, 1812 (Albrecht Adam).

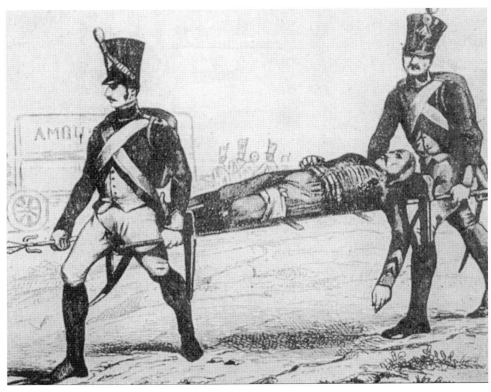

8. *Infirmiers* in action.

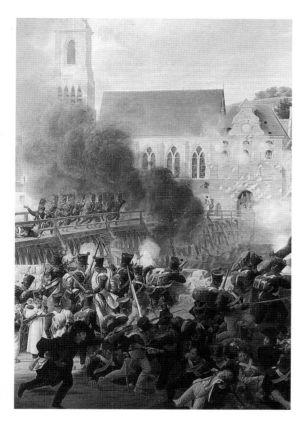

9. A surgeon rushes to assist a wounded man at the Battle of Landshut (1809).

10. The Battle of Eylau (1807) by Gros. Percy is on the extreme left behind the soldier with the outstretched arm.

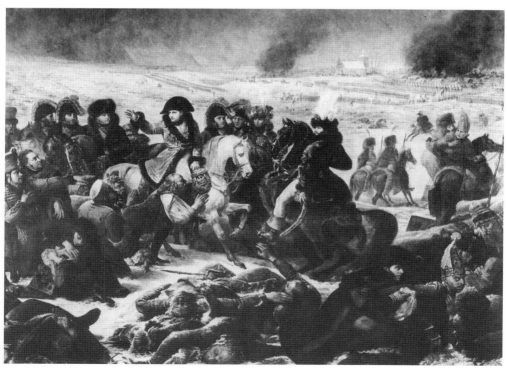

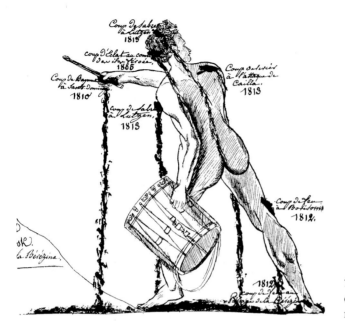

Détail de mes blessures.

11. An old soldier's depiction of his multiple wounds.

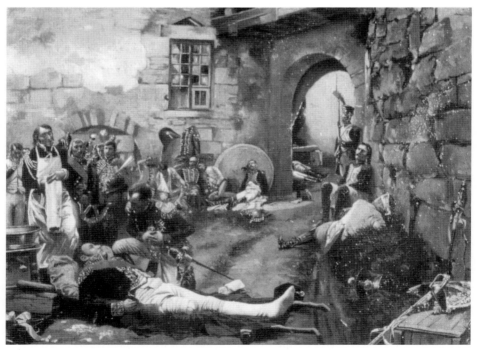

12. Napoleon visits Marshal Lannes after his amputation by Larrey in 1809.

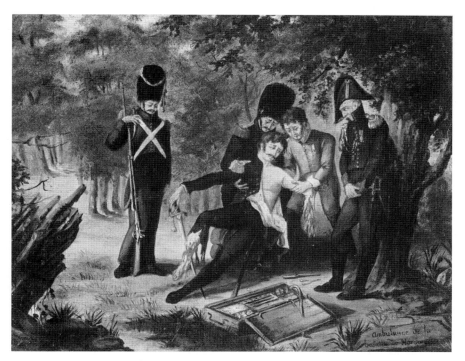

13. Larrey amputates the arm of Captain Rebsamen at the Battle of Hanau (1813).

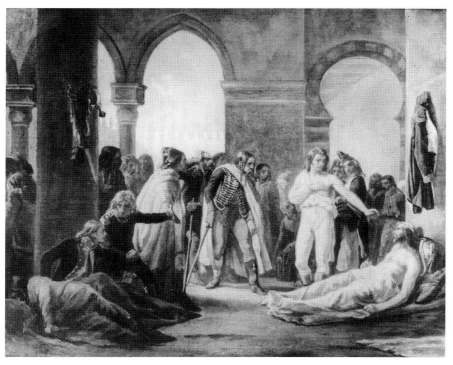

14. Desgenettes inoculates himself with plague.

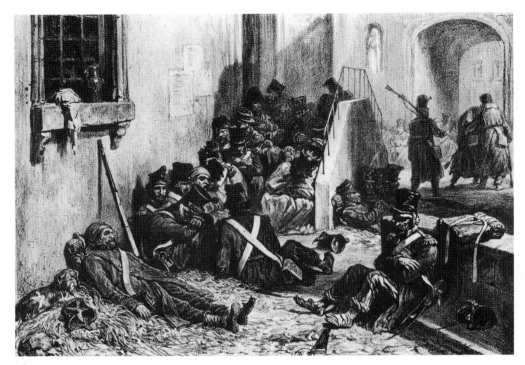

15. Typhus victims at Mainz, 1813.

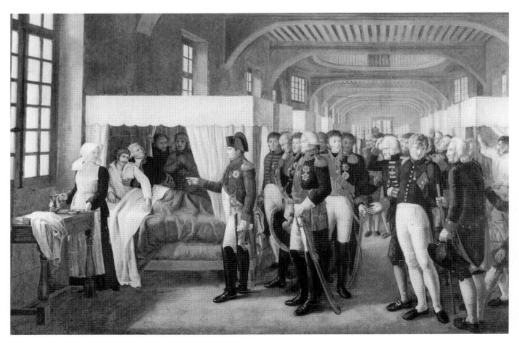

16. Napoleon visits *Les Invalides* in Paris.

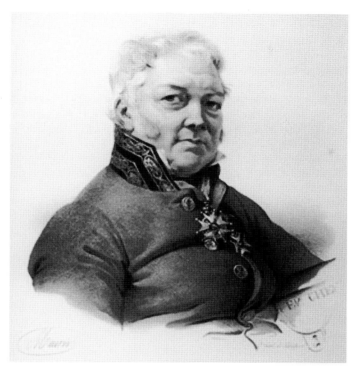

17. René Nicolas Desgenettes.

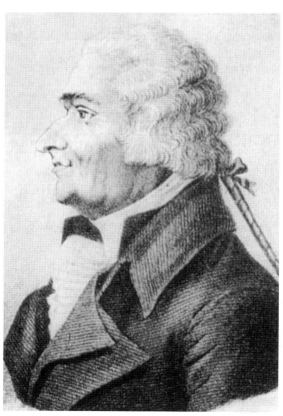

18. Jean-François Coste.

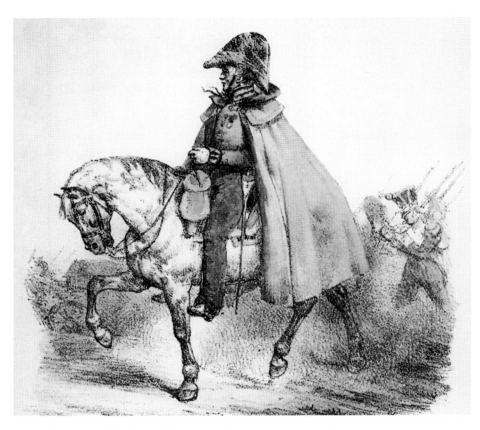

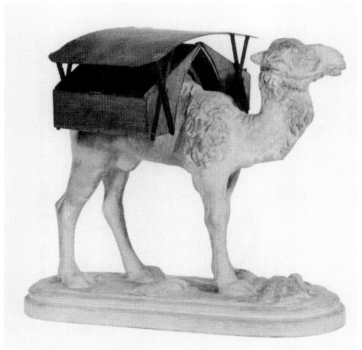

19. A surgeon of the second class 1808.

20. Larrey used camels to carry the wounded in Egypt.

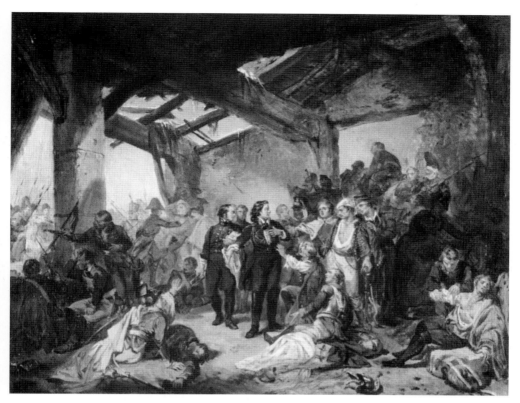

21. Larrey at the Battle of Eylau.

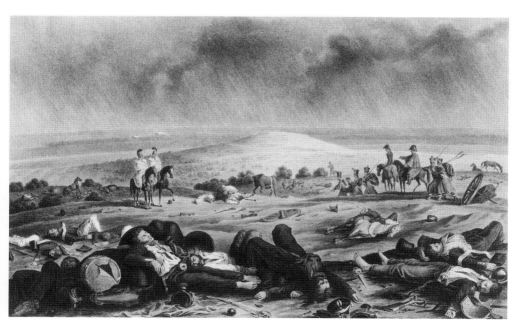

22. The battlefield of Borodino, 1812 (Faber du Faur).

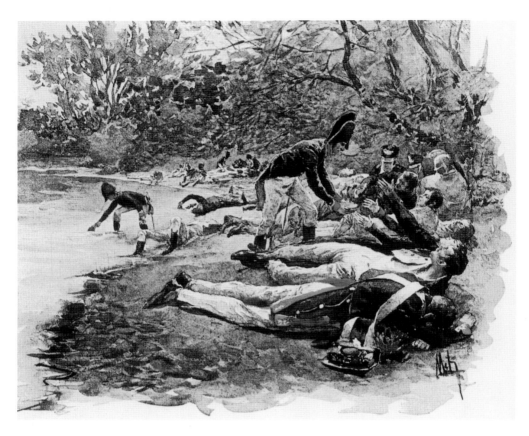

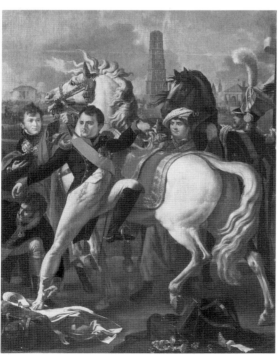

23. Musicians tend the wounded at the Battle of Aspern-Essling (1809).

24. Napoleon is slightly wounded in the ankle at the Battle of Ratisbonne (1809).

Opposite:
25. A soldier has his leg wound dressed.

26. An amputation of the arm.

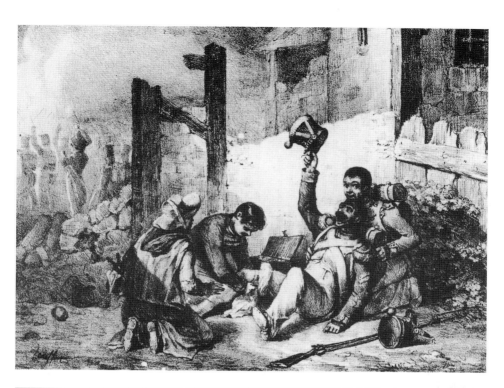

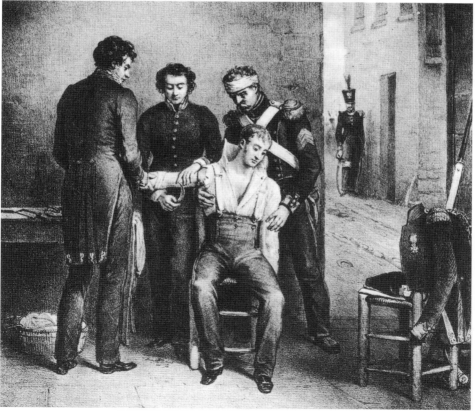

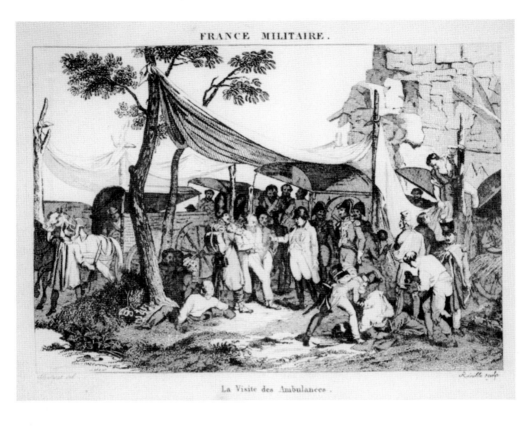

FRANCE MILITAIRE.

La Visite des Ambulances.

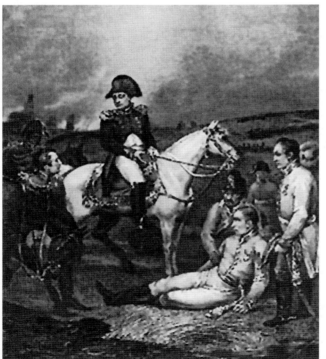

27. Napoleon visits the wounded.

28. Napoleon crosses the field after the Battle of Wagram (1809).

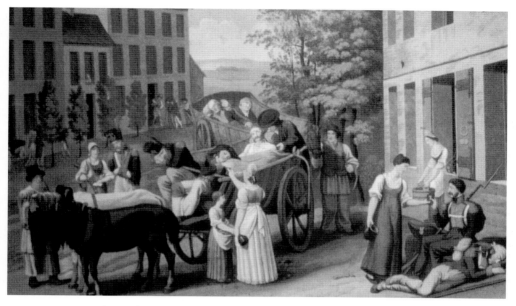

29. Locals help the wounded in Vienna after the Battle of Wagram.

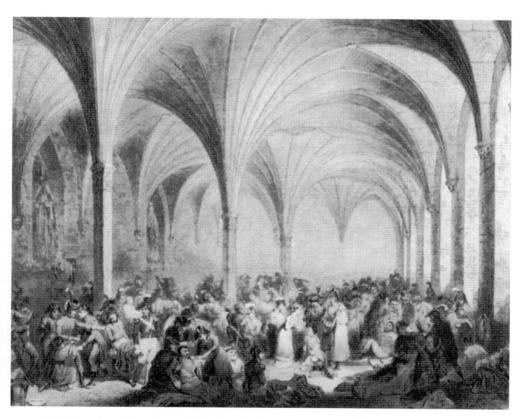

30. French military hospital at Marienbourg in 1807. It housed 500 sick and wounded and Percy describes it as 'stinking'.

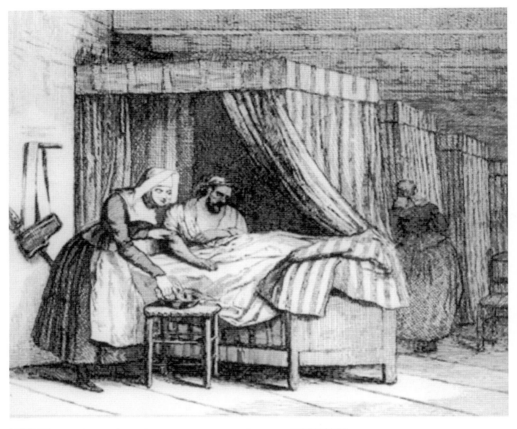

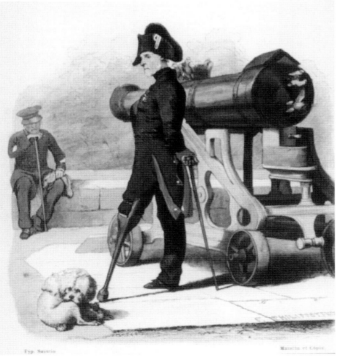

31. Nuns give assistance in a military hospital.

32. A Napoleonic veteran wears his wooden leg with pride.

Denis Davidov, an officer of hussars and Russian partisan, witnessed the French withdrawal.

> The whole road was littered continuously with debris. Hundreds of dying horses obstructed our path, as well as ambulances filled with dying or dead soldiers and officers, mutilated in the battle of Eylau. The rush to get away had become so urgent that besides the victims left in the carriages were found many who had been simply dumped in the snow without covering or clothes, bleeding to death. For mile after mile they lay not in pairs but in tens and hundreds. Moreover, all the villages along the route were filled with sick and wounded without doctors or food or the least care.

In contrast to this calamity, the evacuation of the Guard proceeded smoothly. Larrey quickly moved his wounded to the château of Inowraklaw over a hundred miles away beyond the Vistula. His light ambulances coped easily with the snow, ice and floods. He applauded the decision to evacuate from Eylau and claims that the Guard's wounded reached Inowraklaw in good condition with only around one in eleven dying from their wounds. Although he was aghast at the conditions in which the Line troops had been removed from Eylau, Percy later acknowledged that the evacuation was preferable to leaving the wounded in the town to perish from infection or fall into the hands of the enemy.[25]

It has been claimed that the Battle of Eylau marked the start of an irreversible deterioration in the *Grande Armée*'s *service de santé*.[26] Certainly, the scenes of misery around the field after Eylau exceeded anything after Austerlitz or Jena. With the exception of the cosseted Imperial Guard, surgeons, ambulances and medical supplies were all inadequate. Yet this was nothing new. Similar deficiencies had occurred in the campaigns of the previous two years. What was new was the scale of the French casualties. After Austerlitz, the French losses, killed or wounded, were 9,000 at the most. At Eylau, a realistic estimate is 25,000. This means that at Austerlitz 12% of the engaged troops became casualties whereas at Eylau this proportion rose dramatically to 33%.[27] This was not accompanied by any significant increase in the number of doctors with the army – in 1805 the total staffing of the *service de santé*, including the regimental surgeons, was around 2,000 and in 1807 approximately 2,300. It can be argued that the more acute failings of the *service de santé* at Eylau were not caused by any new deficiency but simply by an even greater chasm between the medical provision and the number of casualties. This fundamental problem was exacerbated by a number of local factors including the inhospitality of Poland, the awfulness of the roads, and the fact that the *Grande Armée* was campaigning at ever increasing distances from its own borders.

The troops were now exhausted and mutinous with cries of '*Vive la paix!*' and '*Du pain et la paix!*' replacing the customary '*Vive l'Empereur!*'[28]

There was, however, unfinished business in Poland and, after some respite in winter quarters, a rejuvenated and reinforced *Grande Armée* crushed the Russians at the Battle of Friedland in June 1807. Again, the French losses are not clear-cut but there were probably around 20,000 wounded and 3,000 killed. Many of the ambulance wagons were held up about ten miles distant from the field and Percy notes that the first only arrived at 9 o'clock on the evening of the battle at the very end of the fighting and the remainder only became available during the night. As at Eylau, local barns were the mainstay of the medical service, the word 'ambulance' being scrawled on all the doors. Larrey says that these barns were in a local village and that Percy was able to operate on the wounded 'with convenience'. Despite the lack of suitable instruments – a *chirurgien-major* was seen using an ordinary knife and a workman's saw – twenty surgeons worked through the day and night performing more than 160 amputations. The recovery of wounded from the field was slow and Percy understood the effect of dehydration on men left on the ground: 'Water is the greatest need of wounded who have lost a lot of blood.' The Herculean task of the surgeons was not helped by the complete lack of support staff such as orderlies or *infirmiers*. If the wounded did receive something to drink, this was most likely to be administered by their fellow soldiers. After the battle, the Emperor granted the use of fifty workmen (*hommes de corvée*) and twenty-five gendarmes to assist with the wounded and compensate for the lack of proper employees with the *service de santé*.[29]

Sandwiched between the battles of Eylau and Friedland was the French capture of the fortress of Danzig, the current-day Gdansk. We will briefly review this operation as it provides a good example of the medical arrangements for a siege as opposed to a conventional battle. The siege craft of the era conformed to a standard pattern and was designed to reduce the garrison with minimum risk to the attackers. Once the fortress had been blockaded, it would then be surrounded with rings of trenches ('parallels') and artillery batteries. When the parallels were close enough to the walls and a sufficient breach caused by the artillery, then the final assault would take place. If this sounds logical and scientific, the reality of siege warfare was squalid and dangerous for both sides. Percy, who oversaw the medical services of the French forces besieging Danzig, captured the general mood. 'What a spectacle is a besieged fortress and the surrounding army! The trenches are stained with blood; there reigns a gloomy silence; everybody seems to await death'. He describes the ground and trenches as littered with musket balls, grenades and burst shells.

Whilst the trenches were being dug, Percy placed three surgeons in the vicinity. These were replaced every twenty-four hours. They were initially protected by a small hut but this was soon taken from them to store the sappers' tools with the result that two of the surgeons had to return to a house at the rear. When the assault on the Hagelsberg bastion of Danzig seemed imminent, Percy stepped up the medical provision as much as was possible.

At six o'clock, the 2^e light infantry and the 19^e, 44^e, 72^e and 12^e line had to go to the trenches; others had to also return there as the assault on the Hagelsberg had been decided. I took three surgeons with me who were providing the service that day; the divisions of ambulance at Langfuhr remained at their post and awaited the wounded. Three stretchers had been placed in the trenches. Four surgeons were in the first parallel. The four others remained in a small shack. They had few dressings and little means of providing first aid although an instrument case and some splints had been procured. At this time, there was much firing.

At half past six, I left with Principal Capiomont. All our colleagues were in place: we found them, some in the hut and others in the trenches. The fire continued with cannon balls falling all around us and musket balls whistling and mewing from all directions. We sat next to the Marquis of Baden leaning against a breastwork where the only risk was from the bombs and shells. The wounded had to be carried from the trenches to the only house still standing, a quarter of an hour in the rear, where two or four surgeons were in permanent residence. There should have been six or eight wagons in front of this house to transport the wounded to the ambulances at Langfuhr for dressings and operations but such was the state of our unfortunate service that we did not even have this help. As a result, the wounded accumulated in this house and in some barns which had not been entirely destroyed. After the fighting, the regimental surgeons went to collect their own men [from the house]; the Bavarians took theirs to their own ambulance and the Saxons the same. In this way, the troops were not depleted because the six or eight grenadiers who carried a wounded man on a stretcher did not have to go farther than the house and might soon return to their post with the stretcher which, like them, would have been lost to the service if they had had to go to Langfuhr.[30]

When the besieging forces reached a critical point where the fall of the town was inevitable it was usual for the town's command to commence negotiations. This happened at Danzig where the garrison surrendered with the honours of war. The fighting described by Percy was skirmishing rather than a full-scale assault and there were probably around 1,700 French wounded.

The Peninsular War is often described as Napoleon's 'Spanish ulcer'. If so, it was a bleeding ulcer, the French losing around 250,000 casualties during the seven-year conflict between 1807 and 1814, an average of 100 men per day. There are several good accounts of the Peninsula by French army doctors and they all stress the particular savagery of the war. Surgeon Jean-Pierre Gama notes that this antagonism meant that the *service de santé* had to be more self-sufficient than in the campaigns of central Europe. Ambulances had to be carried on the backs of mules and precautions taken to prevent the wounded on the battlefields falling into the hands of the local peasants and guerrillas.[31]

The army that first entered Spain under the command of General Junot in late 1807 had a medical service that was rudimentary and inexperienced. Many of the more distinguished military surgeons were with the *Grande Armée* in the East. Chirurgien Sous-Aide Eugene Fenech was typical in having his first taste of battle at Roliça in April 1808 and performing his first amputation at the battle of Busaco two years later. The anecdotal accounts of the battles in Spain suggest that the medical provision was worse than in Poland. At Espinosa in November 1808, Victor's French army routed Blake's Spanish forces. The French lost around 1,100 wounded and dead, a paltry number compared with the slaughter of Eylau and Friedland. Percy, who had just taken over control of the *service de santé* in Spain from Larrey, admits that due to administrative bungling there were hardly any surgeons or ambulances on the field. The surgeons posted at Miranda appeared reluctant to make the potentially dangerous march to Espinosa despite knowing that there were wounded of their corps who needed attention. The difficulties of the *service de santé* were exacerbated by a number of French military reverses in Spain and Portugal, particularly at the hands of the British. At Vimeiro, the first major test of Wellington's army, most of the French wounded were captured by the British and, according to French sources, received poor quality care with many dying.[32]

Larrey offers a characteristically upbeat view of his medical experiences in the Peninsula. At Somosierra in November 1808, Napoleon's Polish cavalry sensationally dislodged the Spanish from a mountain pass with the loss of around sixty men killed or wounded. According to Larrey:

> This affair may be considered as one of the most brilliant that occurred during the war. The wounded were instantly dressed and operated on near the rough road that winds around the mountain. The carriages of our ambulances then conveyed them to Buytrago and then to Saint-Martino near Madrid.[33]

Eye-witness accounts suggest that Larrey glossed over many insufficiencies in the service, even within the Guard. Colonel Niegolowski, who suffered a head wound in the battle, says that the wounded were evacuated to a neighbouring village and deposited in some abandoned houses. 'If some inhabitants had stayed in the village, perhaps moved by pity they might have given us a glass of water to relieve our feverish thirst, but there were only some ambulance orderlies all drunk with wine and forgetful of the care they owed to the wounded.' Aide-de-Camp Philippe de Ségur had received multiple musket ball wounds. He confirms Niegolowski's observations but his account also highlights the privileged treatment given to one of Napoleon's favourites. After having his wounds dressed on the field by the Emperor's personal surgeon, Yvan, he was then carried in the Emperor's carriage to Buytrago where he had his own medical attendant. Despite his relatively cosseted care, the debilitated officer still felt vulnerable to the Spanish with their 'glances full of rage and hatred'.

Morvan refers sarcastically to Larrey's account of a 'perfect' medical service, pointing out the crippling shortage of ambulances and medical supplies and the frequent destitution of the wounded. The enemy fared no better. After Talavera in 1809, the 4,000 Spanish wounded were simply shut up in a church above the town and ignored. The following year, at Busaco in Portugal, where the French failed to push Wellington's army from a strong defensive position on a ridge, the medical service was again improvised and insufficient. The more fortunate of the wounded were evacuated to Coimbra carried by their comrades on stretchers made out of tree branches and the straps of haversacks. For the more severely wounded an awareness of the limited means of evacuation brought a sickening fear of being abandoned on the field to suffer a lingering or brutal death. Captain Nicolas Marcel says that he put his hands over his ears to shut out the cries of the men he knew personally. Fortunately for the French, not all the Spanish were antagonistic. Monks from a nearby convent collected the survivors from the field and cared for them.[34]

Napoleon's crushing victory at Friedland allowed him to occupy Tilsit and dictate peace terms to Alexander in a dramatic meeting on a raft in the Niemen river. Russia and Prussia were now official allies but Austria, humiliated at Austerlitz, had been rebuilding its army under the leadership of the Archduke Charles. By April 1809, it was confident enough to invade Bavaria and Italy. Napoleon responded robustly and the first major battle of the campaign was fought around the villages of Aspern and Essling near Vienna on 21 and 22 May. To understand the problems faced by the medical services it must be appreciated that the French forces were effectively split into three parts: on the south bank of the Danube around Ebersdorf, on the island of Lobau in the river, and on the north bank between Aspern and Essling. The bridges built between Lobau and the two banks were crucial both for the movement of troops and the evacuation of wounded which it was envisaged would be to the south to Ebersdorf and to Vienna. Following fierce fighting in Aspern and Essling and surprisingly stubborn resistance from the Austrians, Napoleon was forced to withdraw his forces back to Lobau. In what was ultimately an indecisive battle, the French had around 5,000 killed and 14,000 wounded and the Austrians probably slightly greater losses. As Percy had been forced to quit the *Grande Armée* due to a chronic eye disorder, the overall medical control was in the hands of Desgenettes and Heurteloup with Larrey, who has left the best account, responsible for the Guard's service.

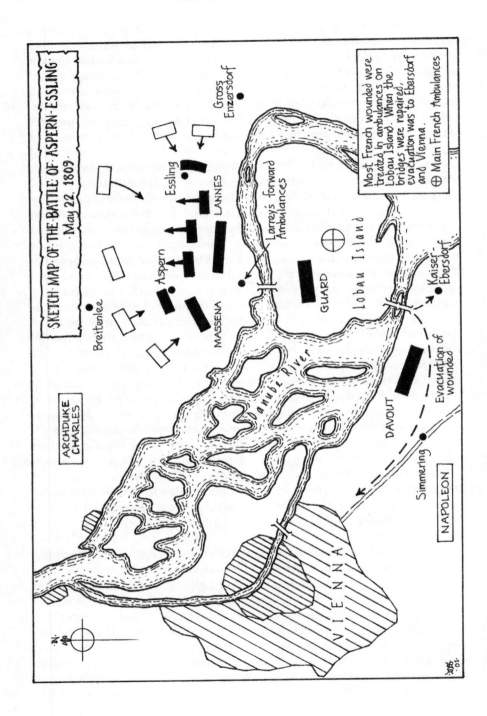

SKETCH MAP OF THE BATTLE OF ASPERN-ESSLING·
May 22. 1809·

ARCHDUKE
CHARLES

Breitenlee

Aspern

Essling

Gross
Enzersdorf

MASSENA

LANNES

Larrey's forward
Ambulances

GUARD

Lobau Island

Danube River

Kaiser-
Ebersdorf

Evacuation of
wounded

DAVOUT

Simmering

VIENNA

NAPOLEON

N.

Most French wounded were
treated in ambulances on
Lobau Island. When the
bridges were repaired,
evacuation was to Ebersdorf
and Vienna.
⊕ Main French Ambulances

At the outset of the fighting, Larrey set up his most advanced ambulances near a small forest on the north bank of the river. Here, he operated on the more seriously wounded whilst those whose wounds were lighter and who could travel more easily were taken back to Lobau where other ambulances were in waiting. At the culmination of the battle the great bulk of French wounded were on the island where they became stranded by the breakage of the bridges. After attending the seriously injured Marshal Lannes, Larrey rushed back to Lobau.

> As far as possible, I separated the wounded of the Imperial Guard from those of the Line but we gave the same care to all without distinction. I brought the surgeons of the different corps of the Guard to assist the medical officers of the ambulances and we did not rest until all the wounded on the island had been operated upon and dressed. Happily, we had all the instruments necessary and a sufficiency of dressings which I had taken care to have brought up by the ambulance orderlies … In spite of the promptitude and efficacy of our measures the wounded were in an ill plight, stretched out on the earth and either collected in groups on the river banks or dispersed in the interior of the island where the soil at this time was dry and arid. The heat was very great in the daytime and the nights damp and frosty. The winds, which are frequent in these regions, constantly covered the wounded with clouds of dust and the branches of a few trees or the leaves of the reeds gave only poor shelter from the sun. The breaking down of the bridges and the want of boats to bring provisions added still more to our misfortunes and we all suffered, particularly the wounded, from the lack of food and drink. I was obliged to order broth made of horseflesh which, from want of salt, was seasoned with gunpowder. Yet, this broth was not black but cleared on boiling and was quite pleasant. On the third day, we fortunately received all sorts of provisions and were able to issue rations regularly. On the fourth day, the bridges were rebuilt and all the wounded conveyed to hospitals prepared for them by Inspector General Heurteloup at Ebersdorf and Vienna.[35]

Charles-Louis Cadet de Gassicourt, a pharmacist on the Emperor's staff, confirms Larrey's account. He says that to make the soup, Larrey commandeered a general's horses and killed them. Being short of cooking pots, he heated the soup in the metal cuirasses of the cavalry placed over fires. Cadet de Gassicourt observed that, 'lots of things that figured in the bulletins were less important than that.' Larrey claimed that there were 'sufficient' dressings but at least some wounded were dressed with tow or other coarse fabrics. Other eye-witnesses claim that as many as half the wounded died without any attention. The inexperience of some of the surgeons was reflected by the fact that senior surgeons had to make chalk marks on the legs and arms of the wounded to show their aides where they should operate.[36]

Most contemporary accounts of Lobau refer to the terrible thirst. Musician Philippe-René Girault and his colleagues did all they could to find water and provide other relief for the wounded.

> During the night, we dressed around twenty wounded but our much greater task was to give these unfortunates something to drink. The thirst was making their tongues come out of their mouths. We had no other containers than our tin cans which we used alternately to dress their wounds and give them muddy water to drink.

Girault alleges that there was effectively no ambulance cover on the island. The best description of what it was like to be wounded at Aspern-Essling has been left by an officer named De Peslöuan. With his regiment near the church in Aspern village, he borrowed a telescope from a fellow officer, Lieutenant Béraud, to better observe the approaching Austrians.

> At the moment that I returned the telescope, a cannon ball struck me near to the shoulder. Béraud said to me, 'Pig, you have spat in my mouth.' It was my flesh and bone that he tasted; he spotted this before me, saying, 'Oh! My friend, you have lost your arm.'

With the help of a sapper, De Peslöuan walked the mile and a half to some regimental ambulances on the north bank of the river. By now he had lost a considerable amount of blood and he collapsed onto the grass.

> I waited for a surgeon to come and dress me; I saw one of them close to me but he did not respond to my call … I swore at and threatened the surgeons with butchery as they were letting me bleed to death. I scraped the ground with rage. The surgeons replied to my curses, saying that the wounded of their own regiments had to be dressed before me. I replied to them that the most severely wounded should be dressed first.

The surgeons of De Peslöuan's regiment were evidently employed elsewhere. Eventually, Heurteloup himself operated on the wounded officer, sitting him on a wounded horse and removing the debris of the humerus from the shoulder joint before ligating the artery. Restored by a little brandy, De Peslöuan was then carried by a drummer of his regiment across the remaining small bridge onto the island of Lobau. Here he spent four days and nights before being evacuated by boat to the hospital in a large building in Ebersdorf. As this was full, he was initially dumped in the courtyard. Later, he moved first to a garden where he lay in a lettuce patch and then into an abandoned house. He was finally carried to the civil hospital in Vienna by four Austrian prisoners. De Peslöuan says that many wounded on the river banks were not allowed back onto Lobau and that it was only his status as an officer and the personal intervention of Marshal Bessières that gained him access.[37]

The medical problems at Aspern-Essling were exacerbated by the severing of the bridges which compromised the movement of men and supplies and undermined the original evacuation plans. Napoleon had underestimated both the difficulty of fighting over the Danube and the durability of the Austrian army. Only six weeks later, a more carefully prepared second crossing resulted in the Battle of Wagram, the last great victory of the Empire. The *Grande Armée* paid a significant price with 5,000 killed and 28,000 wounded. Larrey relates that he followed the movements of the Guard with his flying ambulance dressing the wounded on the ground as quickly as they were brought in. As the casualties mounted, he had to set up a temporary hospital in the nearest village where he treated 500 men, not only the wounded of the Guard but also 'many officers of the line'. This raises the question of the fate of the vast majority of the wounded, the ordinary infantry soldiers. The simple answer is that they were left on the field to fend for themselves, their treatment, in the words of one historian, 'a disgrace'. There was little evidence of an organised ambulance system for the line. This is unsurprising as the shortage of resources was exacerbated by a lack of real planning. Laurillard-Fallot, physician to a division, should have been given directions for the movement of the ambulances but he acknowledges that he often heard nothing and wandered about completely lost. It was only the Guard's ambulance that moved 'with one voice, at the same time, in the same direction'.[38]

Siméon Lamon, chasseur in the Old Guard, remembers that at first the wounded were carried by their comrades to the few available ambulances but that this depleted the ranks too much as it took two soldiers to lift one wounded man. Accordingly, they were later simply deposited about twenty paces in the rear. Those who escaped the fires in the hay were often left unattended for several days, only surviving by drinking their own urine. Dezydery Chlapowski rode over the field after the battle, '… here and there I found wounded men who had not yet been treated by the medical services … Our surgeons were doing what they could but were unable to help them all.' In the absence of an adequate *service de santé*, a bewildering array of staff pitched in to try and help the wounded. It was traditional for musicians to give first aid to the battalions but should the *Grande Armée* have had to rely on postal workers and administrators of the *Conseil d'État* combing the field for survivors six days after the battle? Inspector Boulanger of the postal service found a cuirassier lying wrapped in his cloak and offered to place him on one of the postal wagons. The man opened his cloak revealing a shattered leg crawling with maggots. 'Monsieur,' he said, 'if they had carried me to the ambulance the day after the battle they could have cut off my leg and, as I am strong, I would have survived. Now, as you can see, it is too late.'[39]

The repeated failings of the *service de santé* on the battlefields of the Empire between 1805 and 1809 were acknowledged and understood by its senior doctors. It was transparently clear that the line regiments required a militarised surgical service equivalent to that of the Imperial Guard. Any new organisation would have to be approved by the Emperor. In April 1807, in Poland, Percy had presented his written plan for a *chirurgie de bataille* to Napoleon using General Duroc as an intermediary. In his covering letter, Percy first noted that some components of his plan were already in place in the army and that the remainder would not be difficult to organise. He stressed the vital role of the surgeons in the 'active' army compared with the physicians and pharmacists who, he believed, were better placed at the hospitals in the rear. He then described the detail of his proposed battlefield surgical service.

It is thus an entirely military service which must be formed at the front of the army. In naming it *'chirurgie de bataille'* Your Majesty will define its use and will prevent all jealousy and provocation on the part of other *officiers de santé* who, not sharing in its dangers and work, will not be able to complain about its prerogatives. This *chirurgie de bataille* must be so formed that it is entirely self-sufficient and so that it can take responsibility for everything concerned with the health of an army on campaign. It must have its own internal administration and be provided with soldier *infirmiers* of adequate number and quality to escort the evacuees and wounded, guard the ambulance wagons, remove the wounded from the field of battle, bury the dead, care for the sick in the hospitals on campaign and execute orders relating to the cleaning, tidying and healthiness of the camps, hospitals etc. In establishing the *chirurgie de bataille*, Your Majesty will be sure of keeping in the line all those soldiers who will no longer be able to leave the fight on the pretence, too often invalid, of taking their wounded comrades to the ambulance. It will get rid of the confusion and disorder which the competition of several administrations and the plurality and conflict of different authorities introduce into a service which, to work well, must have natural leaders and be submitted to a single will and be made up of similar parts placed under their guidance and given an immediate and direct impetus. In the body of a surgical service ennobled by your kindness and rewards, you will find Sir, men who have the talent, character and quality necessary to conduct with success and administer with order the new *chirurgie de bataille*. To bring all the necessary parts together and to give it the necessary credibility I believe it is at once fair and indispensable to form it as an absolutely military corps, following the example of the engineers.

PLAN

Article 1: The surgical service of the army will be formed into military corps under the distinctive title of the *Corps Militaire de Chirurgie des Armées*.

Article 2: The *Corps Militaire de Chirurgie des Armées* will be composed of: a *chirurgien-major général des armées*.

Article 3: Of 3 *chirurgiens-majors inspecteurs généraux de service de santé des armées*.

Article 4: Of 16 *chirurgiens-majors supérieurs* having the rank of lieutenant-colonel.

Article 5: Of 260 *chirurgiens-majors* having the rank of *chef du bataillon* or captain of the 1ère, 2e or 3e class according to the length of their service which, apart from the first grade which they have legally held, will be counted in five years.

Article 6: Of 260 *chirurgiens-aides-majors* having the rank of lieutenant of the 1ère class or 2e class according to the length of their service which, apart from their legal commission, will be counted in five years.

Article 7: Of 800 *chirurgiens-sous-aides* having the rank of *sous-lieutenant* and of 400 cadets (*aspirants*) who will be enlisted militarily with the rank of *adjutant-sous-officier* and who will be only given paid appointments in time of war as they become *sous-aides*.

Article 8: The surgeons making up the *Corps Militaire de Chirurgie des Armées*, except for those of the first two grades, will be distributed in the armies, the regiments, hospitals, forts, etc. They will be under the policing of general officers and commandants and under the immediate direction and supervision of their own chiefs.[40]

There were a number of practical and political drawbacks to Percy's grand plan. As Duroc pointed out, it did not embrace the whole of the *service de santé*, the hospitals being largely outside its remit. It was probable that the administration, accustomed to having a substantial influence over the army's doctors, would oppose the new autonomous organisation. Even greater antagonism could be anticipated within the *service de santé*. Despite Percy's protestations, it was very likely that the 'other *officiers de santé*', the physicians and pharmacists, would be jealous of an initiative which overtly increased the prestige of the army's surgeons whilst relegating them to a distant supporting role in the rear. In his interpretation of the *chirurgie de bataille* project, Eugene Fenech notes that the physicians and pharmacists would be '*supprimés*', literally translated as 'cut out' or 'abolished'.[41]

Despite these reasonable objections, there was an obvious need for a *chirurgie de bataille* or a very similar structure. Professional conflict could easily have been avoided by accommodating the other *officiers de santé* within the organisation. However, Percy's plan was doomed to failure. Napoleon, who so often paid lip service to the suggestions of his senior doctors, again showed only an abstract interest when Percy presented him with the documents. Throwing a quick glance at them, he slipped the papers into his pocket with the non-committal comment 'We shall see'. The Emperor only appeared to remember the suggestions for a proper ambulance service six years later. Percy was always treated with kindness and respect by Napoleon but the rejection of his project left him resentful and frustrated. At Friedland, he watched soldiers leaving the line to take the casualties out of cannon range, at least six for each wounded man. In his journal he rants: 'Why not give us *servants de chirurgie de bataille*?.. Our service is dreadful; it is barbaric.' There are references to active divisions of *chirurgie de bataille* in Percy's writings but these units were quite different from his great scheme which never came to fruition on the battlefield. They were small groups of surgeons – for instance, one *chirurgien-major*, one *aide* and three *sous-aides* – who were mounted and attached to each army corps to supplement the regimental surgeons. They were initially formed in 1806 and there were around twenty divisions.[42]

Percy did have some success in setting up formal companies of '*infirmiers*', one component of *chirurgie de bataille*. These were men who acted as medical orderlies or 'servants' to the medical staff. Within the armies, they gave simple first aid on the field and evacuated the wounded to the waiting surgeons whilst in the hospitals they assisted the *officiers de santé* in the management of wounded and sick. It was not a new concept. *Infirmiers* had made sporadic appearances in the early years of the wars but their organisation was ad hoc and they were likely to be summarily moved to other sections of the army. In Spain, where the local population was often antagonistic and unwilling to assist the French medical services, the complete lack of French *infirmiers* was keenly felt and, in late 1808 Percy appealed to Berthier to allow the enrolment of slightly wounded soldiers as *infirmiers*. He wanted them to be well organised, distinctly dressed and ably led by good officers. On this occasion, Percy's efforts bore fruit and Napoleon sanctioned the creation of companies of *infirmiers*, referred to as '*soldats d'ambulance*' or '*infirmiers d'hôpitaux*'. Percy excitedly set to work and combed Madrid for suitable uniforms and equipment for the first thirty men.[43]

A decree announcing the more formal creation of ten companies of *infirmiers* across the Empire appeared in April 1809. It was specified that each company was to be overseen by a '*centenier*' and '*sous-centenier*' to be chosen from among retired or unfit officers or the most senior employees of the hospitals. There were some lower ranking officers and then ninety-six '*infirmiers ordinaires*' recruited from men who had been judged unfit for conscription as soldiers or from among the other hospital employees. Medical problems compatible with service as an *infirmier* but not as a soldier included the loss of an eye and the loss of fingers or toes. The legislation, which was penned by Percy in conjunction with Commissaire des Guerres Mathieu Favier, specified that each company would have a total of 125 men. The first of these units was formed in Vienna in September 1809. Ultimately five were formed in Austria, three in Spain, two in Italy and an additional one in Holland, the last to be created in November 1811.

The *infirmier* companies had an unhappy history. The formations in Spain and those entering Russia were largely destroyed in the course of these brutal campaigns. Those that continued to function were held in low esteem by the soldiers, their staff regarded as 'pallbearers' rather than as essential members of the *service de santé*. The wounded veterans drafted into these posts were often thin-skinned and quick to reach for their sabres at the slightest insult from the serving soldiers. Napoleon's low opinion of the *infirmier* companies can be deduced from the fact that only a solitary *Légion d'honneur* was awarded to the 2,000 or so men who served in these formations.[44]

The *infirmiers* were a laudable initiative but they solved none of the major problems of the *service de santé*, least of all the difficulties in promptly evacuating wounded men from the field. Percy was cognisant of this and refined his original ideas, introducing the post of '*brancardier*' or '*despotat*'. These two terms were used indistinctly to describe men within the pre-existing *infirmier* companies who were fit enough to load the wounded onto stretchers and carry them to the nearest field hospital. Percy anticipated that each company would contain thirty-two *brancardiers* who would be armed with pikes which could be used in the construction of the stretchers. We do get the occasional glimpse of *brancardiers* in action. At the Battle of Borodino, Surgeon La Flize of the 2ᵉ Grenadiers recalls:

> The *brancardiers* received the orders to construct stretchers. These men, working in pairs, removed the straps of their haversacks, unscrewed the iron from the pikes, ran the poles through a knot formed with the straps and then attached their cloth belts. In an instant they had about forty stretchers.[45]

This convincing account contradicts the claim made by some historians that the *brancardiers* never existed. However, their role was probably very limited. They were not included in any formal decree and when Corvissart praised Percy's ideas in 1814 he talked of the *brancardiers* as a potential project rather than as a reality. Like so many other well meaning initiatives in the *service de santé* they appeared more on paper than on the battlefield.

Notes

1. Gallaher, J G, *The Iron Marshal. A biography of Louis N. Davout*, pp. 100, 226; Connelly, O, *Blundering to Glory. Napoleon's Military Campaigns*, p. 73.
2. Tulard, J, *Dictionnaire Napoléon*, Vol. I, p. 898.
3. Lemaire, J-F, *Les blessés dans les Armées Napoléoniennes*, pp. 48, 55–6, 43, 40–1, 84–8.
4. Exteberria, F, *Surgery in the Spanish War of Independence (1807–1813); between Desault and Lister.*
5. Horácková, L and Vargová, L, *Bone remains from a common grave pit from the Battle of Austerlitz.*
6. Percy, Baron, *Journal de Campagnes de Baron Percy*, pp. 67, 71; d'Héralde, J-B, *Mémoires d'un Chirurgien de la Grande Armée*, pp. 94, 87.
7. Pigeard, A, *Dictionnaire de la Grande Armée*, p. 622; d'Héralde, p. 91.
8. Larrey, D J, *Mémoires de Chirurgie Militaire et Campagnes 1787–1840*, pp. 369–70; Horácková, p. 12.
9. La Flize, Dr, *Souvenirs de la Moskowa par un chirurgien de la Garde Impériale*, p. 421; Larrey, p. 462.
10. d'Héralde, pp. 89–91.
11. Percy, p. xii.
12. Richardson, R, *Larrey. Surgeon to Napoleon's Imperial Guard*, p. 100.
13. Larrey, p. 370; Brice, Docteur and Bottet, Capitaine, *Le Corps de Santé Militaire en France*, p. 152; d'Héralde, p. 94; Lejeune, Baron, *Memoirs of Baron Lejeune Aide-de-Camp to Marshals Berthier, Davout and Oudinot*, Vol. I, p. 33.
14. Morvan, J, *Le Soldat Impérial*, Vol. II, p. 308; d'Héralde, p. 94; Brice, Bottet, p. 153; Baldet, M, *La Vie Quotidienne dans les Armées de Napoléon*, p. 165.
15. Connelly, pp. 95–102.
16. Larrey, p. 462; Barrès, J-B, *Memoirs of a French Napoleonic Officer*, p. 89; Brice, Bottet, p. 192; Percy, p. 85; Damamme, J-C, *Les Soldats de la Grande Armée*, p. 241.
17. d'Héralde, p. 105.
18. Pigeard, p. 667.
19. Triaire, P, *Dominique Larrey et les campagnes de la Révolution et de l'Empire*, p.242.
20. Larrey, pp. 480–1.
21. Percy, pp. 158, 143, 163; Soubiran, A, *Le Baron Larrey chirurgien de Napoléon*, p. 202.
22. Percy, pp. 163–6.
23. Morvan, Vol. II, p. 317; Percy, pp. 172–3, 180.
24. Lemaire, p. 144; Percy, pp. 175, 178–81.
25. Davidov, D, *In the Service of the Tsar against Napoleon. The Memoirs of Denis Davidov 1806–1814*, p. 44; Larrey, p. 482; Percy, p. 191.
26. Kouchnir, S L L, *Considérations sur l'évolution du service de santé militaire de 1789 à 1814*, p. 40.

27. Chandler, D, *The Campaigns of Napoleon*, p. 1118.
28. ibid., p. 550.
29. Percy, pp. 295–6, 291–3; Larrey, p. 502; Morvan, Vol. II, p. 321.
30. Percy, pp. 249–50.
31. Brice, Bottet, p. 210.
32. Morvan, Vol. II, p. 325; Fenech, E, *Mémoires d'un Officier de Santé Maltais dans L'Armée Française (1786–1839)*, pp. 33, 51; Percy, p. 404.
33. Larrey, p. 586.
34. Masson, F, *Aventures de Guerre 1792–1809*, p. 166; Ségur, General Count de, *An Aide-de-Camp of Napoleon*, p. 398; Morvan, Vol. II, p. 331; Fenech, p. 51; Marcel, N, *Campagnes en Espagne et au Portugal 1808–1814*, p. 99.
35. Larrey, pp. 601–2.
36. Brice, Bottet, p. 206; Morvan, Vol. II, p. 338.
37. Masson, pp. 175–6; Lucas-Dubreton, J, *Les Soldats de Napoléon*, pp. 287–91.
38. Larrey, p. 635; Laurillard-Fallot, S-L, *Souvenirs d'un Médecin Hollandais sous les Aigles Françaises 1807–1833*, p.31.
39. Pigeard, A, *L'Armée de Napoléon*, p. 183; Lejeune, Vol. I, p. 325; Chlapowski, D, *Memoirs of a Polish Lancer*, p. 86; Lemaire, p. 240.
40. Percy, pp. 217–20; Lemaire, pp. 301–3.
41. Fenech, p. 43.
42. Pigeard, *Dictionnaire de la Grande Armée*, p. 161; Percy, pp. 271, 294.
43. Percy, pp. 421–4, 441.
44. Lemaire, pp. 245–9.
45. La Flize, p. 422.

CHAPTER VI

The Battlefield 1810–1815: Decline and Fall

More men died on the field of Borodino in 1812 than in any other day's fighting in the 19th century. The total was only surpassed by the first day of the Somme in 1916. This relentless growth of casualties in the later years of the wars was paralleled by desperate efforts to sustain the *Grande Armée* and increasing evidence of Napoleon's fallibility. The losses from the calamitous Russian campaign, approximately 400,000 men, are well documented. But this was not the end of the suffering for the *Grande Armée*. When the campaign for Germany began in August 1813, Napoleon had approximately 440,000 men under arms, a remarkable achievement in view of the almost complete destruction of his army in Russia. By November, only 75,000 men were still with the colours, an alarming loss of 365,000 troops in only three months. This equated to an average attrition of over 4,000 men per day from all causes. The Emperor was keen to play down the scale of casualties in his bulletins and public correspondence. After the slaughter of Eylau, at five o'clock in the evening, he wrote to Arch-Chancellor Cambacérès, grossly underestimating the French losses at 1,500 dead and 4,000 wounded. Only an hour later, in a letter to the Empress, the estimated number of killed had fallen to only one thousand. He was deluding others but not himself. In correspondence with Marshal Ney, dated March 1813, he suggests the formation of five ambulances, each carrying enough equipment to give first aid to 10,000 wounded.[1]

The march on Moscow commenced in June 1812 with the crossing of the Niemen river. Napoleon's multinational force of 430,000 men was opposed by the Russian armies of Barclay de Tolly (127,000 men), Bagration (48,000) and Tomassov (43,000). It had originally been intended that Heurteloup would oversee the medical arrangements for the campaign but, after his unexpected death, Larrey was given this onerous responsibility. Although already lauded as a great military surgeon, this was, nevertheless, a considerable step up for a man who had previously commanded only the elite Guard's service. In that role, Larrey had been relatively protected but now he would have to tackle all the problems of the line's medical services while being dictated to by the army's administration. The challenge of providing adequate medical back up for the Russian campaign was made more daunting by the insufficient state of the *service de santé* on the eve of the army's departure. From a report dated March 1811 on the personnel and administration of the Army of Germany, it is clear that the divisional medical services had been completely run down and that many of the *officiers de santé* and employees had returned to France. Compared with a full complement of sixteen physicians, eighty-eight surgeons, sixty-three pharmacists and sixty-nine employees the actual numbers with the divisions were eleven, fifty-three, thirty-nine and forty-four respectively. Much of the equipment of what should have been six divisional ambulances had been assigned to the army's magazines.[2] At this time, each regiment was only allocated one ambulance caisson, quite inadequate for a prolonged campaign.

Some attempt was made to improve the situation but the preparations were both on too small a scale and too late. Napoleon wrote to Daru in early 1812 specifying the contents of the regimental ambulances and suggesting that the ambulances carry at least ten stretchers and two cases of amputating instruments. On learning of his new appointment, Larrey rushed to Berlin where he improvised six divisions of mobile field ambulances, each with eight medical officers. He notes that: 'Every surgeon exercised his division every day in the practice of operating and bandaging under my instruction. There was the keenest competition and the most perfect discipline among all the surgeons.' He does not comment that the divisional ambulances had three fewer *officiers de santé* than had been the case in 1809. The early days of the campaign saw skirmishing around Kovno, Vilna and Vitebsk. The casualties were counted in hundreds rather than thousands but already the administrative services were malfunctioning and the shortage of medical supplies meant that *officiers de santé* had to use their own shirts for dressings. The general bewilderment that the army was reduced to this condition so close to the start of such a major undertaking is well expressed by Caulaincourt, Napoleon's Master of Horse.

> From a spirit of inexplicable and unpardonable meanness, the provisioning of the ambulances had been inadequate. Even the personnel were too scanty. Never had carelessness been carried to greater extremes by the underlings of the administration; never had the courage of unfortunate men been more abused. The army surgeons and the administrative chiefs, as praiseworthy for their zeal as for their talents, were in despair at the state in which they found the hospitals. In vain did they endeavour to make up, by their care and attention, for whatever was lacking. We had only got as far as Vitebsk, we had not fought a battle, and there was not even any lint!

The shortage of dressings was sorely felt at the first major clash of arms in August at Smolensk 400 miles into Russia. The French lost around 1,200 killed and 3,000 wounded in some stubborn fighting in the suburbs. The wounded were piled up in fifteen large buildings spared by the fire that had ravaged much of the city. The linen was by now exhausted and Larrey was forced to improvise.

> For dressings, I employed paper which we found in the archives build-
> ings which we used as a hospital. The parchments also served us as
> splints. Tow and birch cotton took the place of lint and we also used
> paper as bedding for the patients. But what difficulties we had to over-
> come! What toil and labour did we not endure in this crisis!

The day after the battle, a major of the Guard discovered 180 wounded men untended in a windmill. He alerted the administration but little action was taken and it was only when he threatened to speak to the Emperor that something was done. In the two days of inactivity most had died and the dead had started to putrefy.[3]

It was at Smolensk that Larrey took the fateful decision to leave five of the six light ambulance divisions and all the reserve medical officers in the city. He left for Valutina on the Moscow road with only the sixth division and two of his own pupils. The reason for this action was his own conviction that the victory at Smolensk and the advancing autumn rains made any further significant advance of the army very unlikely. He was to be proved wrong and it was soon common knowledge that the Russian army had taken up positions on the heights of Mojaisk and that a great battle was imminent. 'This news greatly perturbed me, since all my surgeons had been left behind at Smolensk and the ambulance wagons had not yet come up.'[4] Larrey asked for a general order putting most of the regimental surgeons at his disposal. This desperate measure furnished him with forty-five surgeons of various grades whom he attached to the general headquarters. A few ambulance wagons were also able to catch up with the main army but there was still an extreme shortage of surgeons and equipment and it was inevitable that Larrey's decision at Smolensk would be viewed as a misjudgement. This apparent error in the distribution of ambulances and staff prior to Borodino may have been in Napoleon's mind when, three years later, he asked Percy to make the medical arrangements for the Waterloo campaign whilst Larrey returned to the subordinate post of chief surgeon to the Guard.

The Battle of Borodino (*la Moskowa*) turned into a murderous pound-ing match around the Russian entrenchments. In unparalleled scenes of carnage, the earthworks started to disappear under a mass of dead and dying which averaged a depth of six to eight men. Wounded soldiers des-perately tried to get out of the slaughter, in the words of cavalry surgeon

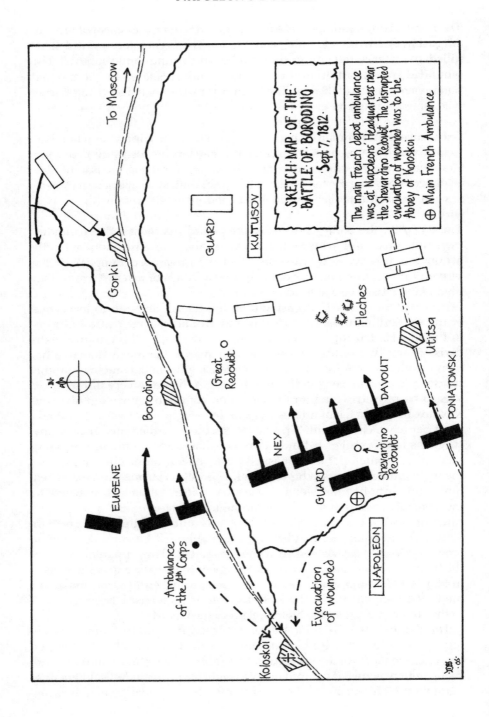

SKETCH·MAP·OF·THE·
BATTLE·OF·BORODINO·
Sept 7, 1812.

The main French depot ambulance
was at Napoleons' Headquarters near
the Shevardino Redoubt. The disrupted
evacuation of wounded was to the
Abbey of Koloskoi.

⊕ Main French Ambulance

To Moscow

Gorki

GUARD

KUTUSOV

Great
Redoubt

Fleches

Utitsa

Borodino

NEY

DAVOUT

PONIATOWSKI

EUGENE

GUARD

Shevardino
Redoubt

NAPOLEON

Ambulance
of the 4th Corps

Evacuation
of wounded

Koloskoi

Raymond Faure, 'hoping to escape death by fleeing the place where she reigned in all her horror.'[5] Napoleon, who appeared ill and uninterested, spurned a chance to commit the Guard and turn a moral victory into a rout. The French lost around 6,500 killed and 21,500 wounded and the Russians roughly 45,000 killed and wounded.

At the commencement of hostilities, Larrey had contrived to assemble thirty-six surgeons. In his memoirs, he talks of the 'disposition of the ambulance materials' and the giving of orders to the corps and divisional ambulances but this matter of fact account cannot obscure the fact that there was a hopeless mismatch between the scale of the casualties and the available medical services. The main French ambulance was set up near the general headquarters tents behind the centre of the French line. This was on the old Kaluga road close to the Shevardino Redoubt. Probably about two thirds of the wounded were dressed at this single headquarters ambulance. On a map of the field drawn, on Larrey's orders, by Chirurgien-Major Sarlandière, the only other ambulance thought worthy of portrayal was that of the 4th corps to the left rear of the French line. Chirurgien-Major La Flize of the Guard describes Larrey's main ambulance as consisting of two tents. Operations and dressings were performed by candlelight in the smaller tent and the wounded were then carried to the larger structure. Larrey says that the shortage of able assistants forced him to do all the major operations himself. 'A great number of men injured by the artillery required amputation of one or two limbs and, during the first twenty-four hours, I performed about 200 operations of this nature.' If this is true, it was a surgical tour de force which can hardly have been equalled in the annals of military surgery.

Larrey comments that his colleagues and the remainder of the service showed great courage and devotion and that the corps and regimental ambulances 'fulfilled their duties perfectly'. Whilst there is no reason to question the devotion of the surgeons, this allusion to the ambulances betrays some wishful thinking. Many eye-witnesses allege paucity or complete lack of medical care. An anonymous officer recalls:

> There was virtually no sanitary service or activity. All the villages and houses close to the Moscow road were packed full with wounded in an utterly helpless state. The villages were destroyed by endless fires which ravaged the regions occupied or traversed by the French army. Those wounded who managed to save themselves from the flames crawled in their thousands along the high road seeking some way to prolong their pitiful existence.

Chirurgien-Major René Bourgeois contradicts Larrey's account stating that, 'there was no real ambulance equipment, no pharmacy where one could obtain the means of preparing the wounded for their operations or their success'. The surgeons were forced to rip up the wounded men's own clothes to use as bandages. First aid was complicated by the severity of the wounds caused by artillery and the Russian musket balls which were larger than the French.[6]

At least some of the regimental *officiers de santé* set up their own small dressing stations at convenient points on the field. Wurttemberger Heinrich Roos established his in a small valley next to a stream. He was soon overwhelmed by wounded French, Saxons, Westphalians and his own countrymen. Many had severe injuries including broken bones. Roos and his aide operated and bandaged until nightfall, occasionally rushing to the stream to rinse the blood off their hands and instruments. He notes that at Borodino, unlike earlier battles, there was confusion as to where the wounded should be evacuated. In practice, many ended up at the abbey of Koloskoi to the south-west of Borodino village. Captain Charles François was involved in fierce fighting at the redoubts.

> I was badly damaged; my shako and coat tails were shot away and I was bruised all over. A ball which passed through my left leg, in addition to the one I had received the previous day, left me so feeble from want of blood that I could neither breathe nor move. When I recovered a little from my weakness, the soldiers led me to the ambulance, where, at that moment, General Morand, who had been hit on the chin, was having his wound dressed. The general shook hands with me and, when he had been attended to, made a sign to the surgeon to look after me. The doctor came to me, put his little finger in the bullet hole and, with his bistoury, made the customary cross-cut at each hole, put in a probe which passed through my leg between the bones, and said, 'A lucky wound.' Then he put on the first dressing and told me to go to the army ambulance at Koloskoi where there were thousands of wounded. The ambulance was at a convent. I was placed in a room where there were twenty-seven officers of my regiment, five of whom had undergone amputation; all lying on straw, and absolutely in want of everything. There were more than 10,000 wounded in this hospital. Eight or ten days after this battle, three-fourths of these poor fellows were dead from want of medical attention and food.

Larrey acknowledges the problems at Koloskoi where the indolence of the administration exacerbated the sufferings of the wounded. La Flize recalls that the Guard received some food but that the remainder of the wounded were famished and reduced to scavenging on horse-flesh, potatoes and cabbage stumps. The overcrowding was such that to get to the first floor it was necessary to climb over men lying on each step of the staircase.[7]

Men of the 8th corps were given the responsibility of removing the remaining French wounded from the field, a task which took several days. Not all were located. Seven weeks later, the troops re-crossed the Borodino battlefield on the retreat from Moscow. Count Philippe-Paul de Ségur describes the chilling scene.

> The *Grande Armée* was filing past this deadly field in reverential silence when a sound of moaning reached their ears. One of the victims of that gory day was still alive! Some of our men ran in the direction of the sound and found a French soldier with both legs broken who had fallen among the dead. For fifty days he had kept himself alive by drinking the muddy water at the bottom of the ravine into which he had rolled and eating the putrid flesh of the dead. The soldiers who claim to have found this man declare that they were able to save him. Farther on, we reached the hospital we had set up in the abbey of Koloskoi where a sight even more terrible than the battlefield met our eyes. At Borodino there was death, but also peace and rest. There, at least, the struggle was over; here it was still going on. Death seemed to have pursued the victims who had escaped from the combat and was attacking them through all their senses at the same time … Nevertheless, despite starvation, cold and the most complete destitution, a considerable number of the wounded had been kept alive in this foul place by a shred of hope and the splendid devotion of the surgeons.

The Emperor ordered some of the stronger men to be evacuated in wagons whilst the weakest were left in the hands of wounded Russian officers. La Flize also re-crossed the field in late October and was puzzled to see a strange coloured pyramid in the middle distance. Curiosity drew him towards it and he was shocked to find that it was a mound of what he estimated to be around 800 French and Russian corpses. The bodies had lost their eyes but were otherwise well preserved by the glacial conditions. The surgeon observed that many had severe sabre wounds and that others had been burnt by exploding shells.[8]

Heinrich Roos, in the midst of the action at Borodino, makes some interesting comments regarding soldiers' differing attitudes to wounding. A Saxon *cuirassier* had received a shell injury which destroyed much of the musculature between his knee and buttock. He showed considerable bravery and optimism, 'Without doubt,' he said, 'my wound is serious but it will be cured because I am healthy in body and my blood is pure.' In contrast, a younger officer of the same regiment who had been hit in the shoulder by a musket ball worried not only about the immediate danger of his wound but about the loss of his horse and luggage, the possibility of him remaining crippled, the fact that he had not been bled and his distance from home. Roos notes that he felt sorry for the young man and admits that if he had been in Germany rather than Russia he would have sent him home to be looked after by his mother. Some of the wounded foreign soldiers of the *Grande Armée* cursed Napoleon. The French generally tolerated their wounds with 'tranquillity and patience'.[9]

This tolerance of wounding by many French soldiers may have been in part due to the status gained in the eyes of their fellow soldiers and countrymen should they survive the injury. When Louis-François Lejeune met his young brother, who was off to join his new regiment at Jena in 1806, he embraced him and wished him three things – a wound, advancement and the cross of honour. By the Battle of Friedland, a year later, all three had been accomplished. Lejeune tells another anecdote which illustrates both the prestige of wounding and the clever psychology employed by Napoleon. In 1809, after the Battle of Ratisbon, the Emperor reviewed the 52nd Regiment.

> He had asked the colonel to order out from the ranks the most deserving of the non-commissioned officers; and as the Emperor passed before them, the brave fellows proudly presented arms, answering his questions and receiving with delight the Imperial baptism, 'I make you an officer.' When he had reached the seventh or eighth sergeant, the Emperor noticed a handsome young fellow with fine but stern-looking eyes and of resolute and martial bearing, who made his musket ring again as he presented arms. 'How many wounds?' inquired the Emperor. 'Thirty,' replied the sergeant. 'I am not asking your age,' said the Emperor graciously; 'I am asking how many wounds you have received.' Raising his voice, the sergeant again replied with one word, 'Thirty'. Annoyed at this reply, the Emperor turned to the colonel and said, 'The man does not understand; he thinks I am asking about his age.' 'He understands well enough, sire,' was the reply; 'he has been wounded thirty times'. 'What!' exclaimed the Emperor, 'you have been wounded so often and have not got the cross!' The sergeant looked down at his chest, and, seeing that the strap of his cartridge pouch hid his decoration, he raised it so as to show his cross. He said to the Emperor, with great earnestness, 'Yes, I've got one, but I've merited a dozen!' The Emperor, who was always pleased to meet spirited fellows such as this, pronounced the sacramental words, 'I make you an officer!'[10]

In the west of the Empire the brutal Peninsular War rumbled on with major French defeats at the hands of the British and their allies in the north of Spain at Salamanca in 1812 and at Vitoria in 1813. These battles effectively ensured a French failure in the Peninsula with subsequent resistance in the Pyrenees only delaying the inevitable. The medical arrangements in the later years of the conflict were not significantly different than those made for the earlier battles in Portugal and Spain. The difficulties and failings of the *service de santé* were exacerbated by military failure and the disarray of the French forces. The *officiers de santé* shared the dangers with their soldier comrades. At Vitoria, Chirurgien-Major Jean-Baptiste d'Héralde saw both his *sous-aides* seriously wounded. He attempted to help one of them who had a fractured hip but was himself struck by a musket ball in the shin. D'Héralde could do little more than mount his horse and join the remainder of the French army in a disorganised retreat.[11]

Napoleon returned to Paris in April 1813 and started to rebuild his army around 50,000 survivors of the Russian disaster. This was not the same *Grande Armée* that had been so carefully assembled eight years earlier. The army was large, over 400,000 at its peak in August, but the infantry was composed of a mixture of jaded veterans and green conscripts and the cavalry was much inferior to that lost in Russia. With this blunt weapon, the Emperor had to confront the combined armies of all the major European powers. The allies opposing Napoleon now included Russia, Prussia, Great Britain and Sweden with Austria awaiting an apposite moment to join them. At the start of the 1813 campaign, the Emperor had 120,000 men under his direct command and was up against a mixed Russian and Prussian army of around 110,000 led by Wittgenstein and Blücher. In May the French crossed the Saale river and marched on Leipzig. As always, the allies were surprised by Napoleon's rapidity and they fell back only sporadically opposing his advance. The first major battle of the campaign was fought at Lützen fifteen miles to the south-west of Leipzig on 2 May where Napoleon won a hard-fought victory over the allies. He was unable to properly follow this up because his cavalry arm was so undependable. French losses were about 18,000 killed and wounded and the allies probably less at 15,000.

This new army of conscripts was not well served by its medical depart-ment. There was a severe shortage of *officiers de santé*. In an alarming report to Napoleon's Chief of Staff Berthier, penned two weeks prior to Lützen, Marshal Marmont complained that not only was his corps depleted and of low quality but that it 'entirely lacked surgeons'. Many *officiers de santé* had died in Russia or had been left with the wounded. Desperate attempts at requisition struggled to raise the necessary number of new doctors as even the despised *chirurgiens de pacotille* were now in short supply. There was also a dearth of horses to pull the ambulances wagons. It was against this background that Larrey was forced to conjure up a service at Lützen. He arrived on the field at 11o'clock in the morning and was directed by Napoleon to take his light ambulances to the nearby town of Lützen to receive the wounded. The number of casualties was such that the town effectively became 'one large ambulance'. As at Borodino, the army's senior surgeon was poorly assisted and, in the first two days and nights after the battle, he again performed most of the difficult operations himself. The strain of providing a decent surgical service was increased by the bloody mindedness of the administration. A surgeon in command of an ambulance division later complained bitterly that he missed the battle because he had been wrongly sent to Merseberg and was then forced to stay there. Supply fourgons were also misdirected by the quartermasters. As was the case after other Napoleonic battles, the sufferings of the *Grande Armée*'s soldiers were alleviated by practical help from the local population. Commissaire des

Guerres Alexandre Bellot de Kergorre asserts that the wounded in Lützen were treated with great kindness by the townspeople.[12]

At the Battle of Bautzen, three weeks later, Larrey arranged the ambulances and performed first aid on the field before returning to the town where he tended the wounded for three days. When he later revisited Bautzen, he found that:

> Two-thirds of them had been moved to Dresden [approximately thirty miles] by the inhabitants who were full of humanity and eager to assist them and, on my advice, they used a kind of hand barrow which is very convenient and much in use in the country for the carriage of goods and merchandise: each house had a number of them. As the road from Bautzen to Dresden slopes downwards there was no obstacle to these barrows and we have seen as many as a hundred to a hundred and fifty filing along it, one behind the other. No means of transport could be better or quieter. This shows how important it is for the Surgeon-in-Chief to study the countries in which armies operate so as to know how to employ the local resources for the benefit of the wounded.

The German civilians also supplied the much needed linen and dressings.[13]

The two battles of Lützen and Bautzen led to 22,000 wounded passing through the ambulances of which approximately a tenth died.[14] One particular type of wound was unusually common. A large number of young recruits, perhaps as many as 3,000, had sustained injuries to their fingers. At headquarters, the senior military officers, Soult and Oudinot among them, were in little doubt that this was an outbreak of self-mutilation which could not go unpunished. They were supported in this opinion by a considerable number of army doctors including Yvan and Desgenettes. The principal surgeon of the 12th corps of the army reported that the wounds of the right forearm and hand in sixty of the young soldiers were typical of self-harm. It was Napoleon's initial intention to shoot these malingerers but, before taking such draconian action, he decided to consult with Larrey. When the latter arrived at Dresden the Emperor accosted him with a series of questions on the differences between the types of wounds suffered at the hands of the enemy and those that were self-induced. Napoleon expected a quick confirmation of the statements of Yvan and Desgenettes but Larrey expressed the view that it was very difficult to tell the difference. Napoleon was taken aback and asked for this opinion to be put in writing. The outcome of this conversation was the creation of a jury, under the jurisdiction of Larrey, which was given the enormous task of examining over 2,000 soldiers who were under suspicion. For each man, the members of the jury had to ascertain several key points: the character of the wound and the disability that had resulted, the most likely cause of the wound, and the circumstances which had accompanied or preceded the wounding.

The jury finally concluded that the great majority of wounds were not self-inflicted. Larrey explained to Napoleon that he believed that many of the hand injuries resulted from the soldiers of the second and third ranks misdirecting their muskets and wounding the men in the first rank. The young conscripts were wholly inexperienced in the handling of the heavy flintlock musket and the tendency to hit their colleagues in front of them may have been increased by the instruction to aim low because of the recoil of the weapon. At Lützen and Bautzen many volleys were fired on the upslope of hills potentially increasing the likelihood of friendly fire accidents which, as Larrey pointed out, had already been described in Poland and Spain. Napoleon listened in silence to this detailed explanation before shaking the surgeon warmly by the hand, 'Adieu, Monsieur Larrey, a sovereign is very happy to have to deal with a man such as you!' The same evening, Larrey received a portrait of the Emperor framed in diamonds, six thousand francs in gold, and a pension of three thousand francs. He was quick to write to his fellow surgeons to underline the fact that they should make no pronouncement on the culpability of men accused of self-mutilation as he believed there was no infallible test or sign to establish their guilt.

Larrey could be arrogant and boastful but this episode alone justifies his reputation as one of the premier military doctors of his time. But, was he correct in his conclusions? Jean-François Lemaire has analysed the events in detail and has concluded that Larrey was probably wrong. It is credible that men in the first rank were wounded from behind but why were all the wounds in the hands? Surely they would also have received musket balls in the back, the neck, head, elbows, buttocks and backs of legs. Many military officers were unimpressed with Larrey's conclusions and remained convinced that the overwhelming majority of soldiers were guilty and that the Emperor had been duped. Jean-Baptiste Barrès, a *chasseur* of the Imperial Guard, accused Larrey of 'knowingly deceiving' the Emperor. He says that every officer in the army believed that the men were guilty of wounding themselves as this had happened in front of them.[15] Marshal Soult was particularly resentful at Larrey's role in the affair and bore the doctor a longstanding grudge. If the jury was wrong, it is likely that Napoleon was a willing accessory to this deceit. By choosing Larrey as the president and allowing him to pick his own team, the Emperor effectively assisted the 'not guilty' verdict. After all, Larrey had already clearly expressed his view that it was not possible to differentiate deliberate self-induced wounds from accidental ones. Napoleon did not wish to be remembered as a general who had executed his own troops for malingering.[16]

The campaign of 1813 culminated in an action at Leipzig fought between 16 and 19 October. This massive battle was the largest of the Napoleonic Wars and was nicknamed 'The Battle of the Nations'. In the course of the conflict, the French forces grew from 177,000 to 195,000 men and the

Allies from 257,000 to 365,000 effectives. Most of the fighting on the 16th was around Wachau to the south of the city. The French held their ground but the approach of more allied reinforcements was ominous. The 17th was relatively peaceful but, on the following day, the Allies launched a major assault against all parts of the French line which was placed around the perimeter of Leipzig. After nine hours of uncompromising fighting, Napoleon decided on a phased withdrawal to the west. The Allies were slow to press home their numerical advantage and the French evacuation would have been successful if a nervous engineer had not blown a bridge over the Elster river prematurely, stranding 20,000 French troops in the city. The defeat at Leipzig effectively brought Napoleon's enemies to the boundaries of France. French losses were 20,000 killed and wounded and the Allies probably had around 30,000 casualties.

The provision of adequate medical cover for a battle which lasted four days, involved close to 500,000 combatants and was fought over an area of a hundred square kilometres was a daunting undertaking. Many French ambulances were placed opportunistically in the villages dotted around Leipzig. Larrey states that the main headquarters ambulance was sited, according to usual practice, behind the centre of the French line in the village of Thornberg in the south-east outskirts of the city. As much of the action on the first day was close to Wachau, ambulances were set up locally. It was probably one of these facilities that William-Theobald Wolfe-Tone, an Irishman serving as an officer in the *Grande Armée*, stumbled across in a village inn.

After climbing to the second floor, I looked down upon a terrifying spectacle. A long table had been placed down one side of the room, the rest being covered with straw and crowded with poor devils who were mutilated and bleeding. A dozen young surgeons, stripped to the waist and covered with blood, were eating and drinking whilst cutting off limbs with all possible speed as soon as the wounded men were placed on the table. They threw the amputated legs, arms, hands and feet into a corner where they formed a hideous pile. The blood ran onto the floor, soaking the straw, before escaping down a staircase.[17]

Adolphe de Gauville, captain of the 54e, received a musket ball injury in the left hip and lay helpless in a cabbage field. Eventually, he was carried on the back of a fellow officer to the nearest ambulance which was placed near a bridge. There were many wounded lying along the road awaiting their turn to be dressed. Others had lost patience and were dragging themselves towards Leipzig itself. Gauville had the necessary surgery and followed the stream of wounded into the city. In the northern outskirts in the small village of Pfafendorf, a Prussian aide-de-camp witnessed appalling scenes as a large building containing French, Polish and Russian wounded went up in flames. Soldiers in the improvised field hospitals were horribly vulnerable to fire and few escaped from this incident alive.[18]

A proportion of the wounded escaped along the Mainz road towards France and at least some arrived home cured. Larrey confirms that most of the casualties of the 16th and 18th were evacuated into Leipzig, the troops of the Guard benefiting from the use of the administrative wagons of the train of the army. He acknowledges that Leipzig was the first battle in which he was unable to calculate the exact number of wounded.[19] The influx of so many men into the city inevitably put a considerable strain on local resources. Hospitals were overflowing even before the battle and there was a shortage of food. Dr Johann Christian Reil's description of the wounded after Leipzig must be one of the most graphic accounts of the Napoleonic Wars. He was professor of medicine in nearby Halle and arrived in the city one week after the fighting.

> In Leipzig I found about 20,000 wounded and sick warriors of all the nationalities involved. The wildest fantasy would be incapable of paint-ing a picture of the misery in as garish colours as I found here in reality … Our wounded had been dumped in places which I should not like to offer the grocer's wife for her sick pig. They lie either in stuffy, damp gin-shops in which even underwater creatures would not find enough oxygen or in windowless schools and vaulted churches where the cold atmos-phere increases as the corruption diminishes until, eventually, individual Frenchmen are pushed into the open air where the heavens are the ceiling and where howling and teeth-chattering prevail. On one side, lack of air kills the sick while on the other it is frost which destroys them. There is a great shortage of public buildings, yet not a single private house has been cleared and turned into a hospital for the rank and file. They lie packed like herrings in barrels, still wearing the blood-stained clothing in which they were carried from the heat of battle.
>
> Among the 20,000 wounded not one has received a shirt, a sheet, a blan-ket, a mattress or a bedstead. These could have been given out to some, though certainly not everybody. No one nation is superior in this respect; all have been wretchedly advised and this is the only thing about which the soldiers have no cause for complaint. They haven't even straw to lie on, but the rooms are strewn with branches from bivouacs and this can only be for the sake of appearances.
>
> All those with broken arms and legs – and there are a large number for whom no place has been found on the bare earth – are lost to the Allied armies. Some of them are already dead, the rest will die yet. Their limbs are dreadfully sore and gangrenous, as if after poisoning, and they lie at all angles from the trunk. Hence the widespread lockjaw [tetanus], which increases in proportion as hunger and cold come to the aid of its principal cause … Many have not been bandaged at all yet, others do not get their

wounds dressed every day. Most of the dressings are of grey linen, cut from Dürrenberg [twelve miles west of Leipzig] salt-sacks, which remove the skin where it is still whole. In one room stood a basket with raw shingles for use to splint broken limbs. Many amputations are neglected, others are carried out by incompetent people who can scarcely manipulate a barber's razor and take the opportunity of gaining experience on the wounded limbs of our soldiers. I watched an amputation which was carried out with blunt knives. The brownish red colour of the sawn-through muscles, which had already almost stopped breathing, and the condition of the man being operated on afforded me little hope that he would recover. Yet he had the advantage that he reached his goal by a short cut.

There is a complete lack of orderlies. Those wounded who cannot stand up have to pass excrement and urine where they lie and then rot in their own filth. Admittedly, open troughs have been put out for the walking wounded, but these receptacles overflow in all directions because they are never carried away. In St Peter's Church, one such trough stood beside another exactly like it which had just been carried in full of soup for the midday meal. The proximity of food and excreta inevitably produced a nausea which only the most ravenous hunger could overcome. The most dreadful scenes of this kind occurred in the cloth-worker's hall. The steps were crowded with a row of such overflowing troughs whose sluggish contents oozed down the steps. I found it impossible to get through the stench of this cascade – the entrance to the underworld could exude nothing more poisonous – and to reach the hospital entrance from the street. Instead, I found another route through the yard and came to a long, dark gallery which was garnished with over two thousand wounded Frenchmen, who, by their groaning and discharges, were making the air equally intolerable for ears and nostrils.

There is no reason to believe that this frightening account is exaggerated. Another local witness, Frederic Shoberl, testifies to the lack of proper medical organisation. Orders had been given to clear out the corn-magazine for 2,500 wounded. Tickets for this hospital were issued at the outer gate of the city but there was little control of their number with the predictable result that there was overcrowding and men expecting admission were turned away at the door.[20]

The destruction of the crucial bridge on the afternoon of the 19th trapped not only four army corps on the wrong side of the river but also the wounded and all of the ambulance equipment. The army's doctors had joined the frantic dash to get out of the city. Larrey managed to get across the bridge with most of the surgeons of the mobile ambulances only a few moments before the explosion. Louis-Vivant Lagneau counted himself lucky that, by pushing through a mass of disorganised troops on his horse, he also crossed just in time and avoided being made a prisoner of war.[21]

The *Grande Armée*'s retreat was blocked at Hanau. In the resulting battle the Bavarians were routed and the army continued its march towards Mainz. It was fortunate that there were few French wounded as the ambulance equipment was still in Leipzig. Larrey and his colleagues used the medical instruments they carried with them and scavenged the haversacks of the wounded men and the first aid panniers for linen.[22] *La Patrie* was now in real danger. For the defence of France, Napoleon had a field army of not more than 120,000 men made up of survivors of the German campaign, new conscripts and National Guardsmen. Arrayed against him were the allied armies of Blücher, Schwarzenberg and Bernadotte, totalling around 400,000 effectives. The Campaign of France became a long series of marches and counter-marches and intermittent battles fought in the region to the east of Paris. Napoleon had regained some of his old brilliance and scored notable victories but, in the end, Allied numerical superiority forced the Emperor's armies back to Paris itself. The capital surrendered to the Allies at the end of March and Napoleon was forced to swap his former European domination for the more humble sovereignty of the Isle of Elba.

Just as the Emperor's army in 1814 was not the powerful *Grande Armée* that had marched from the camps of Boulogne to Austerlitz nine years earlier, the *service de santé*, devastated by the campaigns of Russia and Germany, had contracted to a degree that even the most rudimentary medical provision was under threat. The French historians Brice and Bottet, who describe the medical arrangements of previous campaigns in some detail, simply omit any discussion of the *service de santé* on the battlefields of 1814. 'What is the point of speaking of the Campaign of France?' they ask, 'without organisation or resources it was only a shadow of a *service de santé* … The French army relied on charity in France as it had in all of Europe.' Morvan, whose account of the medical services is, admittedly, an endless catalogue of failures, takes an equally dim view. 'During the Campaign of France the wounded and the sick were abandoned and depended on public charity. Wounded were left to pile up in public buildings where they died of neglect and typhus. Many of the army corps had no available *officiers de santé*.'[23]

Larrey was, of course, inclined to give an overly favourable account of the functioning of the medical services and the fate of the sick and wounded. Nevertheless, his documentation of the 1814 campaign indicates that the French armies were not completely bereft of a *service de santé*. The most detailed portrayal of the battlefield medical arrangements is Larrey's description of the Battle of Craonne fought to the south of Léon in March. The corps of Ney and Victor attempted to dislodge the Allies from a plateau to the west of the town of Craonne and, after a stubborn struggle lasting several hours, a charge from the Old Guard decided the day. The French and Allies both suffered approximately 5,000 casualties. A quarter of the French wounded were seriously injured, largely from artillery fire, and about ninety required one or two amputations. The main French ambulance, presumably the headquarters ambulance, was set up in a windmill situated in Craonne behind the centre of the line. Further ambulances were created in the town itself and what Larrey terms a 'front-line ambulance' was established at a farmhouse near to the centre of the battlefield.

It is clear from Larrey's description that much of the medical care was haphazard and substandard. The ambulances in Craonne were only formed in the course of the battle and significant numbers of wounded appeared to have been completely forgotten. The usually optimistic Larrey was forced to admit that, 'it was only with the greatest difficulty that I could give even the most urgently needed treatment'. The advanced ambulance at the farm was very exposed to the enemy and the doctors working there were in real danger. Peasants from the local villages were rounded up and given the arms of the wounded men to guard the gates of the farm whilst the surgeons operated. Linen sheets, curtains, tow and rags served as dressings. Once the men had had their operations, they were placed in the stables where the peasants gave them food. Back in Craonne, most of the wounded were in deserted private houses where they were tended by a division of surgeons whose actions, Larrey comments, 'could not be sufficiently praised'.[24]

Throughout the campaign, French army doctors were heavily reliant on the help of the local inhabitants. At least they were now dealing with their own countrymen. Nurseryman Henri Tondu-Nangis witnessed the laudable efforts of the locals at the Battle of Montereau in February 1814.

> Despite the exasperation that the Allied occupation had produced and the vexations and poor treatment of all kinds that the Allies had committed, the inhabitants of the town picked up the wounded of both sides without distinction; they were carried to the hospital of the town or to the ambulances and they were all dressed by the military and civil surgeons. Despite the disorder and confusion which reigned at such a moment, the surgeons called upon the goodwill of the locals to provide linen and lint and they soon had a sufficient amount.

This local support was not always unconditional. When the French wounded poured into the capital they received a mixed reception from the Parisians. Napoleon observed bitterly that many of the sick and wounded wandered the streets without any help. In the final days of the campaign, there was still some vestige of a medical service in and around Paris. As the Allied armies attacked the city from the east, Commissaire Bellot de Kergorre took charge of ambulances in the suburbs of Villette and Pantin and requisitioned lint, linen and vinegar from the mayor and other municipal officers. Louis-Vivant Lagneau was also in the eastern suburbs of the stricken city and placed his ambulance in an inn where he was helped by Parisian doctors, including the famous surgeon Dupuytren. When Lagneau followed the army to Fontainebleau, the more severely wounded were left at the inn under the care of surgeons of the divisional ambulances, whilst those who could be evacuated were moved to one of the city's civilian hospitals.[25]

The centre of Empire was about to fall and its army and all its support services, including the *service de santé*, were to be extinguished. However, even in this desperate campaign, after two years of sufferings and losses, the flame of loyalty to Napoleon was still burning. This may have been a faint flicker compared with the halcyon days of Empire but it was still warm. It was this residual sentiment among the army's veterans combined with disillusionment with the new regime which allowed Napoleon to return in triumph to Paris in March 1815 only ten months after his arrival at Elba. There followed the Campaign of the Hundred Days which included the major battles of Ligny, Quatre Bras and Waterloo. This short period must be among the most intensively analysed few months in military history and the campaign has been variously interpreted as an Allied victory, a British victory, a German victory and a glorious irrelevance. It was a crushing French defeat and the true end of Napoleon's hegemony.

In early June, Wellington's Anglo-Dutch army and Blücher's Prussian army were in Belgium, an Austrian army under Schwarzenberg was on the Rhine and a Russian army commanded by Barclay de Tolly was approaching from the east. Napoleon moved quickly, attempting to pick off his enemies one by one, and, by the 14th, the French had concentrated near Charleroi. On the 16th Ney was checked at Quatre Bras by Wellington whilst Napoleon defeated Blücher at Ligny. On the following day, Grouchy set off in pursuit of the Prussians and Napoleon pushed on towards Wellington's army which had taken up a defensive position near the village of Waterloo. In the decisive battle on 18 June, Napoleon was unable to break Wellington's resistance and an Allied victory was assured by the timely arrival of the Prussians on the French right flank. The Emperor's last battle thus ended in the final destruction of the *Grande Armée* and a disorderly retreat from the field. French losses from these battles exceeded 30,000 killed or wounded.

Percy was appointed surgeon-in-chief for the campaign. This was a considerable blow to Larrey's self-esteem and the sulking surgeon was only persuaded to take command of the Guard and headquarters' medical services after a personal appeal from Napoleon. At Ligny, Larrey had yet to arrive and Percy was incapacitated by heart disease. Not helped by the absence of these two guiding spirits, the medical provision was poorly organised. Dressing stations were not well sited, casualty evacuation was inadequate, and the wounded of the line relied on the help of Belgian peasants who, fortunately, were well-disposed towards the French. Details of the medical arrangements at Quatre Bras are sketchy. The account of Physician Joseph Tyrbas de Chamberet, who was attached to a divisional ambulance

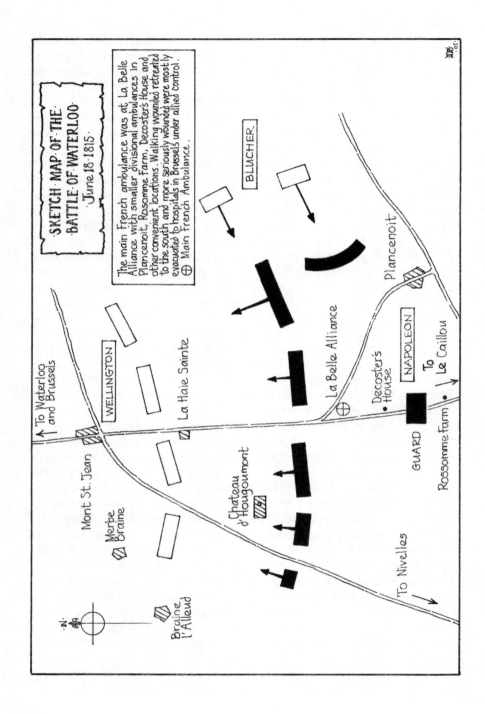

SKETCH·MAP·OF·THE·
BATTLE·OF·WATERLOO·
·June 18·1815·

The main French ambulance was at La Belle
Alliance with smaller divisional ambulances in
Plancenoit, Rosomme Farm, Decoster's House and
other convenient locations. Walking wounded retreated
to the south and more seriously wounded were mostly
evacuated to hospitals in Brussels under allied control.
⊕ Main French Ambulance.

BLÜCHER

Plancenoit

NAPOLEON
To
Le Caillou

La Belle Alliance

Decoster's
House

GUARD

Rossomme farm

WELLINGTON

La Haie Sainte

To Waterloo
and Brussels

Mont St. Jean

Merbe
Braine

Chateau
d'Hougoumont

To Nivelles

·N·

Braine
l'Alleud

of the second corps, suggests hasty improvisation. A regiment of French cavalry fled from the field and rode over his ambulance as the surgeons were bandaging and operating. All the wagons and surviving wounded fell into the hands of the enemy and he and his colleagues were left with only the equipment and instruments in their haversacks and pockets.[26]

On the night before Waterloo, Tyrbas de Chamberet joined the army's other *officiers de santé*, perhaps around three hundred in total, in trying to find shelter from the driving rain. He was depressed at having lost all the contents of his ambulance but found some compensation in an abandoned house on the Brussels road where he feasted on some excellent cheese and slept soundly on the floor. The French medical service at Waterloo was organised in much the same way as for the previous major battles of Empire. At the front, the regimental surgeons set up dressing stations to give crucial first aid on the field whilst, a little to the rear, the major ambulances were set up at key points. In practice, many of the French were wounded during the repeated frontal attacks on the Allied line and, as their units retreated back over the same ground, they were abandoned with little chance of receiving any medical care. Percy had been forced to remain at Ligny due to ill health and Larrey, as so often before, took responsibility for the placement of the larger ambulances. The main headquarters facility was at the farm of La Belle Alliance and divisional ambulances were, in all likelihood, active in other buildings behind the French line at Plancenoit village and at the farms of Rossomme and Le Caillou. Eye witness accounts suggest that the majority of French wounded who were fortunate enough to get off the field ended up at La Belle Alliance.

The fluctuating nature of the battle with frequent cavalry charges and the ceding of ground interfered with the functioning of the ambulances and as the day wore on even the headquarters ambulance came under threat. Surgeon Lagneau had to get his wounded out of the farm of La Belle Alliance as Prussian skirmishers bore down on it from a nearby wood. He states that the Guard's ambulance had been set up by surgeons Zinck and Champion in a barn but he does not give the exact location. He implies that all the surgeons gradually had to fall back as the French forces came under increasing pressure.[27] This is supported by Tyrbas de Chamberet who found himself at La Belle Alliance surrounded by a large number of physicians and surgeons of all grades. Larrey and Desgenettes were also in attendance, as were 'swarms of *commissaires des guerres* and *ordonnateurs* in smart uniforms'. At this stage the wounded were arriving from all directions and were lying on straw in the yard and in the barns, stables and cowsheds. Napoleon was standing on a small mound only a short distance from the ambulance looking through a telescope, no doubt observing the Prussian advance to his right.

Through a combination of good luck and the help of grateful soldiers, Larrey had never been made a prisoner. At both the crossing of the Berezina and at the calamitous flight from Leipzig he had made near miraculous escapes. Now, at the death of Empire, the surgeon fell into the clutches of the Prussians. However, his luck had not entirely run out. After being ruthlessly disarmed, stripped and sentenced to be shot, he was fortunate to be recognised by a Prussian regimental surgeon who had attended his surgical lectures in Berlin. Larrey was first taken to General Bülow and then sent on to Marshal Blücher who gave him a sympathetic reception as the surgeon had treated his son in Austria. Most of the French surgeons accompanied the rest of the army in a rout similar to those seen after the battles of Vitoria and Leipzig. Tyrbas de Chamberet is the best witness.

> After having marched for two or three hours without stopping in this increasingly disorganised crowd on the Charleroi road, I found myself in front of a farm where the ambulance of the 2nd corps was stationed. Bagueris, senior physician of this army corps, had set up the ambulance. He was astonished at the panic and the shameful flight from the field and was standing in the middle of the road, sword in hand, trying to rally some of the soldiers. After making some useless efforts to slow the torrent of men, he came up to me with emotion, 'Tell me where you've come from … What is the cause of this panic? … What is the cause of this terror?'

The two doctors made some further futile efforts to stop the avalanche but soon bowed to the inevitable and got on to a wagon to Charleroi. Despite his best intentions, Tyrbas de Chamberet was himself infected by the atmosphere of fear and ended up running through the mud, fleeing from an invisible foe. Jean-Pierre Gama, acting as *chirurgien en chef* to the 2nd corps, confirms that the wounded who could not march were abandoned at the ambulances in the villages around the field. Many were well treated by the Belgians and transported to Brussels and Louvain in country carts.[28]

In the last battle of the wars, the *service de santé* was dissolved in the body of the *Grande Armée* and simply swept away. It can hardly be held to account for the shortcomings in the treatment of casualties. It was not always so, and we have seen that, even in the most auspicious circumstances, the wounded often received either poor or non-existent care. To what degree was this an inevitable part of the warfare of the period? To what extent can we regard Napoleon himself as culpable for this deficiency? The Emperor's general attitudes to the army's doctors and medical services and his ultimate betrayal of the *service de santé* have already been discussed (see Chapter III). In considering Napoleon's specific role in battlefield medicine, in assessing how much his own beliefs and decision making impinged on the care of the army's wounded, it is worth emphasising two points. Firstly, his view of battlefield medical provision probably changed during the period 1805 to 1815. In the earlier years he shows little interest in any type of formal surgical service on the battlefield. His advocacy of Larrey's revolutionary flying ambulance was casual and he passed up the opportunity to extend its use to the regiments of the line. Percy's rational and feasible *chirurgie de bataille* project received lip service but the Emperor was not prepared to provide more than a few detachments of *infirmiers*. Allusions to battlefield medicine in Napoleon's correspondence of this period reveal an ad hoc and opportunistic approach. Typical is his letter to Daru, written in Poland in December 1806, suggesting that local wagons be commandeered to remove the wounded at the end of a battle. Better than nothing but hardly a substitute for an organised and adequate ambulance service.[29]

The later years of Empire may not have brought real improvements in battlefield medicine but there is a change in the tone of Napoleon's correspondence. Letters written in 1812 are more realistic and reveal an unprecedented element of pre-planning for casualties. In October he writes to Berthier from Moscow with some hard-headed calculations regarding the fate of the wounded three months after a battle – if there were originally 6,000 wounded then, at this stage, there would be only a thousand to evacuate as 2,500 would have returned to their units and 2,500 would be dead. Another letter to Berthier, written a month earlier from Mojaisk, is unusual in that he considers the management of the wounded before a battle, giving instructions as to the placement of ambulances and entrusting the safeguarding of the wounded to Junot, one of his closest lieutenants.[30]

The correspondence which most clearly reveals Napoleon's change of heart is from the German campaign of 1813. The following was written to Daru from Bunzlau in May.

Order for the formation of a bataillon d'équipages militaires d'ambulance

Monsieur le Comte Daru,

Please produce a plan for a bataillon d'équipages militaires d'ambulance. This battalion will be composed of twelve companies. Each company will be composed of fifty wagons and one forge. Each wagon will be organised as in the ambulance of the Guard: one man and two horses to each wagon; which will make for a company, sixty men, 120 horses (including those unhitched), fifty wagons and one forge; and for twelve companies, 720 men, 1,440 horses, 600 wagons and twelve forges. These wagons are principally intended to remove the wounded from the battlefield. However, there will be on each wagon a small case containing linen for bandages, a little lint, a choice of instruments, a small amount of brandy and, finally, the equivalence of the ambulance on the back of a mule which I have granted to each battalion. Each of these wagons will be able to carry four men. I will thus have the means of carrying 2,400 wounded, but, to avoid increasing the size of the army and to avoid further expense, we should be able to convert one of the battalions being organised in France, such as the 4ᵉ which still has no wagons or a similar battalion. It is necessary that this battalion is under the orders of the army's surgeons and that one company is granted to each army corps. There will be six available for headquarters. Some infirmiers on foot will be attached to this battalion so that, immediately a man is wounded or cannot march, he is put in one of the wagons. In attaching fifty of these wagons to one army corps we will thus be able to attach twelve to each division.[31]

Six years after his brisk rejection of Percy's *chirurgie de bataille*, Napoleon appears to have reinvented the project himself. By now it was little more than a pipe dream. In military terms, the Emperor was reacting to events rather than dictating them and there was neither the time nor the resources to set up such an organisation. The moment had passed.

The second point which warrants emphasis is that, despite his declaration in the above letter, Napoleon was in direct opposition to his senior doctors as to the optimal timing of evacuation of wounded. The army's doctors, notably Larrey, repeatedly stressed the need for quick evacuation to allow early surgery and the avoidance of fatal complications. Conversely, Napoleon routinely forbade early retrieval and applauded injured soldiers who stayed at the front, stubbornly refusing to attend the ambulances. A case in point is that of General Valhubert who was seriously wounded by a shell at the Battle of Austerlitz. When his aide-de-camp and some grenadiers tried to remove him from the field, he fended them off with his sabre, reminding them of the Emperor's order that the wounded should only be collected after the battle. Napoleon attempted to immortalise Valhubert's example by commissioning a painting of the scene for exhibition in Paris.[32] The reference to rapid evacuation by ambulance in his letter to Daru of May 1813 probably represents some softening of Napoleon's attitude but this should not obscure a fundamental difference between the Emperor and his doctors. Napoleon's warfare was based on speed, adaptability and a comprehensive mastery of the terrain. Nothing could be left to chance and non-combatants could not be allowed to get in the way. Military necessity dictated that the right time for the ambulances to enter the field and for the casualties to be collected was at the end of the fighting. Whatever the views of his doctors, the Emperor would have to have his victory before the wounded became a serious consideration. He did not plan for defeat.

Notes

1. Zamoyski, A, *1812. Napoleon's fatal march on Moscow,* p.536; Bowden, S, *Napoleon's Grande Armée of 1813,* p. 201; Lemaire, J-F, *Les blessés dans les Armées Napoléoniennes,* p. 166.
2. Brice, Docteur and Bottet, Capitaine, *Le Corps de Santé Militaire en France,* p. 218.
3. Brice, Bottet, p. 220; Larrey, D J, *Mémoires de Chirurgie Militaire et Campagnes 1787–1840,* pp. 728, 740; de Caulaincourt, General, *With Napoleon in Russia. The memoirs of General de Caulaincourt Duke of Vicenza,* pp. 67–8; Morvan, J, *Le Soldat Impérial,* Vol. II, p. 349.
4. Larrey, p. 744.
5. Zamoyski, p. 281.
6. La Flize, Dr, *Souvenirs de la Moskowa par un chirurgien de la Garde Impériale,* p. 421; Austin, P B, *1812 The March on Moscow,* p. 318.
7. Roos, H de, *Avec Napoléon en Russie,* pp. 80–2; François, C, *From Valmy to Waterloo. Extracts from the diary of Capt. Charles François a soldier of the Revolution and Empire,* pp. 239–40; Morvan, Vol. II, p.353.
8. Ségur, Count P-P de, *Napoleon's Russian Campaign,* pp. 158–9; La Flize, p. 425.
9. Roos, pp. 81–2.
10. Lejeune, Baron, *Memoirs of Baron Lejeune Aide-de-Camp to Marshals Berthier, Davout and Oudinot,* Vol. I, pp. 67, 238–9.
11. d'Héralde, J-B, *Mémoires d'un Chirurgien de la Grande Armée,* p. 193.
12. Bowden, p.65; Morvan, Vol. II, p.359; Richardson, R, *Larrey Surgeon to Napoleon's Imperial Guard,* p. 191; Bellot de Kergorre, A, *Journal d'un Commissaire des Guerres pendant le Premier Empire (1806–1821),* p. 101.
13. Dible, J H, *Napoleon's Surgeon,* p. 208.
14. Brice, Bottet, p. 225.
15. Barrès, J-B, *Memoirs of a French Napoleonic Officer,* pp. 171–2.
16. Lemaire, pp. 186–96.
17. Pigeard, A, *L'Armée de Napoléon,* p. 185.
18. *Campagne de Saxe à Campagne de France, Lettres et Souvenirs (1813–1814),* p. 36; Brett-James, A, *Europe against Napoleon. The Leipzig Campaign 1813,* p. 189.
19. Dible, p. 216.
20. Brett-James, pp. 244–6; Shoberl, F, *Narrative of the Remarkable Events which Occurred in and near Leipzig,* p. 30.
21. Dible, p. 217; Lagneau, L-V, *Journal d'un Chirurgien de la Grande Armée,* p. 171.
22. Larrey, p. 952.
23. Brice, Bottet, p. 230; Morvan, Vol. II, p. 364.
24. Larrey, p. 963.

25. *Campagne de Saxe*, p. 130; Morvan, Vol. II, p.364; Bellot de Kergorre, pp. 130–1; Lagneau, p. 183.
26. Richardson, p. 215; Tyrbas de Chamberet, J, *Mémoires d'un Médecin Militaire*, p. 155.
27. Lagneau, pp. 193–4.
28. Tyrbas de Chamberet, pp. 159, 165; Brice, Bottet, p. 268.
29. Lemaire, p. 139; Morvan, Vol. II, p. 314.
30. Lemaire, pp. 158, 160.
31. Brice, Bottet, p. 182.
32. Lemaire, p. 238.

CHAPTER VII

Hospitals: Les Sépulcres de la Grande Armée*

(* The Tombs of the Grande Armée)

In 18th-century France, the word 'hospital' carried a broader connotation than it does today. It was used to describe a range of charitable institutions which cared not only for the sick but also for the disabled and dependent. Some were hospitals in the true modern sense of the word but others were hospices or asylums used to house a variety of unfortunates. Many of the small-town institutions more concerned with care than cure were administered by religious orders. In the cities and larger towns, hospitals were largely under municipal control.[1] The conditions in most of these civil hospitals in the later years of the 18th century were grim. A report on Paris's *Hôtel-Dieu* in 1788 opens as follows.

> The general policy of the *Hôtel-Dieu* – a policy caused by the lack of space – is to put as many beds as possible into one room and to put four, five or six people into one bed. We have seen the dead mixed with the living. We have seen rooms so narrow that the air stagnates and is not renewed and that the light enters only feebly and charged with vapours. We have seen convalescents together with the sick, the dying and the dead, forced to go barefoot to the bridge in summer and winter when they want fresh air. We have seen a room for convalescents on the third floor which could be reached only via the smallpox ward. The ward for the insane is next to the one for unfortunate postoperative patients who cannot hope for rest in this neighbourhood which is full of outcries day and night.

The authors continue to detail the hellish existence of the patients. Those awaiting surgery were forced to watch others receiving their operations in the centre of the room. Cases of contagious diseases such as fever and syphilis were indiscriminately mixed with surgery patients and with pregnant women. The predictable conclusion of the report was that the

Hôtel-Dieu was 'the most unhealthy and most uncomfortable of all hospitals and that, of nine patients, two die'. However, the other Paris hospitals were no better and perhaps even worse. At the *Bicêtre*, several patients shared each bed with no regard to their disease or sex whilst, at the *Concierge*, described by one witness as 'the most horrifying hospital in the world', the patients stagnated in beds placed along the walls of corridors. Apart from the misery for the occupants, such overcrowding provided ideal conditions for the spread of infectious diseases and the contamination of operation wounds.[2]

The Revolutionaries, who had originally vowed to abolish hospitals, ultimately improved them and made them the core of medicine. In 1794 all civil hospitals were taken over by the state. Many of the older institutions were turned into military hospitals and new ones were built. The Convention passed a decree that every hospital patient should have his own bed and that the beds should be separated by at least three feet. These efforts to improve civil hospitals continued under the Consulate and Empire. Thus, in 1801, following further criticism, steps were taken to divide patients between the Paris hospitals dependent on the type and chronicity of their disease. Improved standards were reinforced by an increasingly strong link between the hospitals and medical education and a proliferation of hospital courses of instruction and teaching facilities such as the 'amphitheatres'. Unsurprisingly, Napoleon was keen to encourage a particular interest in soldiers' afflictions – when a chair of medicine was created at the *Charité* in 1802, the professor was instructed to focus on diseases which were 'the most similar to those which are common in the armies'. The Revolutionary and Napoleonic Era, 1789–1815, did not lead to the solution of all the problems of France's civil hospitals but Napoleon left them in a better state than they were in at the end of the *Ancien Régime*. This is underlined by the fact that the key changes in their administration and finance remained largely unchanged in France and conquered countries such as Belgium, Holland and Switzerland, in the years after the Emperor's fall.[3]

France's military hospitals of the 18th century were also subject to deficiencies and abuses. A senior *officier de santé*, writing in 1793, declared that the military hospitals of previous decades were hotbeds of corruption with the administration in the hands of 'brigands'. He concluded that there had been little progress over the previous fifty years[4]. Despite this, the military hospitals compared favourably with their civilian counterparts. In the inspections of the 1780s, which revealed such shocking scenes in the civil hospitals of Paris and the provinces, the military hospitals escaped relatively unscathed. The *Invalides* in Paris, a military facility housing 3,000 sick or disabled soldiers, received no specific criticism. This superiority is supported by the much lower mortality rates in the military compared with civilian institutions. A study performed between 1782 and

1787 showed a peacetime mortality rate of around 1 in 40 in military and naval hospitals, a figure confirmed by Coste in 1789. At this time, the civil hospitals had a mortality rate of 1 in 3. This did not necessarily mean that ill soldiers always got a better deal than civilians as soldiers were commonly admitted to the military wards of civilian hospitals. The dividing line between military and civilian medicine was blurred.

The Revolutionary politicians of the early 1790s were agreed that, as citizens, the soldiers of their armies were entitled not only to the gratitude of the nation but also to the best possible hospital care. For the sick and wounded, this meant the guarantee of a bed and appropriate medical attention. In a report on military hospitals written in 1791, a government officer lays down three principles: that the medicines should always be of a high quality, that there should be adequate food, and that each soldier should have a bed to himself. The early years of the Revolutionary Wars were characterised by a rapid expansion in the number of hospitals as the only means of accommodating the escalating military casualties and epidemics of disease. Reinforced by popular demands that the Republic's soldiers receive every attention, medical men and politicians competed in their efforts to open new hospitals. Whilst some soldiers still returned home for treatment, and others might be housed in the military wards of civilian hospitals, most were to be taken to the nearest *hôpital militaire*. These dedicated military hospitals were favoured by the army as, in contrast to civilian hospitals, the men remained soldiers during their period of treatment and were subject to strict military discipline. Their diet could be regulated, visits supervised and desertion minimised. Such institutions were not always welcomed by the local community who regarded them as dangerous sources of contagion.[5]

In 1792, at the time of the invasion of the frontiers by the First Coalition, the National Assembly decreed that there should be both static and mobile hospitals attached to the French armies.[6] Further legislation two years later dictated four different types of hospital. The first category, the military hospitals (*hôpitaux militaires*), were themselves divided into two sub-categories. The mobile hospitals (*hôpitaux ambulants*) were attached to the army divisions and were to evolve into the ambulances and field hospitals discussed in Chapter IV. The larger fixed hospitals, the subject of this chapter, were for soldiers of all arms and were usually established in large towns or garrisons. They were sub-divided into three classes according to size. The other three categories of hospital were the *hôpitaux d'instruction*, where particular emphasis was placed on education, 'special' hospitals for venereal and skin diseases, and spa hospitals (*hôpitaux d'eaux minerals*) which treated both soldiers and civilians. In 1796 a more general division of military hospitals into permanent and temporary (*provisoires*) was introduced. With respect to the larger hospitals, this meant there were still permanent fixed hospitals in vital locations such as garrisons but also more short-term *hôpitaux sedentaires* which were designed to receive the evacuations from the more mobile ambulances.[7]

The Egyptian Campaigns of 1798–9 well illustrate this hierarchy of hospitals with the fixed facilities, *hôpitaux sedentaires* and ambulances all much in evidence. Fixed hospitals in the major cities received soldiers evacuated from the smaller units and acted as depots for the wounded. They were also the portals for repatriation of troops who were too sick or badly wounded to remain on campaign. In and around Cairo, Bonaparte opened several fixed hospitals ranging in size from a hundred to a thousand beds. During the siege of St Jean d'Acre in Syria, three similar institutions were set up to serve the 13,000 men.[8]

The larger fixed Revolutionary hospitals were subject to both central and local administrative arrangements. Changes made early in the Revolutionary years tended to bring the hospitals under increasing state control although, in practice, they remained much reliant on free enterprise for supplies. In 1796 the general administration of military hospitals was entrusted to six senior administrators or directors who were jointly responsible for economic management, equipment and personnel. Within each fixed hospital, the administrative staffs were composed of a director, an admissions commissioner, a commissioner of accounts, one or two clerks, a supply quartermaster, a paymaster and a quartermaster, who was in charge of the weapons, equipment and patients' belongings. The precise nature of these arrangements was to change through the 1790s but, in general, the *officiers de santé* of the hospital were accountable to an administrative committee. Senior military officers in the locality were encouraged to visit the hospitals to 'taste the soup' and take note of the number of hospital employees – any irregularities were to be reported to the chief administrator of the division. Careful account was also kept of the number of patients as military physicians and surgeons were often accused of being 'disgustingly liberal' in allowing malingerers to accumulate in their hospitals. To try and stop this abuse, it was decreed in 1796 that each sick and wounded soldier had to have a valid hospital ticket or certificate detailing his illness or disability. If a soldier was found guilty of forging a certificate he was to be shot whereas an *officier de santé* issuing fraudulent papers was to be clapped in irons for two years.[9]

The military hospitals of the Revolutionary and Napoleonic periods differed fundamentally from modern hospitals in that they rarely occupied purpose-built buildings. Accommodation was acquired opportunistically. Many were hastily converted monasteries and other ecclesiastical structures. Within France, there were the stately homes which had been abandoned by their former aristocratic owners. The level of medical staffing was determined by size; in 1796 it was stated that each hospital should have *officiers de santé* of all three specialities and that there was to be one physician for hospitals with fewer than 200 sick, two for 200–400, and three for 400–600.[10] With this level of legislation and the relatively favourable quality of military medical care that had been inherited from the pre-Revolutionary period, it might have been hoped that the sabot-wearing soldiers of *La Patrie* would be well served by their hospitals. The reality was much different. The French discovered, as did the British in their Flanders campaign of the same period, that, despite the best of intentions, maintaining high quality fixed hospitals in time of war was a considerable challenge.[11] Whilst standards were quite well sustained in some of the hospitals in France's interior, those facilities nearer the front were soon overwhelmed by the combination of battle casualties and disease epidemics. Well qualified medical staff were in short supply. There were severe shortages of pharmacists and of trained nursing staff, often referred to as *infirmiers*. Hospitals lacked essentials such as mattresses, straw, sheets, linen, beds, food and medicines.

In the military hospitals at Perpignan, the Convention was informed that there was complete disorder. The wards were filthy and the administrative and medical staffs were completely out of their depth. The inspector concluded that most of the patients were doomed, 'the unfortunates who went there in the hope of restoring their health simply languished and ended up leaving behind what small part of their lives remained'. At Maubeuge, the hospital set up in a château in late 1792 was planned for sixty men but there were nearly 400 patients, a mixture of fevers and wounded. The hospitals in Belgium and Germany were worse. At Liège, men lay on the hard floors of the lice-ridden buildings without blankets or mattresses. Disease was bound to thrive in these conditions. In an eight-week period in the summer of 1793 in the hospitals around Bayonne every nurse who started work on the wards died from typhus, joining the three physicians, fourteen surgeons and eleven pharmacists who also succumbed. General Dugommier, commander of the Army of the East Pyrenees, acknowledged that his hospitals were in a 'fearful state' and that the sick were being treated as 'spoilt goods'. Percy's journal of 1799 provides numerous further examples of shockingly poor hospitals. The inadequacies of staff and supplies were often exacerbated by the unsuitability of the accommodation. The enormous monastery at Koenigsfelden contained 800 patients cared for by only ten surgeons, three of whom were sick themselves. The rooms were cramped and dirty, the ceilings too low and the windows scarce and small. At Zurich, in a converted warehouse, nearly all the sick died within a few days. There was a lethal combination of poorly ventilated wards, infected latrines and a 'cesspit' in the courtyard. Percy notes that, on occasions, a happy combination of good administrative and medical staff, adequate supplies and a more healthy location did lead to a better outcome. He was constantly searching for well ventilated buildings in elevated positions which he could commission as his next hospital.[12]

Percy wanted hospitals to be not only of high quality but also as safe as possible. It was this sentiment that led him to propose that military hospitals should be considered neutral and inviolable. While serving in the Army of the Rhine in 1800, he drew up a draft document with the approval of General Moreau which rationalised the need for the hospitals of both sides to be treated as sanctuaries for the wounded and sick. The hospitals were to be clearly indicated by signs and, wherever possible, combat troops were to avoid them. If hospitals fell into enemy hands, they were to be continually supplied and the staff either allowed to continue their duties or safely escorted back to their own army. This groundbreaking concept was not realised because the Austrian General Kray felt that it would interfere with his military operations.[13]

The key regulations for the military hospitals of the Consulate, contained in the decree of 24 *thermidor* year VIII, also appeared in 1800. Comprising 493 separate articles, this detailed decree subdivided hospitals into three fundamental types: permanent, temporary and ambulant. The latter were essentially the ambulances which followed the army. Most of the permanent facilities were in France itself. In 1800 there were only sixteen; in Paris, Saint-Denis, Metz, Strasbourg, Brussels, Liège, Aix-la-Chapelle, Mainz, Lille, Rennes, Toulouse, Bayonne, Alexandria, Huningue, Ajaccio and Porto-Ferrajo. In peacetime, these hospitals were regarded as little more than a nuisance by the locals and there was pressure to close them. This policy proved short-sighted as in the subsequent wars there was a need for a chain of hospitals linking the new borders of France with the interior of the country, as had been the case in the 18th century. The temporary hospitals were set up in time of war on the rear and flanks of the army and were intended to receive troops from the ambulances. Apart from those specialising in venereal and skin diseases, there were hospitals of the first, second and third line, for which the term *hôpitaux sedentaires* was still sometimes used. The first line hospitals were closest to the field of battle. Many of these temporary hospitals were created in cities and larger towns accessible to the fighting, for instance, in Brünn after the Battle of Austerlitz, in the town of Jena after the battle of the same name, and in Vienna after Aspern-Essling and Wagram. The number of temporary hospitals required was decided by a senior administrator, *l'ordonnateur en chef de l'armée*, with advice from the senior *officiers de santé*. Levels of medical staffing were determined by the number of beds. A larger hospital of 450–600 patients usually had three physicians, twelve surgeons and eight pharmacists.[14]

This basic arrangement was to persist throughout the wars, although the decree of 9 *frimaire* year XII (December 1803) took the unfortunate step of removing the *hôpitaux d'instruction* which were not seen again until late 1814. It also diluted the hospitals' medical staffing. It was instructed that, whilst there would still be a physician and a senior surgeon and pharmacist responsible for the service, there would be much greater reliance on the surgeons of the corps of the garrison and from the nearest camps in the locality. This initiative increased the role and status of surgeons in the hospitals but it also risked denuding the army of surgeons in the field.[15] The regulations of 1800 and 1803 set the tone for the whole period. Legislation in 1806 altered the administrative arrangements, the local hospital 'directors' being replaced by an inspector assisted by a clerk, but these were minor organisational issues and the Empire is marked by a dearth of significant legislative change pertaining to the military hospitals.

How were the temporary and permanent hospitals viewed by the ordinary soldiers of the *Grande Armée*? Jean-Baptiste Barrès, *chasseur* of the Imperial Guard, expresses the common opinion: 'Woe to those who go into hospital on campaign! They are isolated and forgotten, and tedium slays them rather than their sickness.' Heinrich von Brandt, a Polish officer who fought with the *Grande Armée* in Spain and Russia, recalls meeting a wounded man dragging himself along the road near Moscow.

> I advised him to go and stay in the hospital. He told me that 'by not leaving the regiment I have some chance of saving my skin; if it comes to the worst, at least my comrades will bury me. If I go to the hospitals I'll be gobbled up by the wolves whether I am dead or alive ...'

Soldiers approached the hospitals with dread, fearing this isolation from friends and home as much as the considerable chances of dying from their wounds or disease. It was commonplace for the hospital's patients to be deprived of letters and outside financial help. A soldier writes to his father back in France of his experiences in a military hospital: 'I remained very dangerously ill for two months without any real hope of being cured; during this time I would cry day and night without being able to see my father and mother, brother and sister.'[16] Compared with a slow lingering death in hospital, a swift end on the battlefield held relatively little fear for many *grognards*.

To understand why so many soldiers saw the army's hospitals as mortuaries rather than as places of salvation – there are innumerable anecdotes similar to those just quoted – it is necessary to explore the functioning of the hospitals in some of the major campaigns between 1803 and 1815. At the beginning of this period, as the *Grande Armée* was being formed, two military hospitals were opened in the camp of Boulogne. They were organised slowly and contained few beds and the local civil hospital (*hôpital de charité*) and civilian physicians provided most of the care. The first great challenge for Napoleon's military hospitals was therefore in the Ulm and Austerlitz campaigns of 1805. From the earliest stages of the *Grande Armée*'s march east, it became apparent that many of the military hospitals established en route were of doubtful quality. Percy is an excellent witness as he was both much involved in the supervision of the hospitals and entirely honest in his assessments. In the hospitals around Ulm, he says that disorder reigned and that it was a 'sad service'. There was no straw, little food, no *infirmiers* and no French employees. Hospitals were often in unsuitable and overcrowded buildings – this was to have devastating consequences after Austerlitz when typhus raged through the hospitals of the line and a quarter of the wounded died. Only the better ventilated and provisioned hospital of the Guard escaped.[17]

In the Jena campaign of the following year, the army's doctors contrived a hospital service from the resources of the country. Percy fully exploited both the local civil hospitals and Germany's religious buildings. At Würzburg, where he had to accommodate 2,000 sick, he used the 'magnificent' civil hospital, an abandoned convent and a Benedictine abbey. These buildings received 200–300 patients and he was still desperately short of beds. After the Battle of Jena, he visited the hospitals in the nearby town. There were enough surgeons, a rare event, but many wounded had not received any food. Further hospitals were opened in Potsdam as all evacuations were hindered by impracticable roads and devastated villages. When the French entered Berlin, where the Emperor had ordered 400 hospital beds to be reserved, Percy made the arrangements directly with local Prussian officers. 'In this way, we will have no French administration in the town and the service will be the better for it …' Relations between the French and German doctors were generally good and local medical staff provided valuable help in the military hospitals. By early November 1806, there were 17,000 sick dispersed in the hospitals of Weimar, Leipzig, Spandau and Kustrin.[18]

In December Napoleon moved into Poland to tackle the Russians. Pharmacist Jacob entered Warsaw on the 11th and found no fewer than twenty-three separate hospitals which had all been opened within the previous four weeks. A wide range of buildings had been pressed into use including an arsenal, barracks and the larger houses of the aristocracy. Unfortunately, many of the *service de santé*'s doctors were still in the hospitals formed in Prussia and at the hospital in the arsenal Jacob was the only French *sous-aide*.[19] Most of the hospital's employees were enrolled from the local inhabitants. As the Polish campaign of 1807 progressed, it became increasingly difficult to provide a decent hospital service. The resources of the country were limited, the roads often impassable, and the weather dreadful. Percy's evocative description of the hospitals serves as a powerful antidote to the ubiquitous glamorising accounts and imagery of Napoleonic warfare. At Pultusk in January:

> At the Benedictine abbey, eighty wounded lie on a little straw with no proper supplies. Their comrades have procured them a few old blankets and other effects, which, already dirty and disgusting, have become more so due to the grease, pus, blood and spit with which they are soiled.

A few amputees are cured despite this miserable state of affairs and some fracture cases are doing well. When the civilian commission provided the food it was good enough; this undertaking was returned to the French and, from then on, everything has been spoilt and of low quality. There has been much to complain about; this continued until news of the arrival of His Majesty at Pultusk. Then they have been given better wine; they have changed the straw, got linen and bandages etc.

Another Pultusk hospital in a nunnery was equally unsatisfactory, 'on entering there, one is struck by a smell of rotting cheese which announces the suppuration of the wounds'. The nuns provided the drugs but made no effort to fumigate the wards.[20]

In a dirty hospital near Danzig there were crude beds made from wood from the local forests but there was a shortage of blankets and sheets and the patients, some unclothed, suffered from the cold. The institution was run by a simple clerk, most of the doctors were sick, the food was poor, and there were no proper utensils for drinking or urinating. These unavoidable shortages and near insurmountable difficulties were aggravated by the corrupt behaviour of the hospital administrative staff and employees. For instance, at Koenigsberg, where Percy is again the unwilling guide:

The stink of the hospital makes me sick. The sight of the detestable food which they are giving to these brave men is upsetting. Our surgeons complain and try to remedy this evil but cannot put right the damage already done. The hospital clerk is a miserable individual who gets drunk three times a day; the unfortunate sick are moaning; there are no *infirmiers*, only help from the surgeons who cannot do everything. The *régisseur general*, an upright and good man, never enters the hospitals; this is one cause of the abominable crisis of which they are the theatre. But what service can one expect from the crowd of bandits, adventurers and bankrupts sent from Paris to be employed in our hospitals by His Excellency, the '*ministre directeur*'? Can one hope to find among such people the sentiments of humanity, piety and sensitivity which should distinguish the employees of hospitals? They have come to the army to do their business and, unfortunately, they only succeed in assassinating the poor sick. Oh, ungodly race!

Percy accuses the hospital administrators of plundering vast amounts of money from the service, stealing with 'as much audacity as impunity'.[21]

The thousand sick in the hospital at Kustrin, the grain-store of the kings of Prussia, fared no better.

The service is detestable; the courtyard is poisoned by the toilets which open into a ditch which is open and overflows. At 10 o'clock, I saw 200 bodies crammed onto a wagon, a terrible spectacle for the sick who are eyewitnesses of it and disgusting for everybody; they load up in this way at the foot of the staircases of the main wards; the bodies release evacuations and make a dreadful smell. The wards are poorly maintained, all the sick are unhappy at the stink, the supplies are dirty and each mattress has seen the death of ten or twelve unfortunates without having been cleaned; there are no *infirmiers* when there should be 200 for such a large hospital.

Food was also in short supply and of poor quality. This was in large part due to the roguery of the local administrators who, according to Percy, enriched themselves at the expense of the helpless patients. 'This happens almost everywhere; His Majesty knows it, he swears, he loses his temper and the evil continues.'

Battling against overwhelming odds, Percy worked hard to try and find suitable locations for the hospitals, at times touring an entire city at breakneck speed. At Danzig:

> I rushed to find some places. I believe we will take house no. 395 ... *l'hôtel des assises* is superb and can take 300 sick ... The money exchange offers resources from which we may profit ... I have inspected the arsenal ... it is there that we will make a magnificent hospital ... The main church is immense ...

Because of the devotion of Percy and other like-minded medical officers, there were a few good military hospitals in Poland which bucked the general trend. In the town of Marienwerder, the two hundred and fifty sick were in a large house where they were provided with wooden bedsteads, mattresses, sheets and new blankets. Similarly, at Dirschau, Percy was very happy with the state of the hospital in a church and adjoining house which was in the capable hands of a *chirurgien-major*. In describing the hospital at Rosengarten, Percy reveals his opinions on the optimal design of such buildings.

> It is in a superb wooden house with a first floor and good windows and it is very well arranged. In the ward on the lower floor there are four rows of beds, which is too many. There are only two rooms on the higher floor and it is healthier. The kitchen is also of wooden construction. The pharmacy and the administrative offices are in a large and beautiful house. I tasted the wine and food; everything is good. The beds are of simple design; the coverings consist of a mattress, two sheets, a sack of straw and a good woollen blanket.

On occasion, wealthy locals voluntarily supplied beds and other crucial commodities. At Danzig, the better off residents were ordered to provide

400 sets of bedding within forty-eight hours for the first wards of the hospital in the city's arsenal.[22] A revealing report by Intendant General Daru for the period between October 1806 and October 1808 suggests that, in Prussia and Poland, there were over 421,000 cases of sickness or wounds with 32,000 deaths. The average number of men in hospital at any given time was 16,500 and the average stay twenty-nine days. Despite the frequent miserable conditions, it appears that as many as ninety per-cent of admissions ended in the soldier being discharged and rejoining his regiment.[23]

If the French received limited help in Poland, they often met outright antagonism in Spain and Portugal. These were not circumstances in which it was going to be easy to maintain a hospital system of high quality. Many hospitals were needed as the French suffered considerable attrition from both arms and disease and it was either not feasible or undesirable to evacuate back to France. As in Poland, Percy's journal is a startlingly honest portrayal of dirty and poorly managed facilities designed to spread disease and kill the debilitated inmates. A few of his examples will suffice as in the Peninsula there are many other strident voices. In the horribly overcrowded hospital in a large convent at Vitoria in northern Spain there was widespread filth and all the *officiers de santé* were ill. Instead of the 500 sick which it should have contained, there were 1,100 patients. The doctors' appeals for more hospitals fell on deaf ears. Percy noted that in hospitals such as this the atmosphere became so polluted that meat arriv-ing from the butchers rotted in only a few hours. In most hospitals, there was a heavy dependence on the local Spanish to perform administrative tasks and act as *infirmiers*. The buildings themselves were often wholly unsuitable. At Burgos, both of the hospitals were characterised by long wards with only occasional windows to allow the entry of light and cir-culation of air.

In these circumstances, there was only one way out for many of the patients. At the hospital of Pamplona, 237 men died in the first ten days of November 1808. Percy regarded the mortality levels in the hospitals of Spain to be 'frightening' and 'out of all proportion'. He comments that the Pamplona hospitals would soon have been emptied if the dead had not been immediately replaced by new victims. They died in their turn, all swept away by the 'overcrowding, the most detestable administra-tion, the ignorance of the authorities and the greed of speculators'. The young recruits, many only 20 years of age, arrived at the hospitals already exhausted by the combination of poor accommodation, little food and sleep, vermin and forced marches.[24]

If Percy's accounts of the hospitals of northern Europe and the Peninsula are monotonously grim, they are no less true. Other *officiers de santé* con-firm his view of events. Physician Laurillard-Fallot describes the chaotic arrangements at the hospital at Ciudad Rodrigo in 1810. Housed in a large church, the hospital lacked the most basic resources and the sick were randomly placed on the floor, the steps and the altars. Laurillard-Fallot had good cause for complaint: 'To give some idea of the disorder which reigned in the medical service, my two colleagues, Cornac and Blanchefon, remained at Salamanca doing nothing while I was crushed by the workload at Ciudad Rodrigo.'[25]

In the hospital at Burgos, Larrey found 4,000 wounded and sick lying on rotten straw without medical help or food. He makes no mention of the hospital at Alagon where Heinrich von Brandt was unlucky enough to be admitted in December 1808.

> I was seized by a violent fever, complicated by dysentery, and had to be carried to a military hospital which was more like a den of thieves than a place of healing. The hospital was located in a filthy monastery whose monks had fled to Saragossa and were, no doubt, inflicting the wounds we were coming here to die of. Typhus was rampant as all the area around had been infected by the stench of the corpses left so long unburied after the Battle of Tudela. For the first few days, whilst I was still conscious, I could follow the details of the burial of the many sick who succumbed. They were thrown from the windows stark naked and they fell, one on top of the other, with a muffled thud just as though they were sacks of corn. Then they were piled onto carts and taken to the huge pits that were being dug unceasingly only one hundred yards away. The Spanish who had been charged with this duty undertook it with a diabolical glee. They pointed out to me the countless mounds of earth that marked the completed and covered graves and made signs which indicated there would be no lack of future work.

During his illness, Brandt was delirious and, during one bout of fever, he wandered into the ward of the 'ordinary soldiers', a clear indication that the men were segregated according to rank. Although so ill as to become unconscious, he eventually recovered.

> At the time of my departure, the Spanish gravediggers assured me that the number of corpses had already passed two thousand and I do not believe that they were exaggerating. The commandant, it is true, was an excellent man, full of energy, and the chief surgeon had an excellent reputation. But, as they were overloaded with duties, they were forced to rely on less scrupulous and unsupervised subordinates for a host of essential details. I often recalled, in my military career, the French proverb which says that 'the subordinate is the real master'.[26]

There were a few good military hospitals in Spain. Where this happened, it was usually attributable to the efforts of exceptional individuals; soldiers, civilians or doctors. In Burgos, where we know that many of the hospitals were of execrable quality, General Thiébault claimed to have created a 'model hospital' for five hundred sick. Apparently, the building was well ventilated for the summer and had stoves for the winter, everything was in ample supply, and the principal physicians, surgeons and pharmacists visited the wards each morning. Thiébault was never slow to promote his own exploits and there may be an element of wishful thinking in this account. In Madrid, Larrey's presence ensured that the largest hospital, able to contain 3,000 sick, was well organised. He improved the building by adding latrines and facilitating the supply of water to the second and third floors. Local help was a welcome bonus and Physician Lixon believed that the best hospitals were often those staffed by the nuns of the country. Spanish administrators and doctors were capable of running good hospitals when they were disposed to. Percy describes a hospital for 200 men at Valladolid which was locally administered and was clean and well supplied.[27]

More commonly, support from the local population was strictly conditional or completely lacking. French doctors and administrators had to negotiate with officials and religious orders for buildings and supplies. At Valladolid, Percy persuaded the local priest to allow him to use the convent as a hospital in exchange for a promise that the French would not later send any troops or prisoners of war there. He was not always so successful. At St Jean de Luz, the local convent was owned by the master of the post who refused to rent it out – surprisingly, he was not compelled to do so and the sick were instead dumped in a draughty rope factory. These were minor problems compared with the overt enmity that the French met in many parts of the Peninsula. A cruel guerrilla war was being waged against them and the hospitals were not exempt as targets. The security of hospital buildings and the safety of the staff and patients was a constant source of anxiety. Surgeon Gama graphically describes guerrillas attacking isolated hospitals and massacring the doctors, employees and patients, 'glorifying in an exploit from which the trophies were pieces of bodies'. Attempts were made to move the sick and wounded to the most secure buildings available – in 1808, when the French were threatened in Madrid, Napoleon ordered the wounded to be transported to the Retiro palace where additional defensive works had been put in place.[28]

When the *Grande Armée* suffered reverses, and in the Peninsular War these were commonplace, there was the dreaded possibility that the hospitals would fall into enemy hands. Whereas the British were expected to act honourably, the 'vengeance of the Spanish' was much feared. In Madrid in 1807, Pharmacist Jacob and his colleagues drew lots to select those who would remain behind if the city had to be evacuated.[29] In the event, few hospitals actually fell to foreign troops as this was regarded as shameful, an unequivocal sign of military failure. Napoleon himself had commented to General Foy: 'For an army to lose a hospital is like losing a flag. I have never lost a hospital in war.' One notable example of a French military hospital falling to the enemy was that of Coimbra in Portugal in 1810. Marshal Masséna was much criticised for this action, but isolated in a belligerent country more than a hundred miles from his base without sufficient supplies or means of transportation, he had little choice. The hospital, in the convent of Santa Clara, contained 3,000 sick and wounded and was barricaded and given a small garrison for protection. The staff left to the mercy of the attackers included one physician, twenty-eight surgeons, nine pharmacists, twenty employees and three administrators. Colonel Trant assaulted the building with his 4,000 Portuguese militia. The French garrison of around 200 infirm soldiers put up stiff resistance but had to capitulate having inflicted some thirty casualties. What happened next is controversial, but it seems that, despite Trant's promise of protection, more than ten French soldiers were massacred and other wounded men were forced to march over sixty miles in four days.[30] One presumes that he might have been more lenient if the hospital had been less vigorously defended.

Many of the failures of the French military hospitals in Spain and Portugal are easily explained by the brutal nature of the surrounding conflict and the alienation of the population. However, some of the wounds were self-inflicted. Corruption was rife in the administrative services. The hospitals in Madrid can be quoted as examples of relatively good practice, but even here the efforts of dedicated medical staff were undermined by the double-dealing of grasping administrators and a minority of dishonest doctors. Physician Tyrbas de Chamberet, who served in the large hospital described by Larrey, acknowledges that the building was in many ways ideal and the supplies superficially abundant, but he also describes a deeper malaise. For instance, when the physician prescribed eggs for his dysentery patients he was later disappointed to find that they had not received them. After this happened several times in a week, he enquired why and was told by the senior administrator that there were no eggs available in the city, a singularly unlikely event in the capital of Spain. The real reason was more prosaic. On passing the kitchen of the director of the hospital, Tyrbas de Chamberet spotted piles of egg shells.

> At 11 o'clock in the morning or 5 o'clock in the afternoon, I was able to see through his apartment window, a splendid table of twelve to fifteen places, at which were dining honourably the *commissaires des guerres*, the *commissaires ordonnateurs*, various functionaries and senior military officers. All were living the high life at the expense of the sick.

The hospital's senior pharmacist was equally culpable, making fraudulent prescriptions in the doctor's name for wine and other luxuries which he used to entertain his friends.[31] With the hospitals' senior officers and some doctors setting such a loathsome example, it is predictable that the more junior hospital employees, be they French or Spanish, also lined their pockets. Joseph Vachin, a soldier from Mende, complained that he had been reduced to penury during his stay in hospital in 1808 as the orderlies stole from the weak and delirious patients. Tyrbas de Chamberet concedes that it was difficult for individual doctors or honest administrators to oppose this institutional corruption. His fellow physician, Lixon, who served in Spain between 1808 and 1810, voices the dilemma of many.

> If he does his duty, following the impulse of his heart and conscience, and decries the food or other supplies of low quality he antagonises the very authority on which he relies on a daily basis. He is forced to betray his sick or be exposed himself to every possible misery; what a cruel choice![32]

The hospitals of the remaining campaigns of the wars will be more briefly reviewed as the harrowing scenes in Poland and Spain were repeated and the underlying deficiencies and problems – poor hospital buildings, staff shortages, inadequate supplies, dreadful roads, antagonistic locals, chaotic and corrupt administration – remained essentially unchanged. At the Battle of Aspern-Essling, the wounded were transferred to the civilian hospitals of Vienna. These buildings were large and well laid out but their 36,000 sick and wounded patients were indiscriminately mixed together. Napoleon ordered that the French wounded should be divided up by regiment but this was unrealistic. Staff were thin on the ground and Sergeant Routier, who had been admitted to a hospital converted from the stables of the Austrian Emperor, had to dress his own wound with the sheet from his bed. The full extent of the administrative disorder is revealed by a desperate letter from Napoleon, written in June 1809, asking for the whereabouts of the hospitals holding the wounded from the Battle of Raad. As in earlier campaigns, occasional good hospitals emerged from the mire. The facility at Ratisbonne was well kept with the 400 wounded amply supplied and having the sheets on their beds changed every eight days.[33]

The Russian campaign put an intolerable strain on all parts of the *Grande Armée*'s infrastructure and the hospitals were no exception. At Smolensk, Ségur describes the surgeons overwhelmed with work in the fifteen hospitals. For three days, a hospital containing a hundred patients was completely forgotten and it was only by chance that it was rediscovered. In Moscow, the French were able to use the Russian civilian and military hospitals. These hospitals were in good buildings but were not enough and it was necessary to also use private houses. A few wounded were left in Moscow at the Foundling hospital but most were evacuated to Smolensk, perhaps three quarters dying en route. Little had been planned for the retreat. Lieutenant Vossler says that, because of the desolation left behind by the Russians, from Smolensk onwards 'it would have been impossible with the best will and the best organisation in the world to establish hospitals for the sick and exhausted'. Many of the survivors of the retreat ended up in Vilna where there were forty makeshift hospitals in monasteries and country houses. Larrey notes that he left behind in the town 'sufficient surgeons for the care of all the wounded' and also comments that many of the sick were ill-treated by the locals and Cossack bands. Physician Lemazurier has left a more damning account of the Vilna hospitals.

> In the poorly covered unheated wards were seen the sick in the last stages of emaciation and feebleness, lying mixed up with the dead. They were devoured by vermin and covered with their own excrement. Those who still had a little strength threw themselves on pieces of flesh to relieve their hunger. The floors of the wards and the yards of the hospital were full of bodies, the cold slowing their putrefaction.

General Sir Robert Wilson, the British government's liaison officer at Kutusov's headquarters, confirms this account. At the hospital of St Bazile:

> Seven thousand five hundred bodies were piled up like pigs of lead over one another in the corridors; carcasses were strewn about in every part; and all the broken windows and walls were stuffed with feet, legs, arms, hands, trunks and heads to fit the apertures and keep out the air from the yet living.

Several eyewitnesses state that the patients had to resort to cannibalism. With typhus raging, as many as 30,000 men died in Vilna in a couple of weeks.[34]

It may have been thought that such visions of hell could hardly be repeated but the campaign in Germany, the following year, yielded many more examples of the abject failure of the *service de santé*'s hospitals. The hospitals in Mainz in October 1813 were perhaps even worse than those of Russia. The principal physician, Bartoli, later admitted that he could only remember these 'with a shudder'. They were lacking in all essential supplies, the *infirmiers* were few and of the poorest quality ('... they only fulfilled their duties with the greatest repugnance and under threat'), and the sick had to share the beds. Senior surgeon Kerkhoves served at the hospital established in the municipal Octroi building and had to walk about on tiptoe to avoid sinking up to his ankles in filth. Mainz was not exceptional. Similar scenes are described by doctors and soldiers in the hospitals at Leipzig and Torgau. In the latter city, the number of deaths exceeded 8,000 in the month of November alone. It was necessary to climb over the dead to reach the sick.[35]

In the Campaign of 1814, affluent locals were exhorted to help the wounded soldiers in a belated attempt to rekindle the old Revolutionary spirit. The city fathers of Alençon, more than a hundred miles west of Paris, were instructed to provide accommodation and supplies for 500 wounded being moved from hospitals nearer to the front. Some wounded would be lodged in private houses but the demands were still considerable: 250 wooden beds with a mattress, a bolster and a coverlet; also 1,000 sheets, 1,200 night shirts, 1,000 night caps, 1,200 napkins, 400kg of linen bandages and 200kg of lint. The tone of the directive to local leading citizens was threatening – they would not like what was going to happen to them if they did not contribute their fair share. The hospital was organised promptly in a local convent.[36]

In Paris, the Emperor wrote to Daru ordering him to organise hospitals for six or seven thousand. 'By this means, the capital will not have under its eyes the spectacle of negligence towards the sick and wounded.' Some occupied the city's abattoirs, a grim irony in view of the slaughter of men that was occurring in the *Grande Armée*'s hospitals. Napoleon was understandably concerned that the insufficiencies of his medical services should not become common knowledge. In fact, the state of the hospitals was used as a weapon against him in a small pamphlet entitled *Les Sépulcres de la Grande Armée*, an interesting example of an army's poor medical care being used as propaganda. On an early page, we find: 'At Erfurt, there were seven hospitals. Within twenty-four hours, there was not a bowl of soup, not a glass of wine, not a piece of bread, not a bandage, not an ounce of lint!' There is much in the same vein and the author concludes that the hospitals had become the 'tombs' of the *Grande Armée* and the poor patients 'the martyrs of Bonaparte'. He criticises not only Napoleon but also Daru, the Intendant General, who allegedly denied the young soldiers any bread.[37] The writer of this inflammatory, but largely accurate, piece of literature was Augustin Hapdé, the director of hospitals in the *Grande Armée*. When Napoleon returned from Elba, Hapdé wisely took refuge in England.

After the Campaign of the Hundred Days, the destruction of the army and its support services meant that the French wounded were cared for in Brussels and surrounding towns in hospitals under the auspices of the British and Belgians. Initially, the wounded of all nations were mixed together but most of the French ended up in *Le Corderie* in Brussels, a hospital able to accommodate 1,500 men. An English witness describes the beds arranged in four rows along the whole 1,300 feet of the building. He thought that the French wounded were mostly more severe cases than their allied counterparts and that the death rate in the French hospital was higher.[38]

In addition to the general hospitals, set up in numerous locations during the various campaigns, there were also the specialist hospitals. Some of these were designed to take only patients with venereal and skin diseases. Percy makes a number of references to these facilities in his journal. The specialist hospital at Kustrin in Poland in 1806 was able to house up to 2,000 of these cases whilst the specialist hospitals around Danzig were able to accommodate a further five hundred. Maltese *officier de santé*, Eugene Fenech, alludes to a hospital for venereal diseases in a convent in Lisbon in 1808 but, like Percy, he gives no detailed description. From the tone of Percy's journal, we can deduce that the large number of soldiers with these relatively trivial but debilitating diseases were regarded as a nuisance and were moved sideways when the opportunity arose. When anticipating a large battle in Poland, Percy generated some space for the expected 6,000 wounded by shifting several hundred skin and venereal cases to a neighbouring town. On finding forty or fifty skin disease patients occupying a precious good quality general hospital in Danzig in 1807, he again forced them to leave.[39]

There were also hospitals intended specifically for convalescents. Men were discharged from the general hospitals into the convalescent hospitals for a period of recovery prior to rejoining their regiment. These hospitals were often placed in larger barracks. The soldiers were under the supervision of senior military officers and the medical service was provided by the physicians of the local hospitals or army corps. In the convalescent unit at Cairo in 1799, most of the patients only required a short admission of three to six days before being regarded as fit enough to return to duty. Four years later, at the Camp of Boulogne, three large convalescent depots were able to house a total of 2,300 men. Legislation in 1806 dictated the formation of further convalescent depots, notably in the cities of Chambéry, Strasbourg and Mainz. This type of hospital could potentially speed the full recovery of the sick and wounded and reduce readmission rates to the general hospitals. Equally, some convalescent hospitals of the wars became sanctuaries for malingerers – the British hospital at Belem in Lisbon was notorious for its sizeable population of 'Belem Rangers' who kept well out of the way of the fighting. Marshal Davout evidently believed that the advantages outweighed the risks, as he specifically requested the formation of extra convalescent depots in 1811. To supplement these larger buildings there were also smaller stopping off points for men returning to the army from the hospitals, the so-called *'gîtes d'évacuation'*.[40]

Soldiers with more trivial wounds or illnesses were routinely treated in their own regimental hospitals. Percy was a great supporter of this approach which had the advantages of keeping men with the army and allowing them to be treated by their own doctors. The key regulations for the regimental infirmaries appeared in 1803. The regimental surgeons were encouraged to treat all lightly wounded in houses, barracks and tents. The *chirurgien-major* of the corps was to be given a sufficient amount of money to provide all the dressings and medicines necessary for the management of patients who could be cared for outside the main hospitals. Each regiment had an ambulance caisson to help carry these vital commodities.[41]

The regimental infirmaries played a more minor role on campaign and the bulk of sick and wounded trawled up in the despised general hospitals. The medical officers of the *service de santé* were aware that these hospitals were the nadir of their organisation and there were well meaning efforts to produce systematic improvement. Hospitals were inspected both by doctors and military officers. Both Percy and Larrey were continually visiting military hospitals in the vicinity and making suggestions for improvement. Eugene Fenech accompanied the principal surgeon of his army corps on a hospital inspection in Spain in 1808. The young *sous-aide* took notes which were later to be presented to the General-in-Chief. Inspections by informed and influential military officers were potentially beneficial as they reassured the patients and pulled the local administrators into line. When Masséna visited the hospital at Huningue in 1799, he praised the medical staff and cheered the soldiers. Conversely, when the Emperor sent some generals to inspect the hospitals in Burgos in 1808, Percy complains that 'they promised, they scolded, they proposed and the misery continued'. Pharmacist Jacob recalls an unfortunate visit by Grand Chamberlain Talleyrand to a hospital in Poland in 1806.

> This exquisite gentleman held a perfumed handkerchief to his nose with one hand whilst using the other to give each wounded man a gold coin, saying to each in a monotonous voice, 'This is what His Majesty has asked me to give you'.

The senior dignitary's air of repugnance angered both patients and staff. Not all military officers appreciated the problems of the *officiers de santé* and the hospitals and their intervention could be harmful. In Spain, Tyrbas de Chamberet had to endure a 'derisory' inspection of his hospital by a general. The military officer ordered the beds to be placed closer together to increase capacity. When the physician tried to point out that this was against the regulations and would encourage the spread of typhus and other infectious diseases, he was shouted down.[42]

In many cases, the lot of soldiers in the *Grande Armée*'s hospitals could have been greatly improved by only modest changes. Tyrbas de Chamberet's list of five items, which he vainly requested from the administrators in Spain, is simple enough: fresh straw, buckets, baths, chamber pots and more *infirmiers*. The administrators responded with impatience and even anger, 'You are not in Paris! – The sick cannot be cared for as they are in France! – Limit yourself to making visits!'[43] Whilst ordinary military doctors like Tyrbas de Chamberet struggled to make any impact at ground level, the more senior *officiers de santé* were also considering how the hospital service could be improved. Foremost among them was Jean-François Coste who, towards the end of the wars, wrote a substantial article on military hospitals for the *Dictionnaire des Sciences Médicales*. If nothing else, this article proves that men like Coste were well aware of the shortcomings of French military hospitals and that they understood the need for change. In a work which owes much to the pioneering work of the British army doctor John Pringle in the previous century, Coste systematically details the need for better ventilated, spacious hospitals with clean beds and sheets and adequate latrines. He particularly stresses the need for the medical staff to regularly visit the wards to maintain strict discipline and to carefully divide up the patients according to the nature of their disease. This enlightened piece of writing gave hope for the future but it appears curiously detached from the actual experience of soldiers who had suffered and died in French military hospitals over the previous two decades.[44]

To avoid the general hospitals of the first line becoming overwhelmed, it was necessary to constantly evacuate men unfit for action away from the front. The formation of these sick convoys was a major task as, at any time, there were significant numbers of sick and wounded winding their way along the roads of the Empire. Responsibility for this daily undertaking was in the hands of the *commissaires des guerres*. It was they who had to ensure adequate numbers of wagons and horses not only for the sick and wounded but for the surgeons, employees and military escort. *Officiers de santé* made lists of those men who required evacuation and indicated whether they required a wagon or were fit to march. The movement of sick men remained a constant headache for the *Grande Armée*'s doctors. Percy's account of events in Poland in 1807 is unremarkable but well illustrates this daily chore.

> We found General Walther and two strong detachments of *grenadiers à cheval* of the Guard at Neumarkt; this town is extremely miserable. Between Neumarkt and Löbau we met more than fifty wagons of wounded, each hitched to two horses of the artillery train of the Guard; they were going to Neumarkt and the horses could get no farther. It is General Lariboisière who has taken this effective measure to evacuate the wounded that were piled up in the town of Löbau where he is in cantonment with the Guard artillery; but how will these unfortunates be looked after at Neumarkt? I quickly sent two surgeons there. Tomorrow, this general will, in the same way, send off all the remaining wounded and sick at his headquarters, which will soon fill up again unless we can get twenty-five or thirty wagons on the road every day.[45]

As for many aspects of medical care, evacuations were particularly difficult in Spain and Portugal. The carts provided through official channels were often in short supply or unsuitable. Percy describes the vehicles used for transport of wounded to Madrid in 1808 as being so high with such raised sides that it took at least four soldiers to get a man with a fracture into them. Accordingly, it was necessary to resort to the crude ox-carts of the country or any other available transport. Eugene Fenech accompanied an improvised sick convoy in Spain in 1811. The sick were carried in wagons, on artillery caissons, in the small carts belonging to the *cantinières* and on stretchers born by soldiers. In tough terrain donkeys were invaluable. Captain Nicolas Marcel was distressed to receive an order to slaughter his. A cartoon which had made the rounds of the bivouacs showed a miserable wounded soldier sitting on a donkey. The inscription underneath read 'The saviour of the Army of Portugal'.[46]

Conscientious *officiers de santé* accompanying the sick and wounded convoys worked hard to ensure continuous medical care. Fenech dressed his patients twice daily. However, it was frequently impossible to give good quality treatment. The hospitals can be criticised for their poor standards but in many cases the sick reached them already in a pitiable state. Percy witnessed such a convoy of wounded after the Battle of Espinosa in northern Spain in November 1808. They had travelled approximately one hundred miles to reach Burgos.

> I was just about to set out from the town when I discovered that more than eighty wagons of wounded were making their way towards the Conception Hospital; I cancelled my plans to go and care for these unfortunates. Around ten surgeons rushed to assist me (those of the first corps, from which these wounded had come, were not to be seen except for two who were with the evacuees). I set about carrying the wounded and giving orders for their carriage in such a way to harm them as little as possible. The wagons had served both as their transport and beds and most of them had not left the wagons for five days; their straw was rotten; some had mattresses which were soiled by their wounds and excrement; they were covered with scraps of carpet, with curtains, with bits of damask and the poor quality sheets of the peasants. We got them down, not without great difficulty, and as some of them wanted to open their bowels, we had to hold them up to allow it. These miserable and extremely disgusting tasks took about two hours. There was an almost unbearable stink. The wounds had hardly been dressed for several days and several were already gangrenous.[47]

Not all the wounded arrived at their destination. The guerrillas were a constant threat and sick and wounded convoys and their doctors were regarded as soft targets. Surgeon Jean-Baptiste d'Héralde accompanied a convoy of seventy-eight wounded in Andalusia in 1810 – twenty were able to walk, fifty-five were mounted on mules or donkeys and three had to be carried. The convoy was protected by four companies of soldiers but it was still incessantly attacked in the mountains by the local guerrillas. Nine wounded were killed and several others received additional wounds.

Without fortuitous help from the 63ᵉ Line it is likely that the whole convoy would have been massacred. D'Héralde stresses that it was crucial to carry the wounded with them as if they had been left in any town or village, 'these barbarians would have made them die a thousand deaths'. Abandonment was the greatest fear of wounded or sick men. There are several instances of this in the Peninsular War and it was a particular feature of the retreat from Moscow. Napoleon ordered Mortier to evacuate all the sick and wounded from the Russian capital, even instructing him to overload the wagons if necessary as he was optimistic of finding empty supply wagons at Mojaisk. He was to give preference to officers and to Frenchmen. The horses dragging the wagons soon died and the wounded were left on the side of the road. There were no *officiers de santé* and they could not rely on help from their comrades. In the words of Lejeune, 'as we rode away, we turned aside our heads so that we did not see their despairing gestures'. Eugene Labaume, who wrote his campaign journal in ink made from gunpowder and melted snow, also heard the 'lamentable cries' of the abandoned sick and wounded but he acknowledges that, in the horror of the retreat, it was every man for himself.[48]

The difficulties of land evacuation made travel by water relatively attractive and this was more widespread than is generally believed. During the Prussian campaign of 1806, Percy evacuated sick and wounded along the Main and Rhine rivers. Although there were severe food shortages he judged this a successful operation. The following year, in the quagmire of Poland, the rivers and canals were extensively used, especially between Koenigsberg and Berlin. The local boats were not always ideal but were much preferable to the wagons of the country. In the course of a single week in the summer of 1807, four boats carried over 800 patients between Tilsit and Koenigsberg. Rivers were also exploited in the Peninsula. Surgeon Gama recalls several hundred wounded being evacuated in boats along the Dax after the Battle of Orthez in 1814. Unfortunately, the severity of the Russian winter made river transport impracticable during 1812.[49]

Napoleon's views on the evacuation of his sick and wounded soldiers are well represented in his correspondence and are predictably inconsistent. He appears genuinely concerned for the wellbeing of the convoys. In Egypt in 1799, the young Bonaparte is reluctant to abandon his wounded. He is willing to improvise, to use horses, camels and donkeys according to circumstances. His directive to segregate the sick from the wounded is well founded and we find this repeated in the Prussian campaign seven years later. However, by this stage, Napoleon was more calculating, viewing the evacuation of non-combatants as a necessary evil which could not be allowed to hinder the rapid movement of active units or damage the morale of impressionable new recruits. Thus, writing to the administrative department of the army from Berlin in 1806, he declares that evacuations are 'disasters' for the sick and wounded but, if absolutely necessary, they had to be directed along strictly specified routes. In subsequent years, the Emperor's solicitude for his sick and wounded is still in evidence but his orders regarding their movement are more often at odds with reality, as is well illustrated by his abortive attempt to evacuate from Moscow in 1812.[50]

Notes

1. Rosen, G, *Hospitals medical care and social policy in the French Revolution*, pp. 131–2.
2. Ackerknecht, E H, *Medicine at the Paris Hospital 1794–1848*, p. 16; Vess, D M, *Medical Revolution in France 1789–1796*, p. 32.
3. Rosen, p. 148; Lemaire, J-F, *Napoléon et la Médecine*, p. 193; Tulard, J, *Dictionnaire Napoléon*, Vol. I, pp. 968–9.
4. Tissot, C J, *Observations générales sur l'administration des hôpitaux ambulans et sedentaires des armées*, p. 1; Vess, p. 33.
5. Sèze, V de, *Rapport et Projet de décret sur le service de santé des Armées et des Hôpitaux Militaires*, p. 14; Vess, p. 190; Forrest, A, *Soldiers of the French Revolution*, pp. 144–5.
6. Brice, Docteur and Bottet, Capitaine, *Le Corps de Santé Militaire en France*, p. 54.
7. Pigeard, A, *Le Service de Santé de la Révolution au 1er Empire 1792–1815*, pp. 7–9.
8. Milleliri, J-M, *Médecins et Soldats pendant l'expédition d'Égypte (1798–1799)*, p. 165.
9. Brice, Bottet, pp. 60–1; Vess, pp. 179, 110.
10. Pigeard, p. 10.
11. Howard, M, *Wellington's Doctors. The British Army Medical Services in the Napoleonic Wars*, p. 93.
12. Forrest, p. 146; Vess, pp. 83–98; Percy, Baron, *Journal des Campagnes de Baron Percy*, pp. 44–5.
13. Percy, pp. xliv, 55–6.
14. Pigeard, pp. 11–13; Brice, Bottet, p. 122.
15. Brice, Bottet, p. 125.
16. Barrès, J-B, *Memoirs of a French Napoleonic Officer*, p. 56; Brandt von, H, *In the Legions of Napoleon. The memoirs of a Polish Officer in Spain and Russia 1808–1813*, p. 225; Forrest, A, *Napoleon's Men. The soldiers of the Revolution and Empire*, p. 121.
17. Brice, Bottet, p. 137; Percy, pp. 68–9; Morvan, J, *Le Soldat Impérial*, Vol. I, p. 309.
18. Percy, p. 74; Brice, Bottet, p. 195.
19. Jacob, P-I, *Le Journal Inédit d'un pharmacien de la Grande Armée*, p. 93.
20. Percy, pp. 145–6.
21. ibid., pp. 232, 360–1.

22. ibid., pp. 388–9, 258, 230, 269, 356, 267.
23. Petre, F L, *Napoleon's Campaign in Poland 1806–1807*, p. 26.
24. Percy, pp. 401, 407, 421, 498.
25. Laurillard-Fallot, S-L, *Souvenirs d'un Médecin Hollandais sous les Aigles Françaises 1807–1833*, p. 55.
26. von Brandt, pp. 51–2.
27. Lemaire, J-F, *Les blessés dans les Armées Napoléoniennes*, p. 258; Larrey, D J, *Mémoires de Chirurgie Militaire et Campagnes 1787–1840*, p. 527; Lixon, L J M, *Médecin a l'armée d'Espagne en 1808, 1809 et 1810*, p. 207; Percy, p. 461.
28. Percy, pp. 397, 479, 435; Brice, Bottet, p. 210.
29. Jacob, p. 193.
30. Pelet, J J, *The French Campaign in Portugal 1810–1811*, pp. 206–8.
31. Tyrbas de Chamberet, J, *Mémoires d'un Médecin Militaire*, pp. 92–3.
32. Forrest, *Napoleon's Men*, p. 124; Lixon, p. 210.
33. Lemaire, pp. 152–3; Baldet, M, *La Vie Quotidienne dans les Armées de Napoléon*, p. 168; Morvan, Vol. II, p. 341.
34. Ségur, Count P-P de, *Napoleon's Russian Campaign*, p. 48; Vossler, H, *With Napoleon in Russia 1812*, p. 59; Brice, Bottet, pp. 223–4; Wilson, General Sir R, *Narrative of Events during the Invasion of Russia by Napoleon Bonaparte*, p. 354; Zamoyski, A, *1812. Napoleon's fatal march on Moscow*, p. 529.
35. Brice, Bottet, p. 229; Kerkhoves, J R L, *Observations médicales faites pendant les Campagnes de Russie en 1812 et Allemagne en 1813*, p. 68; Prinzing, F, *Epidemics resulting from Wars*, p. 312.
36. Elting, J R, *Swords around a Throne. Napoleon's Grande Armée*, p. 288.
37. Lemaire, p. 176; Hapdé, J B A, *Les Sépulcres de la Grande Armée*, pp. 15, 60.
38. Simpson, J, *Paris after Waterloo*, p. 6.
39. Percy, pp. 114, 263, 377, 126, 251; Fenech, E, *Mémoires d'un Officier de Santé Maltais dans l'Armée Française (1786–1839)*, p. 31.
40. Milleliri, p. 165; Pigeard, p. 16; Brice, Bottet, p. 219; Percy, p. 74.
41. Percy, p. xxix; Brice, Bottet, p. 127.
42. Fenech, p. 25; Percy, pp. 41, 409; Jacob, p. 94; Tyrbas de Chamberet, p. 102.
43. Tyrbas de Chamberet, p. 101.
44. Lemaire, J-F, *Coste. Premier Médecin des Armées de Napoléon*, pp. 313–21.
45. Percy, p. 202.
46. Percy, p. 434; Fenech, p. 58; Marcel, N, *Campagnes en Espagne et au Portugal 1808–1814*, p. 106.
47. Percy, p. 414.
48. d'Héralde, J-B, *Mémoires d'un Chirurgien de la Grande Armée*, p. 137; Zamoyski, p. 370; Lejeune, Baron, *Memoirs of Baron Lejeune Aide-de-Camp to Marshals Berthier, Davout and Oudinot*, Vol. II, p. 210; Labaume, E, *A circumstantial account of the campaign in Russia*, p. 339.
49. Lemaire, pp.263–9.
50. ibid., pp.127–8, 139.

CHAPTER VIII
Surgery: The Cutting Edge

Surgery in 18th-century France was a crude business far removed from the sophisticated medical speciality of today. In large parts of the country, operations were routinely performed by barbers and barber-surgeons whose expertise was based on a short apprenticeship, perhaps with their father or uncle, and a willingness to learn at the patient's expense. By far the most popular operation was the removal of bladder stones (lithotomy) – presumably because the pain of the stone was so severe that even a botched operation was preferable. Amateur lithotomists slashed away and left a trail of dead and dying in their wake. Parisian surgeons regarded themselves as superior to their country brethren and they had at least discarded the razor in favour of the scalpel.

In contrast to the previous stagnation of civilian surgery, the first decade of the 19th century witnessed real progress. Not only did the wars provide an endless supply of instructive case histories, but the status and practice of surgery was elevated by its unification with medicine and the incorporation of surgical teaching into the Paris medical curriculum. The new professors of surgery urged their students to 'read little, see a lot, do a lot'. This new spirit of practical improvement and optimism was expressed by the *Charité* surgeon Baron Boyer at the start of his classical treatise on surgical diseases in 1814: 'Surgery has made the greatest progress in our time and seems to have reached, or almost reached, the highest degree of perfection which it seems able to attain.' In reality, technical advances were of limited value without anaesthetics and antisepsis and the new surgery was still murderous. In the decades during and after the Napoleonic Wars, the mortality statistics for Paris hospitals make depressing reading. In 1832 twenty-one patients underwent uterine surgery and all died either during or immediately after the operation.[1]

In military surgery, the difficulties were increased by the magnitude of the casualties, the severity of the injuries, the shortage of equipment, and the crudity of the ambulances and hospitals. Success was dependent on simplicity and speed. More experienced surgeons did not elaborate and performed major surgery remarkably quickly. When Dominique Larrey amputated at the shoulder on a *chasseur* who had received a severe sabre wound complicated by gangrene, he noted that the operation 'was performed in a minute according to my plan'. Napoleonic surgeons also had to be great improvisers. Pierre-François Briot, an experienced army surgeon of the Revolutionary and Napoleonic period, pays homage to his colleagues.

> If genius is doing great things with small means, then one can say that surgery has never shown it more than in the late wars. Often lacking the most crucial articles, the military surgeon knew how to turn everything that came to hand on the battlefield into a means for a cure; he had turned the first piece of cloth that he found into lint, bandages and compresses; a simple bistoury was all he required for every type of incision and almost any operation. A probe was enough to find and often extract musket balls, bone splinters, bits of weapons, clothing and other foreign bodies ... A finger applied to a bleeding vessel stopped it long enough until the surgeon was able to secure it with a ligature. Simple bandages skilfully applied served several purposes at once. The wounds were simply washed with water and this often led to the cure of severe wounding in a short period of time. Helped only by his innate talent, the military surgeon was able to see and judge instantly, in a single glance, the number of wounded, those who needed the quickest help, the most appropriate type of treatment, and how he would procure it. When lacking lint and linen, he resorted to moss, grass and leaves: short of normal meat, he used horsemeat for soup which he salted with gunpowder. He practised surgery just as the soldiers practised war.[2]

Of course, not all surgeons achieved this ideal and, despite the efforts of the best, battlefield surgery remained chaotic and brutal. Ordinary soldiers who wandered, sometimes inadvertently, into the operating areas of ambulances and field hospitals were stunned by what they saw. A musician, who helped with the care of the wounded at the siege of Colberg on the Baltic in 1807, recalls that his job was to pick up the limbs after amputation.

> I had the air of a butcher ... I was covered in blood from head to feet ... I saw a leg on the straw and went to collect it and put it in the pile with the others, but there was still a body connected to it. Under the straw I found an unfortunate who had been there since the morning and who was sleeping deeply. He was dead drunk and had a broken arm which was only attached by a piece of skin.

The man tolerated his amputation with no complaint and later walked back to the ambulance, refusing to wait for a wagon.[3] Such scenes were to be repeated innumerable times in the makeshift operating theatres of the *Grande Armée*.

The surgeons had a daunting workload. The number of casualties which could be expected after a major battle has been detailed in previous chapters. Whereas Larrey's claim to have performed two hundred operations within twenty-four hours of Borodino might be exaggerated, there is no doubt that prodigious surgical feats were performed. This was despite the frequent practical difficulties of undertaking any surgery. There was often no suitable furniture. In the Egyptian campaigns, the wounded received surgery on the hard ground, on sand, on a simple table or sitting in a chair or on a stool. Operating in dirt, often exposed to the elements, the surgeon could struggle to see what he was doing. Heinrich Roos describes performing surgery in the depths of Russia with only the illumination of some burning wood shavings. The surgical memoirs of the wars contain allusions to the shortage of good quality surgical instruments. To hold and cut through tissue and bone, to secure bleeding vessels and close wounds, Napoleon's surgeons required many of the basic surgical tools that are used today – these included saws, knives, forceps, probes, scissors, needles and tourniquets. In 1800 Bonaparte was forced to write to Berthier:

> I am reliably informed, Citizen Minister, that the chests sent to the various armies by the general hospital administration in Paris contain defective instruments and saws which lacerate soldiers who have to have operations. I invite you to put an end to this abuse without delay and to punish those responsible.

When crucial instruments were lacking, the surgeons at the front had to make the best of things. Percy records in his Danzig journal in May 1807 that he had assisted a surgeon who was amputating at the thigh. Lacking a retractor, an instrument designed to expose the operation site, the surgeon had little choice but to continue. The operation was conducted 'in a disgusting and embarrassing manner'.[4]

From a modern perspective, the most appalling aspect of the surgery of the Napoleonic Wars was the lack of any effective anaesthetic. Surgeons were motivated to operate quickly to minimise the agony of the victim. The muscle spasms and protestations of the patient complicated the operation; as Bernard Shaw pointed out in typically perverse vein: 'Chloroform has done a lot of mischief. It has enabled every fool to become a surgeon.' Percy showed interest in the concept of 'artificial sleep' and there were some inconsistent attempts made to prepare the patient – French country practitioners relaxed the great muscles of the legs and abdomen by inserting a strong cigar into the rectum – but most soldiers were fortunate if their senses were a little dulled by alcohol or opium. Few army surgeons make reference to the pain of surgery, but La Flize was an exception.

It is impossible to imagine what a wounded man feels when the surgeon has to inform him that he will certainly die unless one or two limbs are removed. He has to come to terms with his lot and prepare himself for terrible suffering. I cannot describe the howls and the grinding of teeth produced by a man whose limb has been shattered by a cannonball, the screams of pain as the surgeon cuts through the skin, slices through the muscle, then the nerves, saws right through the bone, severing arteries from which blood splatters the surgeon himself.[5]

General Marbot required surgery to his foot after Eylau, the surgeon removing the dead tissue as if it was 'the rotten part of an apple'. He was held down by four assistants and he tolerated the operation well until the bistoury reached the live skin and he admits that he struggled to escape their grasp. There were conflicting views as to the worst part of an amputation. Captain Jean-Casimir Jouan required amputation of his arm.

I had always heard that it was most painful when they sawed the bone. I am not sure that I am built any differently from other men but, during my amputation, I hardly felt the cutting of the bone compared with the cutting of the flesh.

Many soldiers must have feared surgery more than wounding. Some 18th-century military surgeons, notably Faure, believed that the sight of their comrades receiving painful surgery would demoralise the remaining wounded and hasten death. Larrey vigorously opposed this view, insisting that the wounded often encouraged each other through operations and that they gained confidence from seeing the surgeons in action on their behalf.[6]

In describing the main types of military surgery of the era, we can rely in part on anecdotal accounts by soldiers and surgeons. Much more detail is contained in a number of contemporary surgical texts and, among them, Larrey's memoirs are supreme. His writings contain much rationalisation for his views on surgery and are littered with countless case histories designed to illustrate key points. Larrey's surgical practice had no limits. Although most famed for battlefield surgery, he operated with equal confidence on patients with tuberculosis, hydrocoeles, fistulae and herniae. When his daughter accidentally stabbed her eye with a bread knife, he replaced the protruding iris himself. His surgical opinions may not have been in complete agreement with those of senior colleagues, but in researching the surgery of the wars we must always turn to Larrey first. Percy is a better witness of the daily life of the *service de santé* but his surgical works, most notably his *Manuel du Chirurgien d'Armée* published during the Revolutionary period, are modest in comparison.

Gunshot wounds of the limbs were among the commonest injuries of the wars and, contrary to popular belief, they were often managed conservatively. If it was not possible to easily extract the ball, the injured soldier commonly had to face a prolonged period of debility. This is well illustrated by the case of Lieutenant Arnaud who was struck in the thigh by a musket ball at the Battle of Bautzen. He was aide-de-camp to General Bertrand and the general keeps us informed of the patient's progress in a series of letters to his wife. Initially, the wound was thought to be not dangerous and Arnaud started to mobilise on splints but suppuration soon set in and, three weeks after the battle, the surgeons made incisions above and below the wound in an abortive attempt to remove the ball which they had hoped would spontaneously rise to the surface. Bertrand was optimistic of his aide-de-camp's quick recovery but, a month later, the wound was only a little better. Following further set backs, Larrey operated in early August, three months after the injury, but still the ball proved elusive. The discharging wound only dried up after another two months and the lieutenant eventually returned to duty with his leg intact but after a prolonged and dangerous recovery lasting over six months.[7]

With wounds evolving in this way, it is easy to understand why surgeons were so keen to remove balls and other foreign bodies at the time of wounding. In the Revolutionary period it was routine practice to make incisions around the edges to allow dilatation of the wound itself. This facilitated probing for foreign bodies and might permit any 'poisons' to be evacuated. The surgeons were encouraged in their efforts by the obvious improvement in the patient's morale in seeing a musket ball extracted and also by the common belief that a ball left in situ might move about and damage a vital organ. Such aggressive management caused its own problems, not least haemorrhage, and in the Napoleonic era wound dilatation was less in vogue. Surgeons did, however, routinely explore for and extract balls with fingers, probes and forceps either on the battlefield or when wounds became complicated in the ambulances and hospitals. When Louis-Jacques Romand of the *fusiliers-grenadiers* of the Guard was hit in the side by a musket ball, his comrades fashioned a stretcher from two muskets and carried him to the regimental *chirurgien-major*. The surgeon searched for the entry wound and then removed the lead ball with his finger, a procedure that Romand estimated as lasting more than two minutes and during which he transiently lost consciousness.[8]

For any deeper extraction, instruments had to be used. Larrey describes the management of a grenadier with a wound in the thigh. When the wound began to discharge brown offensive matter, Larrey attempted, as he did in the case of Lieutenant Arnaud, to remove the offending foreign body. On this occasion he had more success. After locating the presumed ball close to the bone with a probe, he widened the wound with an incision and gripped it with forceps. Unexpectedly, it was not a musket ball but a nine centimetre piece of copper ramrod which had been fired accidentally. Percy was also prepared to open wounds when there were complicating factors. In the case of the colonel of the 44ᵉ Line, wounded in the shoulder at Danzig, he advised the *chirurgien-major* to plunge a bistoury into a swelling which had developed around the entry site and which he presumed to contain not only the ball but also bony fragments, bits of clothing and blood.

There are many anecdotes of strange and unexplained bodies in wounds – coins, teeth, bits of equipment, etc. – but two instances recalled by Larrey and Heinrich Roos deserve mention. During the Austrian campaign of 1809, Larrey encountered an artilleryman who related being hit by a bouncing cannon ball which, he insisted, had subsequently also killed one of his comrades. He had suffered a severe leg injury but complained only of an 'inconvenient weight in the limb'. On seizing the leg to amputate it, Larrey found it unusually heavy and discovered the 5lb ball still lodged in the thigh. The case described by Roos, also of a soldier in the Austrian campaign, is perhaps even more remarkable. He was dressing a serious wound in the right chest when the patient suddenly complained of a dragging sensation below his left arm. After some exploration, the surgeon discovered a large hard lump in the armpit just below the skin. On making an incision, he was able to easily extract a 6lb cannon ball. The man survived the initial operation but he later became jaundiced and died of haemorrhage and convulsions, an almost inevitable outcome in such extensive wounding.[9]

The types of wound dressings used changed over the course of the wars, in part because of changing medical opinions and in part due to necessity. In the early years of the Revolutionary Wars, there was a preference for complicated dressings comprising plasters immersed in various types of oils, ointments, alcohol and other solutions. This approach gradually became outmoded and there was increasing reliance on more simple dressings with irrigation with cold water alone. Many surgeons became expert at applying bandages, Briot claiming that it was the skill that French army doctors had honed to the greatest perfection. These trends continued under the Consulate and Empire, although proper dressings were frequently replaced by bits of clothes held on by straps or belts and naturally absorbent substances such as moss were often substituted for lint. Not least because it was widely available, water remained the favoured method for moistening these dressings. In Percy's words:

> How many times have the waters of the Moselle, of the Rhine, the Danube, the Lech, the Limmat, the Oder, the Elbe, the Bug, the Vistula, the Guadalquivir, the Ebro, the Tagus etc. been used to freshen the dressings of our numerous wounded? With these waters alone, I have, on many occasions, saved limbs and especially hands and feet which were in such a poor state that it seemed imprudent to postpone amputation.

It may be thought that new bandages were preferable but, in fact, much new cloth was stiff and heavy making it difficult to apply and cumbersome for the patient. Frequent washing made them lighter and more malleable. The dressings of choice, sourced from Strasbourg, were the lightest available with uncut edges and no sewing. These could be washed and reused up to ninety times without becoming rough or developing sharp edges.[10]

Where wounds became infected or complicated, poultices were sometimes applied. Percy describes a variety of these, one consisting of flour sprinkled with camphor and kina, and another of onions. The poultice was usually put on at the time of removal of the first dressing. Larrey was a supporter of wound cauterisation, the application of heat to the affected area. He popularised the use of moxa, an instrument of ancient Chinese origin in which short hollow cylinders of smouldering pith or cotton were held close enough to the wound to induce small circular burns on the patient's skin. The moxa might also be also be resorted to in the treatment of skin ulcers or abscesses. Larrey was not, however, an advocate of more brutal use of the cautery iron which potentially did more harm than good.[11]

Sword wounds could be destructive and complicated dependent on the depth and site but management was generally more straightforward than for gun shot wounds with less concern as to the presence of foreign bodies. Larrey's management of the sabre wounds inflicted on French troops by the British at Benavente in Spain in 1808 highlights the normal surgical practices. The surgeons in the field had attempted to unite the wounds using 'twisted' sutures but this was not successful. Many of the lacerations became inflamed and did not heal. Larrey undid the original sutures and brought the lips of the wounds into exact apposition. He then applied a bandage designed to give additional support. The result, even in the case of complicated wounds of the face, was a complete success.[12]

Troops were caught in blazing buildings and shell explosions and suffered extensive burns. Traditional treatments such as cold ammoniated water, opiate water or vinegar water exacerbated the skin damage. Larrey had an opportunity to experiment with new approaches at the siege of Figueras in Spain in 1794 where an explosion in a redoubt caused severe injuries to many of the French attackers. He dressed the burns with fine linen soaked in saffron and honey. The dressings were left in place for some time before being gradually replaced by dry lint smeared in wax and oil. This carefully conceived strategy both relieved pain and much increased survival rates – sixty Spaniards who suffered shock and burns when their powder magazine blew up during the Battle of Black Mountain in 1794 were all saved by French surgeons. Skin grafts were not known although Briot did manage to successfully replace some small flaps of skin sliced off by sabres.[13]

Fractures were among the most common injuries in Napoleonic battles. We can state this with some confidence both because of contemporary accounts by surgeons and patients and from the evidence of battlefield excavations. In the soldiers' grave at Austerlitz, many of the skeletons showed fractures, some of these being complicated with splinters and multiple bone fragments. In their management of fractures, the *Grande Armée*'s surgeons were able to draw from the extensive experience of the 'bone-setters' of rural France who handed down their skills through the generations. As for so many other aspects of wound treatment, Larrey was the great innovator, rediscovering the full value of immobilisation of fractures. He stipulated that the injury should be infrequently dressed and held in place by his *'appareil inamovible'*, which can be roughly translated as 'fixed appliance', the precursor of modern plaster casts. In Larrey's opinion, this had the advantage of reducing pain, promoting healing and lessening the chance of infection by keeping the wound covered. He rejected complicated materials and constructed his apparatus from widely available components such as straw and bags filled with chaff. The appliance usually remained in place for around seven weeks with the patient mobilising on crutches. Percy also understood that fractured limbs were often best left as they were. In 1807 in Koenigsberg, he elucidates the management of men who had had their legs fractured a month earlier. He stresses the importance of simply redressing the wound and of avoiding the temptation to remanipulate the limb to bring the bone ends in closer conjunction as this would only result in profuse haemorrhage. Many soldiers did survive uncomplicated fractures, a fact confirmed by the grave excavation at the Napoleonic military hospital at Tolosa in Spain where the remodelling of bone around fracture sites proves that the soldiers survived this injury even if they later succumbed to disease.[14]

Complicated or 'compound' fractures, where the bone splintered and pierced the skin and the resulting wound was open, carried a much worse prognosis than simple fractures. In his treatise on gunshot wounds, Surgeon Eugene Fenech includes several case histories of men with compound injuries. Typical is that of a *chasseur à cheval* of the Hanoverian Legion who received a gunshot wound to his left arm in Spain in 1810. Upper limb injuries were generally less dangerous than wounds to the lower extremities but, in this instance, the cavalryman's humerus was severely fractured with numerous bony splinters and the two bone ends displaced in the soft tissues. The wound showed little sign of healing and, after local infection and enormous swelling of the limb, the man died on the ninth day after the original wounding. Modern evidence of a death from a compound fracture was found in the Austerlitz grave pit. One of the adult male skeletons has splintering of the right femur. This was certainly a compound fracture and the lack of any evidence of bony healing indicates that the soldier died shortly after the trauma, probably from torrential bleeding.[15]

The high risk of death following more severe limb injuries such as compound fractures provided the justification for the archetypal surgical procedure of the wars, amputation. In the early phase of the Revolutionary Wars, amputation was widely regarded as an operation of last resort. Military surgeons were influenced by practice in civilian life where only a limb severely damaged by trauma, gangrene or cancer was likely to be surgically removed. This followed the practice of much of the 18th century – an influential monograph of 1762 entitled *On the inutility of the Amputation of Limbs* had been translated into several languages. As the wars progressed there were an unprecedented number of limb injuries and the surgeons in the field soon learnt that the relatively conservative practice of civilian medicine was not necessarily applicable in the heat of battle. There was little time to perform elaborate and laborious surgery on damaged limbs and a quick amputation with prompt evacuation to the rear appeared to give the soldier a better chance of survival. Percy and others continued to resist wholesale amputations, describing the 'pseudo surgeons who counted their battle actions only by the number of arms and legs that they had cut off'. Nevertheless, the indications for amputation gradually evolved and, by 1795, it was widely accepted that there were five situations in which early amputation was judged appropriate: shattered bones; limbs partially or completely shot away; loss of considerable soft tissues or arterial damage; marked disorganisation of muscles, nerves and bone; and where joints were smashed. It was inevitable that many major wounds to arms and legs would meet at least one of these criteria.[16]

The surgical case for amputation was further elucidated by Larrey and other senior surgeons during the Napoleonic Wars. In simple terms, amputation had the great virtue of removing a dirty traumatised limb and replacing it with a relatively simple and clean surgical wound. Infection was still likely but at least this would only affect the healthy tissues at the amputation site rather than a gaping and complex wound inflicted by weapons. The technique used for amputation is graphically described by Larrey in his memoirs. Initially, he used several cuts of a knife in a circular manner to divide the skin and other superficial tissues. These were held back by an assistant whilst Larrey cut through the muscles down to the bone. This part of the operation often took four to five strokes of the knife. The actual amputation was completed by sawing through the bone and the immediate application of a ligature to the blood vessels. Saw marks on the femurs in amputation cases from Spanish Napoleonic War graves confirm that the amputation was performed from the front to back. Other assistants might help by compressing arteries, supporting the amputated limb or by passing knives and saw to the surgeon. With this team effort, major procedures could be performed at remarkable speed. At the Battle of Lützen, Larrey and colleagues effected the amputation of the mangled leg of General Latour-Maubourg in less than three minutes.[17]

The management of the resultant amputation stump was controversial. Many military surgeons of the era, notably the Prussians, Russians and British, tightly sutured the edges of the wound. Larrey fiercely opposed this practice as he considered it to lead inevitably to pain, infection and even gangrene. In support of this view, he quoted the unfortunate experience of the Saxon amputation cases during the 1813 campaign where there was a high rate of complications affecting the stumps and many deaths. He also criticised the British surgeons for their immediate closure of the wounds, the so-called 'healing by first intention', and the use of rigid adhesive bandages, '… this aspect of English surgery lacks the perfection one would expect from such well informed practitioners'.[18] Larrey realised that the wound edges did not need to be drawn tightly together and that good healing could be achieved with a simple dressing of linen supported with a roller-bandage. The wound was cleaned with water and benefited from free drainage of any blood or pus.

The precise site of amputation was also a matter for debate. Where the lower leg was amputated, then the most common location for the cut was about four inches below the knee (or, in anatomical terms, below the tuberosity of the tibia). However, in Egypt, Larrey showed that it was possible to operate very close to the knee joint itself and he made it a rule that it was better to take off the lower part of the leg too high than too low. He did not operate at the thigh unless there was significant damage to the knee. In a skeleton from the Austerlitz grave pit, a thigh amputation was performed only an inch from the top of the femur.[19]

Amputations through major joints, the hip and the shoulder, were particularly challenging. Hip amputations had been previously thought to be unjustified but, in the course of the Napoleonic Wars, there were a few surgeons either brave or foolhardy enough to attempt it where the leg had been almost completely destroyed. Surgeon Briot comments:

> If the amputation at the hip was rarely performed, this was less because of lack of opportunity than because there were few surgeons with the courage and sang froid to carry it out. I admit that, even among the most distinguished surgeons, few had the necessary quality to undertake to save three quarters of a man by removing the other quarter.

Larrey, not a man to shirk a challenge, attempted the procedure seven times in the course of the wars. He was unable to follow up most of the men after their operations but it appears likely that he succeeded in at least one and he retained his faith in this formidable surgery, '… however cruel an operation may be, it is an act of humanity in the hands of a surgeon'. Larrey also pioneered amputations of the arm at the shoulder joint – indeed he probably performed it more than any other surgeon. By disarticulating the limb at the shoulder, he ensured that all parts of the damaged arm were removed and also avoided the need to cut through bone and muscles. Out of fourteen soldiers on whom he performed the operation after Aspern-Essling and Wagram, twelve recovered completely. One of the fatalities was a *fusilier-grenadier* who became depressed by the thought that he would not be able to fend for himself and threw himself out of a window. Conversely, many soldiers regretted not having an amputation at the shoulder as the procedure through the arm itself was frequently painful and useless.[20]

The greatest of all controversies pertaining to amputation was its timing. In the 18th century, military surgeons were not only conservative in their use of amputation but they tended to delay it until the initial 'shock' of the trauma had resolved. Larrey and other experienced surgeons of the Napoleonic Wars, notably his British counterpart George Guthrie, strongly advocated early intervention with an operation within twenty-four hours. In his memoirs, Larrey first pointed out the extremely poor outcomes of amputations in the wars of the previous century; at Fontenoy in 1745, where the amputations were deferred, there were only thirty successful procedures out of three hundred. This contrasted markedly with the experience of the Napoleonic Wars where, with prompt amputation, Larrey expected three-quarters of his patients to fully recover. Early removal of limbs also brought a number of practical advantages on and around the battlefield. It minimised the length of stay in the pestilential hospitals, avoided subsequent aggravation of complicated wounds on crude transport and, if the field fell into enemy hands, French soldiers would already have received their definitive treatment and were less vulnerable to poor surgical care or neglect. Larrey defines eight specific indications for early amputation, all involving significant damage to the soft tissues, bones or joints of the limb. The French surgeon was the most famous proponent of early amputation but Guthrie was the most methodical. His impressive collection and presentation of surgical data from the Peninsular War and Waterloo conclusively shows a much lower mortality for early or 'primary' amputations on or around the field (around 20%) compared with delayed or 'secondary' operations in the general hospitals (around 40%).[21]

Although Larrey favoured early action, he was not extreme in his opinions and he clearly acknowledges a number of situations where it was sensible to delay surgery. He advocated caution where there was ill-defined gangrene or symptoms of tetanus or where the patient was systemically unwell with fever or diarrhoea. Larrey has been accused of being an over-zealous operator with too low a threshold for removing limbs but, in his defence, he makes it clear in his memoirs that there should be definite reasons for amputation and that this should not be regarded as a routine procedure for all severe limb injuries. Of the delayed amputations performed by the French surgeon Faure after Fontenoy, Larrey declares that four should have been amputated immediately but that the other six could have been spared such radical surgery. He concedes that it was often easier to conserve the arm than the leg.[22] Figures derived from Larrey's and Percy's writings and official bulletins suggest that after a typical major battle 5–10% of the French wounded underwent amputations.

The surgeons of the period tried hard to standardise the indications for amputation but, inevitably, it remained an imprecise decision with every wounded soldier presenting a slightly different problem. Percy's natural tendency was to try and preserve the limb but he understood that it was difficult to generalise. In his 1800 journal, written when he was serving with the Army of the Rhine, he agonises over the management of General Montroux who had a severe wound to the knee.

> This type of case is one of the most difficult in surgery and it is necessary to have great experience to master its complexities. Should one amputate? Is it possible to keep the limb? It is a difficult decision. One hesitates to amputate a largely healthy and vibrant leg but, on the other hand, in keeping it one risks losing the wounded man. Which way to turn? If swelling of the thigh soon leaves only the cruel option of amputation and one resorts to this, one is then open to the accusation of leaving it too late.[23]

Such painful dilemmas remain today. In a recent review of the care of wounded American troops in Iraq and Afghanistan, the author acknowledges that 'whether to amputate is one of the most difficult decisions in orthopaedic surgery'.[24] It is unsurprising that there were serious disagreements between the *Grande Armée*'s surgeons. Larrey and Yvan were at loggerheads on more than one occasion. Marshal Lannes was badly wounded in both legs at the Battle of Aspern-Essling and was carried in the arms of his soldiers to the nearby ambulance. Marbot recounts what happened next.

> We carried the marshal to one end of the bridge where the senior surgeons were ready to dress him. These gentlemen first held a secret conference in which they disagreed as to the best course of action. Doctor Larrey advised amputation of the leg which had a broken patella; another doctor, whose name I forget, wanted both legs to be amputated; finally, Doctor Yvan, from whom I learnt these details, opposed any amputation. This surgeon, who had known the marshal for a long time, believed that his good morale would give some chance of cure whilst an operation performed in such heat would inevitably consign him to his grave. Larrey was the head of the army's *service de santé* and his views thus carried the most weight: one of the marshal's legs was amputated![25]

Lannes bore the procedure with great courage and was later visited by Napoleon, a meeting immortalised in a famous painting by Emile Boutigny. Unfortunately, he eventually succumbed to the severity of his injuries. Maltese doctor Eugene Fenech recalls a similar episode before the Battle of Leipzig where Larrey and Yvan disagreed over the correct course of action in the Comte de Lomond who had been struck by a musket ball in the knee. Napoleon ordered his two senior surgeons to care for the aide-de-camp and was not amused by the discordant opinions on amputation. 'I have two of the most skilful military surgeons in the whole of Europe who both have my confidence! One wants to cut the leg off and the other wants to keep it.' On this occasion, in large part because it was he who reported to the Emperor, Yvan got his way and the Count kept his leg. Lomond made a full recovery and, only a month later, Yvan had the satisfaction of presenting his patient to Napoleon. The Count gallantly played his part by asking for a waltz with the Emperor's sister, Caroline.[26]

The accounts of amputation by soldiers and surgeons suggest that the agonising operation was often borne with remarkable bravery and that the amputees frequently showed great powers of recovery. Velite Billon recounts the behaviour of a sergeant of the *chasseurs à pied* of the Guard at Eylau. Placed on the operating table, the old soldier shouted out, 'Monsieur Larrey, to work!' and continued to smoke his pipe during the amputation of his leg. It was only when the saw reached the bone that he exhaled, let out a feeble '*Vive l'Empereur!*' and lost consciousness. Those watching were so moved that 'there was not a dry eye'. Some exhibited incredible toughness. Poussiergues, *chirurgien-major* of the 2ᵉ *Lanciers*, documents the case of Baron Sourd who suffered several deep sabre wounds to the face, chest and arms in the Waterloo campaign.

> The severity of these wounds necessitated the amputation of the lower third of his arm. Despite the weakening effect of the loss of a considerable amount of blood before and during the operation and despite the pain from the numerous bruises he had received from the hooves of the horses during the cavalry charges, Baron Sourd gradually recovered over the course of a month during which he remained at the head of his regiment. He made a journey on horseback of 450 miles, setting out only an hour after his amputation.

The surgeon attributed the cure to the courage and 'force of character' of his colonel.[27]

Those who had both legs amputated faced the most extreme challenge. This grim necessity was accepted by Larrey who advocated that any double amputation should be performed as soon as possible after the wounding. 'Of three men who had both legs amputated during the Battle of Wagram, the first only survived because, in his case, it was done within a few minutes of the injury.' Even with early intervention, the mortality from this radical intervention was high. General Moreau was hit in the right knee and left calf by French fire at the Battle of Dresden in 1813. He was initially believed dead but survived long enough to have both legs amputated by Russian doctors including the Tsar's personal surgeon. When, after the first amputation, he was informed of the need for the second leg to be also removed, he simply requested to smoke a cigar between the two operations. Sadly, he perished the next day after writing a letter of farewell to his wife and daughter. Not all soldiers showed such bravery and the sight of their comrades being mutilated not only by the enemy but also by their own surgeons must have starkly reminded many of their own vulnerability. The army's doctors were aware that multiple amputations were not good for morale. Near Burgos in Spain in 1808, Percy was annoyed to find a pile of arms and legs near the road in full view of the passing troops. They were the remnants of nine amputations performed by a *chirurgien-major* of the light infantry who had not bothered to bury or hide them.[28]

Most wounded men submitted to the amputations judged necessary by their doctors but some refused. This decision is generally portrayed by the narrator, usually the doctor or a fellow soldier, as a preference for death over life without a limb but it is likely that fear of the surgery was a factor in at least some cases. Resistance to amputation could be stubborn or even violent. Commandant de Lenthonnye received a severe gunshot wound in the arm and was forced to return to the hospital of Val-de-Grâce in Paris. The wound had originally been treated by placing coins over the entry and exit sites and when it was undressed in Paris the surrounding skin was yellow, there were plenty of maggots and a dreadful smell. The hospital doctor, Lacroix, removed the coins and decided that the arm must be amputated. Lenthonnye recalls the subsequent events.

> At the end of five days, at 4 o'clock in the afternoon, about thirty medical students arrived in my room, the first carrying a large box of surgical instruments. Master Lacroix, who was wearing a large apron, took my pulse and said to me that he was going to cut off my arm. 'Doctor,' I replied severely, 'If your young men see another operation after mine, I swear to you it will not be in this life.' The poor man flew into a dreadful rage; he pointed out that my wound was gangrenous and that death was inevitable if I did not have the operation. 'Doctor,' I said, 'I prefer death with my two arms than life with one.' Still angry, the doctor replied, 'What are you doing here if you do not let us care for you?' 'I will die doctor, but do not amputate. Don't you know doctor, that I am only twenty-five years old and that I have been made *chef de bataillon* on the field of battle. What importance does life have for me if I can no longer serve?' This only made him more irritated and he was stupid enough to say to me, 'Watch out or I will tie you up.' My haversack was near the head of my bed and my gunner gave it to me. There were two pistols in it. I took one and with an angry gesture, I replied to this brave man, 'I defy you to restrain me; the first who advances will be laid low!' – 'Very

well,' said the doctor, 'since you want to die, die! – I will not give you any care – the priest is close by!'

Despite this exchange, Lacroix did maintain an interest in the commandant's case and the soldier made a slow recovery over the next two years. This was not an isolated episode. When Surgeon d'Héralde suggested amputation to the colonel of the 64ᵉ Line he was forced to retreat under a barrage of insults. D'Héralde observes that the colonel 'was brave but without education'.[29]

It was less common for a soldier to request amputation and the doctor refuse it. Larrey relates the case of Baron Gruyer who, during the 1813 campaign, was wounded by a musket ball in the right arm and asked the surgeon to remove the limb. Larrey declined as he judged the injury not sufficiently severe and the general later recovered in Paris in the care of Larrey's nephew, another army surgeon. Not all the *Grande Armée*'s surgeons were as competent or confident as Larrey and some may have refused to amputate or perform other major surgery because of ignorance or diffidence. There was much learning on the job. Eugene Fenech joined the army in 1803 but only attempted his first amputation at the Battle of Busaco seven years later. It is not clear how well prepared he was to undertake this but he took the precaution of asking the advice of a *chirurgien-major* of a neighbouring regiment. Fenech decided to keep the operation as simple as possible, amputating the leg at a site where he had the least number of arteries to tie. His patient survived and was sent to the *Invalides* in Paris.[30]

With surgeons in short supply on and around the battlefields of Empire, it was inevitable that military officers and ordinary soldiers would be asked to assist with amputations. During the retreat from Russia, Aide-de-Camp Lejeune sat down on a tree trunk near to a young artilleryman who had just been wounded in the arm. Lejeune spotted two doctors passing and asked them to look at the wounded soldier.

> They did so, and at the first glance exclaimed, 'The arm must be amputated!' I asked the soldier if he felt he could bear it. 'Anything you like,' he answered stoutly. 'But,' said the doctor, 'there are only two of us to do it, so you, general, will be good enough to help us perform the operation.' Seeing that I was anything but pleased at the idea, they hastened to add that it would be enough if I just let the artilleryman lean against me. 'Sit back to back with him and you will see nothing of the operation.' I agreed and placed myself in the required position. I think the operation seemed longer to me than it did to the patient.

Lejeune heard the sound of the saw but the operation was indeed out of his vision. After it had finished, he shared some precious wine with the artilleryman who then promptly got up and with the words, 'It is still a long way to Carcassonne', set off at a good pace. At least this wounded soldier had the attention of two *officiers de santé*. Many were left to fend for themselves and some even attempted to manage their own wounds. In an extreme example, a severely wounded Russian officer, left lying in a hole on the battlefield of Friedland, used his sabre to cut away the remaining pieces of skin and muscle which still attached his shattered lower leg to his knee.[31]

For the Napoleonic soldier who survived amputation there was the souvenir of a wooden leg. In October 1806, early in the Jena campaign, Percy saw a crude wagon full of wooden legs and crutches. He says that the troops laughed at it but he adds, '... they should have been spared this spectacle; why bring all these frightening instruments along at the start of a campaign when they are hardly likely to be required until the end?' A regulation of March 1810 formalised the right of a soldier deprived of his limb to a wooden prosthesis. Two of the most famous prosthetic devices are today on display in the army museum at *Les Invalides*. General Daumesnil, who lost his leg at Wagram, wore a light and sophisticated wooden leg which allowed some movement at the knee. When asked to surrender part of Paris to the allies in 1814, he allegedly replied: 'I will give you Vincennes when you give me back my leg.' On display in the same cabinet is an elaborate artificial shoulder manufactured out of steel and wood which was worn by General d'Abouville who was also wounded at Wagram and had an amputation at the joint performed by Larrey.[32]

Wounds to other parts of the body brought their own specific problems and potential solutions. Significant chest injuries often caused the recipients considerable distress. Percy describes soldiers who were 'in dreadful anguish ... short of breath, unable to lie down and forced to remain sitting, having difficulty in spitting up fluids with most painful anxiety and the strain showing on their faces'. In the Revolutionary period it had been standard practice to leave penetrating chest wounds open with the hope that any bleeding would stop spontaneously. Larrey pioneered the simple closure of the wound with the patient nursed lying on the affected side. If an effusion of blood or purulent fluid (empyema) accumulated in the chest, he simply evacuated this by making an incision in the muscles of the chest wall. Where he was convinced that there was a foreign body, he was prepared to try and extract it as he believed that it would otherwise cause pain and fever and ultimately prove fatal. This might involve removal of one of the ribs. Larrey's memoirs contain examples of surprisingly invasive surgery. In 1810 he managed the case of a 30-year-old *chasseur* of the Imperial Guard who had plunged a knife into his own chest after being wrongly accused of a misdemeanour. The man was cold, breathing laboriously, spitting blood and, from all accounts, near to death. The surgeon deduced that he had a pericardial effusion, a collection of fluid in the sac which surrounds the heart. Realising that this would be rapidly fatal, he operated immediately. Cutting through the muscles and ribs he located the distended pericardial sac and punctured it with a probe allowing the offending fluid to escape. During the operation, Larrey actually felt the apex of the patient's heart with his finger. The soldier tolerated this radical surgery poorly, being 'in great agony and ready to expire', but over the next few days he made some recovery. He died three weeks later from a probable infectious disease. Ambitious procedures such as this were the exception and they would not have been attempted by ordinary army surgeons.[33]

At the start of the Revolutionary Wars, gunshot wounds of the abdomen were usually managed aggressively with surgical removal of the ball and closure of the wounds. The results were disastrous with the demise of the victim from infection of the wound and the abdominal contents (peritonitis). It was eventually concluded that men with abdominal injuries were better off left alone. This applied for much of the Napoleonic era although Larrey did recommend selective intervention in soldiers after intestinal and bladder trauma. He thought that abdominal wounds from sword, bayonet or lance had a worse prognosis than gunshot injuries from which spontaneous recovery was possible. Where the intestine was damaged by cold steel the lacerated bowel was either stitched to the adjacent peritoneum to try and avoid the contents spilling into the abdomen or the ends of the intestine were carefully sutured back together. Bladder wounds, only likely when the organ was at least partly filled with urine and therefore a target, were often treated with catheterisation. Percy favoured a conservative approach to abdominal wounds just as he did for limb injuries. Such inaction had notable successes. General de Ségur, wounded in the lower abdomen at Somosierra in Spain in 1808, caused his surgeons some anxiety. When, seven days later, Napoleon asked Percy why the musket ball had not been removed, the surgeon predicted that nature would be the best cure and that the missile would eventually be discharged through the anus. This happened; Ségur fully recovered and lived another sixty-five years.[34]

Surgical practice in wounds of the head and neck mirrored abdominal wound surgery in that some of the more alarming procedures of the Revolutionary Era were applied more advisedly. Trephining (or trepanning), the removal of pieces of skull, was popular in the mid 1790s and was performed indiscriminately for various head injuries and skull fractures. Larry recommended it only when a foreign body had penetrated into the skull, where the broken skull was pressing onto the brain or there was a collection of fluid under the injury. Percy supported this selective use of the trephine, criticising those who rejected it completely. Not even Larrey was willing to dig deep into the brain for foreign bodies but he did perform some remarkably complicated surgery of facial and neck wounds and he also described the use of tracheostomy to facilitate breathing.[35]

Many soldiers died instantly at the moment of wounding or succumbed during operations but others fell prey to the more insidious complications of the wound and subsequent surgery. As much medical treatment was given with scant attention to basic hygiene – the Napoleonic Wars preceded the discovery of antisepsis by sixty years – infection of weaponry and surgery wounds was almost universal. Infection was so routine an occurrence that it was regarded as part of the normal healing process; hence its first appearance was often described as 'laudable pus'. Surgical accounts of the period make frequent allusions to the signs of infection in wounds and surrounding skin, cellulitis being often referred to as 'erisypelas'. In unsanitary conditions, it was not unusual for insects to gain access to wounds, particularly maggots from bluebottle flies. Tyras de Chamberet saw the wounded in Spain being tortured by 'insects of all shapes and colours'. Despite the misery they caused, the horror of the infestations and the intolerable itching, maggots may have cleaned the affected area and stimulated healing.

Other afflictions were unequivocally sinister. Tetanus was well recognised and associated with a very high death rate. This disease, now known to be caused by a bacterium which enters the wound from the soil, was variously attributed to 'violent passions', damp or a sudden change in temperature. Larrey gives the best contemporary account of tetanus, describing the characteristic contraction of the muscles. 'In complete tetanus, the limbs become so rigid and the whole body so stiff that it may be lifted by one of the extremes without bending.' He identified a more chronic form that might be compatible with survival and an acute form that was almost always fatal, the unfortunate victim having increasing difficulty in swallowing and breathing. Treatments were eclectic and unsuccessful. Ingested substances, ranging from mercury to castor oil, made little difference to the course of the disease, at most providing temporary palliation. When tetanus struck following the Battle of Danzig in 1813, Larrey resorted to cautery and amputation of the injured limbs and believed that he had saved a few lives.[36]

Perhaps the most prevalent discrete infection of wounded and surgical patients was a syndrome called 'hospital gangrene (la pourriture d'hôpital)'. This unpleasant disease was, in modern terminology, a bacterial infection carried between cases on the hands of medical and nursing staff and on instruments and dressings. Its appearance in a hospital caused near panic. At the hospital in Tolosa in Spain, 100 out of 130 wounded succumbed in two months, whilst at the Hôpital St Louis in Paris in 1814 there were 500 victims per month. Percy wrote an article on the condition and he describes the previously healthy wound becoming brown and foul smelling. In severe and progressive cases there was considerable destruction of skin and muscles with swelling of the limb and deterioration of the patient who became fevered and delirious. Percy opposed a contagious aetiology but, in the course of the wars, a number of his colleagues in the *Grande Armée* argued cohesively that this was a disease that could be spread by contaminated instruments, dressings and clothes. In a heroic attempt to conclusively prove his point, a young army surgeon campaigning in Spain, Alexandre François Ollivier, inoculated his arm with pus taken from an affected wound. Several days later, an abscess appeared which was fortunately cured with a combination of cauterisation and camphor impregnated dressings.

Ollivier, in a series of surprisingly modern recommendations, supported the isolation of hospital gangrene cases and the careful cleaning of instruments and dressings. He stressed the importance of the surgeon washing his hands between tending unhealthy and healthy wounds. Believing his significant contribution to have been overlooked by the authorities, he later indulged in a prolonged war of words with Percy whom he regarded as the chief culprit in the upper echelons of the *service de santé*. As for tetanus, treatment of hospital gangrene lacked consistency with cauterisation and amputation the last resort. Mortality figures varied widely in different epidemics.[37]

Although there are references to dehydration and the 'shock of the wound' in contemporary surgical accounts, there was little real understanding of the full implications of these states. The administration of water to wounded on the battlefield was designed more to palliate thirst than to allay the underlying damage that dehydration caused. Similarly, 'shock', by which is meant the condition arising from the loss of a significant amount of blood, was explicitly detailed but inadequately acknowledged. Larrey recounts the case of a man suffering from the 'shock of a ball', the blood loss causing, 'his countenance to be pale, his pulse scarcely perceptible'. Later, he notes that such 'commotion or shock' was greater when the patient was standing erect or when the lower limb was injured. However, he tends to underestimate the importance of blood loss from both wounds and surgery – when justifying amputation at the hip he writes, '… as to the loss of blood we have nothing to fear from it.'[38]

Because they failed to understand the fundamental causes of shock, infection and other wound complications, the attempts of army surgeons to prevent these outcomes were misguided and harmful. They resorted to 'antiphlogistic' remedies, a treatment philosophy which will be described in greater detail in the following chapter on disease. In essence, it was believed that if impurities could be forcibly removed from the blood then the surgical patient would be less likely to suffer the harmful effects of inflammation and fever. Accordingly, soldiers who had been wounded and who had received surgery were subjected to regimes of drugs designed to induce vomiting (emetics) and diarrhoea (purgatives) and were also prescribed special diets and bled. There are innumerable examples of these futile interventions in the memoirs of Larrey and Percy. Referring to the management of General Maison who was wounded in the foot in Spain, Percy comments:

I have given him a purgative in some chicken water and this has produced a dozen stools; he had a fever and was much agitated; he is much
more peaceful now. It would be better if all our wounded could be gently
purged; their wounds would only improve; but there is nobody to either
give them a bedpan or empty the commodes.

Elsewhere, Percy employs emetics and specific diets. Larrey also issued a
variety of purging medicines, particularly in patients with fever. After one
such administration he approvingly notes that, 'this was followed by copious effortless vomiting and abundant very foetid bowel movements'.[39]
The widespread practice of bleeding may have been less unpleasant but
it was more dangerous to men who had already lost a substantial amount
of blood from their original injury and surgery. Its use well illustrates that
the *Grande Armée*'s doctors had no appreciation of the true nature of haem-
orrhagic shock. The blood was taken from a convenient superficial vein
or extracted with leeches. Bleeding was especially favoured in wounds of
the chest – in Percy's *Manuel de Chirurgie d'Armée*, a 40-year-old captain
with three thoracic wounds is documented as having undergone nineteen bleedings in one week. Larrey was not a great advocate but he also
practised it in situations where it was only likely to do harm, for instance,
after amputations at the hip. Soldiers had great faith in the powers of
bleeding. General Pépé, wounded in the head during the Italian campaign
of 1799, expresses the common view: 'Fortunately, my wounds were not
very serious and I believe that the copious loss of blood they occasioned
tended greatly to prevent their having any serious result.' At Borodino,
the wounded French General Bonamy was taken prisoner by the Russians
and pleaded with them, 'For God's sake, bleed me or I shall die'.[40]
Some attempts to heal wounded men hint at desperation. Larrey
famously wrapped Marshal Lannes in a warm skin from a freshly slaughtered sheep after he had suffered extensive bruising from his fallen horse
in the Peninsula. Where skins were unavailable, warm horse manure
could be applied instead.[41] It is easy to be dismissive of such medieval
treatments. This reasonable scepticism should not, however, obscure the
significant advances in military surgery that occurred during the wars.
Many overly aggressive and complicated procedures were abandoned
and there was a greater emphasis on simple and rapid intervention. In
the context of the medical knowledge of the period and the dreadful
conditions of war the results obtained by Napoleonic surgeons were
surprisingly good. We have seen that the mortality rate from amputation
varied between 20% and 40% depending on the nature of the injury, the
skill of the surgeon and the timing of the procedure; to express this more
optimistically, we can say that 60–80% of soldiers survived their amputations. These mortality figures compare remarkably well with the wars of
the later 19th century and even the 20th century. Data from the United

States Department of Defense for the lethality of significant war wounds in American troops includes a figure of 39% for the Napoleonic conflict of 1812 – within the range of the known likelihood of death after different types of amputation. Mortality figures for the American Civil War, the two World Wars, and the Vietnam War remain surprisingly consistent between 21% and 33%.[42] These figures are very approximate and are not necessarily directly comparable. They are not limited to severe wounds of the limbs but, particularly for the later conflicts, are likely to include chest, abdominal and head wounds. Medical advances such as anaesthesia, antibiotics and blood transfusion may have been neutralised by the greater lethality of weaponry. Nevertheless, the best results obtained by Larrey and his colleagues are a testimony to the skill of the surgeons and the fortitude of the soldiers of the Napoleonic era. Only in the very recent fighting in Iraq and Afghanistan since 2001 has the aggressive use of 'forward surgical teams' and mobile hospitals reduced the proportion of deaths in those severely injured in combat to around ten percent.

Notes

1. Vess, D M, *Medical Revolution in France 1789–1796*, p. 13; Ackerknecht, E H, *Medicine at the Paris Hospital 1794–1848*, pp. 141, 146.
2. Lemaire, J-F, *Les blessés dans les Armées Napoléoniennes*, pp. 233–4.
3. Baldet, M, *La Vie Quotidienne dans les Armées de Napoléon*, p. 167.
4. Milleliri, J-M, *Médecins et Soldats pendant l'expédition d'Égypte (1798–1799)*, p. 177; Roos, H de, *Avec Napoléon en Russie*, p. 230; Howard, J E, *Letters and Documents of Napoleon The Rise to Power*, p. 346; Percy, Baron, *Journal des Campagnes de Baron Percy*, p. 240.
5. La Flize, Dr, *Souvenirs de la Moskowa par un chirurgien de la Garde Impériale*, p. 421.
6. Marbot, Baron de, *Mémoires de Général Baron de Marbot*, Vol. I, p. 356; Pigeard, A, *L'Armée de Napoléon*, p. 186; Larrey, D J, *Mémoires de Chirurgie Militaire et Campagnes 1787–1840*, p. 637.
7. Lemaire, p. 89.
8. Pigeard, p. 184.
9. Larrey, pp. 654, 651; Percy, p. 239; Roos, p. 182.
10. Vess, p. 122; Brice, Docteur and Bottet, Capitaine, *Le Corps de Santé Militaire en France*, p. 243; Lemaire, p. 182.
11. Percy, pp. 198, 213; Fenech, E, *Mémoires d'un Officier de Santé Maltais dans l'Armée Française*, p. 163; Dible, J H, *Napoleon's Surgeon*, p. 244; Vess, p. 121.
12. Larrey, p. 588.
13. Larrey, p. 62; Vess, p. 123; Dible, p. 10.
14. Horácková, L and Vargová, L, *Bone remains from a common grave pit from the Battle of Austerlitz*, p. 8; Dible, p. 136; Percy, p. 355; Exteberria, F,

Surgery in the Spanish War of Independence (1807–1813); between Desault and Lister, p. 33.

15. Fenech, p. 166; Horácková, p. 9.
16. Vess, pp. 128–30.
17. Exteberria, p. 33; Dible, p. 215.
18. Dible, p. 303.
19. Horácková, p. 10.
20. Lemaire, p. 257; Dible, pp. 130, 123; Larrey, p. 660.
21. Larrey, pp. 431–47; Howard, M, *Wellington's Doctors. The British Army Medical Services in the Napoleonic Wars*, pp. 234–5.
22. Larrey, pp. 452–6.
23. Percy, p. 60.
24. Gawande, A, *Casualties of War – Military care for the wounded from Iraq and Afghanistan*.
25. Marbot, Vol. II, p. 202.
26. Fenech, p. 86.
27. Damamme, J-C, *Les Soldats de la Grande Armée*, p. 260; Lemaire, p. 73.
28. Larrey, p.649; Damamme, pp. 262–3; Percy, p. 407.
29. Baldet, pp. 170–1; d'Héralde, J-B, *Mémoires d'un Chirurgien de la Grande Armée*, p. 149.
30. Dible, p. 229; Fenech, p. 51.
31. Lejeune, Baron, *Memoirs of Baron Lejeune Aide-de-Camp to Marshals Berthier, Davout and Oudinot*, Vol. II, pp. 233–4; Damamme, p. 259.
32. Percy, p. 77; Huard, P, *Sciences Médecine Pharmacie de la Révolution à l'Empire (1789–1815)*, p. 75.
33. Ducoulombier, H, *Le Baron P-F Percy. Un chirurgien de la Grande Armée*, p. 159; Dible, pp. 253–4; Larrey, p. 703.
34. Vess, p. 127; Dible, pp. 260–72; Ducoulombier, p. 158.
35. Vess, p.124; Dible, pp. 245, 253; Percy, p. 262.
36. Tyrbas de Chamberet, J, *Mémoires d'un Médecin Militaire*, p. 95; Larrey, p. 136; Dible, p. 213.
37. Ducoulombier, pp. 369–83.
38. Larrey, pp. 289, 297, 653.
39. Howard, M, p. 148; Percy, p. 440; Dible, p. 247.
40. Ducoulombier, p. 160; Larrey, p. 299; Pépé, General, *Memoirs of General Pépé (1783–1815)*, p. 57; Brett-James, A, *1812. Eye-witness accounts of Napoleon's defeat in Russia*, p. 138.
41. Larrey, p. 583; Ducoulombier, p. 217.
42. Gawande, p. 2472.

CHAPTER IX

Disease: The Greatest Enemy

Despite living through an era of almost unceasing conflict, the citizens and soldiers of Revolutionary and Napoleonic France were much more likely to succumb to disease than meet a violent death. The ideal conditions for the spread of myriad little understood infectious diseases were amply provided both in the towns and villages of civilian life and in the garrisons and cantonments of the army. Even in Paris, the extolled capital of Empire, squalor and poverty were all pervading. One contemporary observer wrote of the poorer areas:

> The extreme overcrowding of residents in certain quarters and the stench of the household animals blended with that of excrement, decaying animal cadavers and rotting food all create extensive atmospheric pollution in which people live and eat. The fetid air is a visible haze that generally covers Paris and there are districts over which it is particularly thick.

Those visiting Paris from afar were shocked at what they saw. There was a serious lack of clean water, most Parisians taking their chances with the polluted Seine. 'You are barbarians,' Stendhal fumed at the post-revolutionary citizens of the city, 'your streets stink aloud … this comes of the absurd idea of turning them into a main sewer'.[1]

These primitive conditions were commonplace throughout France and they destroyed the population's health. There were catastrophic levels of infant mortality. More than a quarter of newborns died in the first year of life and, of the survivors, more than one in five would die in the next four years. On the eve of the Revolution, overall life expectancy was 28 years with those who survived the dangerous first few years expecting to live up to around 44 years. Many deaths were attributable to infectious diseases including tuberculosis, typhus, malaria, smallpox and influenza. Although couched in obscure contemporary terminology, records of causes of death in the Paris hospitals in the years 1809–16 give an insight into the major medical problems affecting the poor sections of the city's inhabitants. We find a high incidence of 'malignant putrid fevers', particularly for the year 1814 when typhus was rife in the region. Large numbers of deaths are more obscurely attributed to 'sudden and apoplectic causes'. Tables of hospital admission statistics detail diseases such as rheumatism and gout, nervous affections, epilepsy, cancers, heart failure, jaundice, scurvy, skin and eye disorders, venereal diseases and drunkenness. Despite this depressing social background and a catalogue of diseases fed by dirt and deprivation, the Revolutionary and Napoleonic years witnessed not only a real growth in the population of France but an increase in life expectancy. This improvement might be attributed to a combination of amelioration of poor sanitary conditions and medical advances such as vaccination.[2]

The overcrowding and filth of civilian life was mirrored and even magnified when the Revolutionary armies took to the field. During the siege of Verdun in 1792, the fearful lack of sanitation caused such a stench that 'one often saw people seized with convulsions and sickness or even suffocated while crossing the streets'.[3] The mortality rates in Revolutionary battles were relatively low and it was infectious disease which cut down the young, patriotic citizen soldiers. As is generally the case in military history, secondary accounts of the wars underestimate or completely ignore the significant impact of diseases which killed in such large numbers as to seriously impair the functioning of armies and change the course of campaigns.

The military hospitals were filling up before serious fighting had begun. In the summer of 1792, up to a quarter of men were suffering from syphilis or gonorrhoea and, more alarmingly, there was an increasing incidence of typhus and dysentery. Sick rates varied from 21% in the Army of the North to 12% in the relatively healthy Army of the Rhine. At the Battle of Valmy in September, the battle casualties appear almost negligible compared with the heavy toll exacted by dysentery which affected both French and Prussian armies. Reports filed with the Council of Health from selected military hospitals in France and Belgium during the winter of 1792–3 show that the incidence of 'fever' increased from 23% of admissions in November to almost 80% in the following February and March. 'Fever' was a general term used to describe a wide range of infectious diseases but it will have included a significant number of cases of typhus and dysentery, diseases which, as will be discussed later, thrived in the cold and wet when the troops huddled together. The mortality from the recorded hospital fever cases during this period was 375 deaths in 1,752 patients or 21%. Further figures are available for the military hospitals at Landau and Metz for June to October 1793. The mortality from fevers (945 deaths in 14,901 cases: 6%) was significantly lower than in the previous winter but, at least from the evidence of these hospital admissions, the impact of disease remained much greater than that of wounds (ninety-five deaths in 4,360 cases: 2%). Venereal and skin diseases were significant causes of debility and misery but they caused few deaths. These broad patterns of disease persisted throughout the remainder of the Revolutionary Wars. Typhus was rampant in 1798–9, killing 14,000 men in the hospitals of Nice alone, whilst malaria wreaked havoc in the army of Holland and in garrisons in Italy. Venereal diseases were ubiquitous. One soldier commented of the Italian women, 'they are beautiful and not cruel, but when they give you a present it is often for a long time'.[4]

Before considering the diseases which affected the *Grande Armée*, it is necessary to understand something of the contemporary views on the classification, cause and management of diseases in general. Classification at the end of the 18th and beginning of the 19th century was far removed from the disease nomenclature recognised today and it now appears over-involved and obscure. Many French physicians of the period relied on the complicated system devised by Philippe Pinel in which there were five classes of diseases: fevers, phlegmasias (inflammations), haemorrhages, neuroses and organic lesions. The ancient authors had subdivided fevers into bilious, mucous, putrid, malignant and pestilential types. Pinel renamed the fevers as angiotenic, meningogastric, adenomeningeal, adynamic, ataxic and adenonervous. This revision implies no greater insight and, although this terminology does appear in the writings of army doctors, we are often more reliant on their descriptions of disease symptoms and signs to retrospectively identify modern disease equivalents. More basic contemporary terms included typhus, intermittent fever (malaria), and simple continued and remittent fever, the latter two entities being a mix of infectious diseases such as typhoid and dysentery. The potential confusion in these various systems is well captured by Larrey's description of the typhus epidemic in Brünn after Austerlitz, '[a disease] which we recognised as a malignant, nervous and putrid hospital fever (adynamico-ataxic) or contagious typhus of the old nosologists'.[5]

The causation of disease remained controversial with more modern views of 'contagious' aetiologies gaining ground at the expense of medieval 'miasmatic' theories. Many army doctors continued to believe that the majority of diseases were caused by 'miasma' or 'miasmata', invisible poisons in the air which were exuded from rotting animal and vegetable material, the soil and standing water. Thus, in a report concerning the fever epidemic in the Army of the Rhine in 1793, Physician Jean Jomard blames the disease on the housing of soldiers in humid barracks during the winter, 'with little ventilation, the stale air prompts a putrid miasma and, when you add to that the bad quality of the majority of soldiers, you find the cause soon enough'. Both Larrey and Desgenettes relied heavily on the miasmatic model to explain the diseases of Egypt. Larrey alludes to the winds being 'loaded with the putrid effluvia of animal and vegetable substances decomposed by the heat in the lakes', whilst Desgenettes invokes the 'pernicious exhalations of animal carcasses and excreta' as being a significant cause of mortality. In Spain, Physician Lixon

uses almost identical terminology to explain the local maladies. Closely
linked to these miasmatic theories was the view that climate and the lie
of the land both played significant roles in determining the types and
incidence of diseases. In his review of the diseases affecting the *Grande
Armée* in Prussia and Poland in 1806 and 1807 Physician Gilbert asserts:
'One cannot give a good history of the diseases which are epidemic in
an army without having first described the medical topography of the
theatre of war and the state of the atmosphere whilst the army was in the
field.' The direction of the wind was believed to have special significance.
In Egypt, Desgenettes claimed that the warm southerly wind favoured
the plague and that the cold northerly wind suppressed it. Percy makes
very frequent references to the weather and its influence on disease in his
journal; in an entry for 6 December 1806 in Poland we find: 'The night has
been quite warm; there is a dominant north-west wind; it rains little; there
are increasing cases of cough, catarrh and fluxes.' Elsewhere, he blames
sudden outbreaks of disease on a change in the temperature.[6]

In many contemporary medical writings, there is an acknowledgement
that the epidemics afflicting the army were, in all likelihood, caused by
an unfortunate combination of factors and that they could be predicted.
Percy, still in Poland, writes:

> If we remain more than fifteen days in this country the army risks being
> attacked by an epidemic as the air is unhealthy, the terrain malarious and
> the water disgusting. There are bodies of men and horses rotting in the
> open air and all is generally miserable.[7]

Even so, Percy judged that the troops were better exposed to the vagaries of
an inhospitable country than being admitted to the army's hospitals where
rampant disease was even more likely. Not all the *Grande Armée*'s soldiers
were at equal risk of falling sick. Lixon writes of the troops in Spain:

> The legions are formed of young men who, having scarcely left home
> and not even having finished their growth, are put on the road, deprived
> of their normal habits and exposed to a new climate and all types of
> privation ... in the hospitals we see the same individuals being admitted
> and discharged until many of them die.[8]

It was obvious to the more acute medical observers that some afflictions, for
instance many types of fever and hospital gangrene, were somehow being
passed from one man to another – in other words, they were 'contagious'.
At the two extremes were those doctors in civilian and military spheres
who vigorously proposed this theory, the 'contagionists', and those who
preferred a more traditional miasmatic version of disease causation, the
'anticontagionists'. Of course, it was difficult to prove contagion as the

doctors of the period had no knowledge of micro-organisms such as bacteria and viruses and their carriers such as mosquitoes, body lice and rats. Despite this ignorance, many were drawn to the contagion theory by their daily experiences. In the military hospitals of Poland, Physician Gilbert saw dysentery spread quickly from one sick man to his neighbour and witnessed *officiers de santé* also falling victim. He ordered the isolation of all dysentery patients. In the West Indies, Moreau de Jonnès, a French staff officer and later a renowned statistician, comments:

> No one doubts the contagiousness of yellow fever ... Several doctors assured everyone that the disease was not communicable ... but even those who voiced this opinion took all possible precautions.

When Larrey diagnosed the outbreak of bubonic plague in Egypt, he wrote: 'One cannot deny that the plague is epidemic and contagious.' Desgenettes, who notoriously inoculated himself with plague to improve the soldiers' morale, had no real illusions as to its true nature, stating in his *Histoire Médicale de l'Armée d'Orient* that the disease was 'evidently contagious'. In practice, some army doctors chose to embrace the contagion theory while hanging on to part of their previous beliefs. Larrey confusingly asserts that, in Egypt: 'There is no doubt that these exhalations [i.e. miasmata] that are more abundant during the prevalence of south-east winds, contributed not a little to the production of contagious disease.' Soldiers could see diseases spreading among their comrades and they feared for their own lives. The authorities of invaded countries expressed dismay at the prospect of diseases being communicated from the *Grande Armée* to the local population, a clear indication that they believed contagion rather than miasmata to be the major cause. When the Majorcan Junta learnt of the decision to dump French prisoners of war on the neighbouring island of Cabrera in 1809 they were shocked as they knew 'the horrors of a single immigrant suffering from contagion'.[9]

Treatment of disease depended on the 'antiphlogistic' regimes also used in wounds and after surgery. In simple terms, the rationale of what was often debilitating and harmful treatment was the removal of 'impurities' which were presumed to be present in the blood and other body fluids. Different diseases were managed with different combinations of drugs and other methods but this basic philosophy remained constant. Bleeding was performed to a greater or lesser degree by most army doctors. Blood could be removed from an accessible vein with a lancet, sometimes with the addition of a heated 'cupping' glass to encourage the flow, or by the application of leeches. When Jean Jomard treated typhoid fever in the Army of the Rhine in 1793, he advocated bleeding to relieve inflammation and improve circulation and recommended a second blood-letting ('venesection') if the fever persisted.[10] Doctors also had great faith in water treatments either applied crudely or in more elaborate bathing rituals. The warm water showers enjoyed by the wounded at the springs at Baden in 1799 were harmless, something which cannot be said of the more violent 'cold affusions'. Larrey describes the use of cold water in a soldier in Austria in 1809.

> The cold bath recommended by some physicians was used. The first two applications of it produced a most distressing sensation and the patient derived no benefit. When he saw the bath a third time, he felt an invincible dread of water and refused to go into it; but he was covered with a sheet and plunged into the water without suspecting it.[11]

This description well illustrates the potentially brutal nature of antiphlogistic treatment. In further drastic efforts to rid the body of invisible disease causing agents, army doctors applied irritant substances to the skin to create blisters ('vesicatories') and resorted to cauterisation as described in wound management. Numerous drugs were used but these were largely those of the 18th-century pharmacopoeia and there were few real advances in medicines – indeed many of the remedies were either inert or poisonous. Hospital inventories show a mixture of benign herbal and vegetable drugs and more aggressive mineral compounds. The military hospital at Brussels in 1793 stocked wine, olive oil, rhubarb, senna and soda but also lead oxide, zinc sulphide and mercury. There was great disagreement over the correct use of these drugs and a tendency to administer many agents simultaneously to achieve a maximum effect. Senior army physicians and surgeons suggested that this might be doing more harm than good. Desgenettes was worried at what he saw in Egypt.

> We should not be afraid to say that medicines are endlessly abused; soldiers tend to like the more aggressive remedies but it is the duty of those who are looking after them to refuse useless drugs; heroic treatment regimes should only be used in difficult circumstances. It is essential to decry those who overload the sick with their polypharmacy.

Percy also favoured a more gentle approach with a predilection for natural substances such as herbal teas and other decoctions. He believed that nature should be supported rather than oppressed with what he described as 'medical poisons'. He also criticised the excessive use of other types of antiphlogistic intervention, attacking German surgeons for their careless employment of bleeding and blistering in pneumonia.[12]

With so much theory and so little real understanding, it is unsurprising that *officiers de santé* sometimes argued over the best drug treatments for their patients. Eugene Fenech recalls an incident in Spain in 1808 where a pharmacist and surgeon had a disagreement over the optimal emetic to administer to a sick soldier. The argument became so heated as to attract the attention of some drunken hussars and the doctors had to flee to avoid injury. Drugs were often in short supply and, in these circumstances, *officiers de santé* prescribed what was to hand. This was certainly the case in Russia where Heinrich Roos was forced to purchase from the local apothecaries. Ironically, this may have helped his patients as the more dangerous inorganic compounds were unavailable and he used the regiment's cooking pots to brew up concoctions of mint, camomile, lemon balm and elder.[13]

A few of the drugs of the early 19th century were efficacious and have survived the test of time. We still use senna as a laxative, ipecacuanha as an emetic and opiates for their analgesic and sedating effects. Quinine, which was derived from Peruvian bark, remains a vital drug in the treatment of malaria. For much of the wars, quinine was in short supply in France as the Royal Navy intercepted shipments from America. In desperation, doctors substituted willow bark, arsenic and sawdust. This situation was exacerbated by ruthless profiteers. Physician Laurillard-Fallot reports that in Portugal in 1810 a guard had to be placed next to an apothecary's shop to protect the quinine, an act he much approved of, 'What a philanthropic measure! What care for the sick!' Ordinary soldiers were keen to receive treatments like quinine, which they could see were effective in intermittent fevers, but they often appear sceptical of their doctors' other therapeutic efforts. Elzéar Blaze repeatedly lampoons his regimental surgeon's attempts to cure his comrades but the following excerpt does have the ring of truth. The surgeon addresses a sick officer:

> 'Listen carefully. The first is a potion of which you must take a teaspoonful every half-hour; the second is a herbal infusion; swallow a soupspoon of it every quarter-hour. If you feel the effects of the teaspoon dose passing away quickly, you can take the soupspoon dose sooner. If, however, the soupspoon dose upsets your stomach you may delay the second teaspoon dose. The remedy is infallible and is indispensable for a patient in your condition. Everything depends on the regularity with which you take it. Remember now what I've told you.'
> 'But, doctor, it is so devilishly complicated. I'll never be able to remember.'
> 'Oh, well,' said the doctor, forgetting his role as charlatan and reverting to his every-day self, 'do it or don't do it, you'll neither get better or worse – all that it's good for is to keep up the patient's morale.'

Disillusioned with the official treatments on offer, many army veterans devised their own pet cures some of which were literally 'kill or cure'. Gunpowder was widely regarded as a panacea.[14]

Having considered the contemporary views on disease, we can now address the specific diseases which afflicted Napoleon's armies in their far-flung and prolonged campaigns. It is appropriate to start in the West Indies as the islands were a death trap for European troops, almost all perishing from yellow fever, malaria and other infections. Yellow fever is caused by a virus and spread by mosquitoes. If the French soldier was lucky, he developed only mild symptoms such as fever and headache which lasted less than a week. Unfortunately, many developed more severe manifestations including jaundice and vomiting of blood (often black in colour) and then delirium, coma and death. Staff Officer Moreau de Jonnès has left a grim account of the yellow fever epidemic which struck the French forces in Martinique in 1802. In the first three months half of the army were lost to the disease. Because the real cause was not understood and it appeared to strike everywhere, almost every activity was implicated in its relentless march. In Moreau de Jonnès' opinion, one only had to,

> ... expose oneself at length to the hot sunshine, be caught in a draught when perspiring, neglect to change one's rain-drenched clothes, undertake a taxing journey on foot or on horseback, breathe the burning air in churches during the great religious ceremonies, be bled needlessly, take excessive baths or drugs, be frightened, depressed, homesick, agitated by a passion such as rage or love or simply experience some strong stimulation that might favour the development of sickness.

He believed that yellow fever first attacked soldiers and sailors who were given to excess and who frequented places of 'ill-fame' and that it then selected the officers, particularly those with onerous duties. Terrorised soldiers deserted their posts and bivouacked in the open, refusing to return to barracks. Officers noted for their bravery suddenly refused to carry out hospital inspections. Superstitious beliefs and paranoid rumours proliferated; it was alleged that the water supply had been deliberately poisoned. The *officiers de santé* tried to fight yellow fever with antiphlogistic regimes but Moreau de Jonnès cuttingly remarks that, 'the number and variety of remedies shows only too clearly that they are useless'.[15]

A similar catastrophe unfolded on St Domingo (Haiti) in the same year. Napoleon had sent an initial force of 20,000 troops under the command of his brother-in-law, General Victor-Emmanuel Le Clerc, to seize the island from the local pretender. Le Clerc's correspondence to his powerful relative was soon dominated not by military events but by the destructive effects of yellow fever. Within three months, he had lost a third of his men to the epidemic.

> A man cannot work hard here without risking his life and it is quite impossible for me to remain here for more than six months ... my health is so wretched that I would consider myself lucky if I could last that time! ... the mortality continues and makes fearful ravages.

In response to these losses, the French simply sent in more reinforcements. By the end of the expedition, yellow fever had claimed the life not only of Le Clerc but also of over half the *officiers de santé* and at least 35,000 soldiers. Le Clerc's original force of 20,000 men was reduced to only a few thousand lucky survivors.[16]

The second great blight of the tropics was malaria. Like yellow fever, malaria is a mosquito-borne disease and at the time of the Napoleonic Wars it was far more widespread than today, affecting many troops in Europe. However, whereas in Europe soldiers generally acquired one of the less severe strains of the disease, in the West Indies the most malignant ('falciparum') form was common. Malaria classically causes an intermittent high fever associated with exhaustion. It is difficult to be certain how many French troops actually died from malaria in the West Indies; in practice, it is likely that Le Clerc's expedition was attacked by a lethal combination of both malaria and yellow fever. Malaria was probably the more prevalent of the two afflictions as immunity was only slowly acquired whereas a single bout of yellow fever left the soldier dead or immune. Both diseases were more common in low-lying swamps where mosquitoes thrived.

Malaria was also commonly seen in the Iberian Peninsula where the mosquitoes were a constant source of irritation. Heinrich von Brandt of the Vistula Legion describes swarms of mosquitoes being blown in from the sea following floods at Mora in Spain in 1811: 'These disgusting insects formed a thick cloud hovering above the ground, a veritable humming and stinging fog.'[17] The malaria that arrived with them may have been less lethal than the tropical version but it still caused high levels of sickness and considerable debility. Captain Nicolas Marcel fell victim to the disease at Truxillo in 1811. Every regiment, he says, had 800 to 900 men sick and in his own battalion there were 400 of the 500 soldiers and twenty-three out of twenty-four officers laid low with fever.

> I had been spared by the epidemic but, on 28 August, my servant and myself were affected by this confounded fever which lasted seven months; despite the most conscientious care of our *chirurgien-major* and despite the quantity of quinine we took, it would not leave us; it would stop for a few days and then return. How many times, lying in the middle of an arid plateau under a violent sun, dying of thirst with not a drop to drink despite the devotion of my men, experiencing the opposite during the night as cold as the day was warm, soaked with sweat, obliged to put my shirt back on still damp from the day before, how many times have I hoped that a bullet would put an end to such a miserable existence. Such tortures can only be understood by those who have endured them.[18]

Different countries brought the army's doctors bewildering new challenges. In Egypt, Bonaparte's force became ill with a disease more commonly associated with the Middle Ages. Bubonic plague, the 'black death' of earlier centuries, is primarily a bacterial disease of rats or other rodents but it can be transmitted to humans via rat fleas. Sufferers develop a high fever, headache, enlarged lymph glands ('buboes') and complications such as pneumonia. In severe cases, delirium ensues and death can occur within twenty-four hours. Plague first appeared in the summer of 1798 at Alexandria, Damietta and Manssurah. These were localised outbreaks but by the end of the year the volume of cases in Alexandria was increasing alarmingly. The state of demoralisation of the French army is clear from the correspondence of General Marmont to his colleague, General Menou: 'For God's sake, my dear general, do not abandon us and send us money … wheat … some help.'[19]

Damietta witnessed a similar escalation of cases and the disease subsequently followed Bonaparte's troops into Syria where it threatened wholesale destruction of the army at Jaffa. There is no doubt that the pestilence was plague. Larrey explicitly describes the symptoms and signs.

> The patient languishes for some time in a state of inquietude and general indisposition … he experiences difficulties in breathing … the pains of the head increase … the patient grows drowsy … the fever then commences, delirium takes place sooner or later. Tumours arise in the groin, arm-pits and other parts of the body called buboes …

Desgenettes supports Larrey's account and also divides the plague into three different levels of severity; those with the most severe or third degree form often died between the third and sixth days. Larrey's description of these deaths explains why the disease was so feared.

> If the patient was marching he fell into convulsions and violent distortions of the face; the lips opened and were distorted and the tongue tumified to such a degree to be forced out of the mouth; thick fetid saliva flowed involuntarily; the nostrils were dilated and discharged a foul smelling mucous. The eyes were opened; they seemed to project from their sockets and were fixed. The skin of the face was discoloured; the patient writhed, uttered some mournful cries and expired immediately.

There was an urgent need for effective treatment but the antiphlogistic remedies were predictably useless. Attempted treatments included emetics, diaphoretic drinks to stimulate perspiration, quinine, camphorated brandy, coffee and vinegar. Captain Joseph-Marie Moiret, who contracted the disease at Gaza in March 1799, could find no doctor and had to resort to a consultation with a local apothecary who also had the plague. 'He advised me to make myself vomit and added that he was about to do the same thing.' Eugene Fenech, who made a study of an outbreak of plague in his native Malta, concluded that treatment was near futile and that only means to limit the spread of the disease were worthwhile.[20]

What was the prognosis for soldiers with the plague? This appears to have varied according to the stage of the epidemic. Larrey states that when the plague first broke out in Egypt, 80% of the patients died. This very high early mortality was repeated in Syria; Etienne-Louis Malus, in charge of the plague hospital at Jaffa, quotes mortality in excess of 90%. As the epidemic ran its course the virulence of the disease waned and Larrey says that two thirds were cured. He generously attributed this improved survival to the 'courage and zeal' of Desgenettes. The latter believed that the plague was not indiscriminate but that it preferentially attacked healthy men rather than women and children.[21]

The outbreak of plague in the French forces in North Africa provides good examples of how an infectious disease could undermine soldiers' morale and how military officers and doctors tried to counteract this. The concept of plague terrorised the army. Troops frequently hid the classic symptoms to avoid being taken to the dreaded plague hospitals. Desgenettes adopted two strategies to try and mollify them. The first was denial: 'I refused to ever use the word plague (*peste*). I believed it correct in the circumstances to treat the whole army as a single sick man in whom it is dangerous to state the nature of the disease when he is critically ill.' This approach was destined to fail as it became common knowledge that plague was everywhere. The army's senior physician then resorted to inoculating himself with plague material to try and convince the soldiers that it was not contagious and therefore less sinister than they believed.

Bonaparte understood the fear of disease and he believed that this mental state increased the vulnerability of his men. 'During the Egyptian expedition, all those whose imagination was struck by fear died of it [plague]. The surest protection, the most efficacious remedy, was moral courage.' His own visit to the plague hospital at Jaffa in 1799 can be viewed as being both heroic and politically motivated. Desgenettes describes the young general helping to lift and carry the 'hideous corpse' of a soldier whose torn uniform was soiled by the spontaneous bursting of a plague bubo. This appears an extremely risky action by Bonaparte and, in a much later conversation on St Helena documented by General Bertrand, the Emperor asserted that Desgenettes had told him that the men were sick but not with plague.[22] As for many of Napoleon's actions relating to the *service de santé*, his real reasons for visiting the plague victims and his true state of knowledge remain obscure.

Plague was not the only devastating disease to dog French troops in Egypt and Syria. Ophthalmia, a disorder of the eyes, was not life-threatening but it was a cause of enormous misery with blindness a possible outcome. From the descriptions of French and British physicians, it seems to have been a mixture of infectious eye complaints including simple purulent conjunctivitis, gonorrhoea, and a more chronic disorder termed trachoma. This heterogeneity explains the range of severity of cases. Most of Bonaparte's doctors were stubbornly opposed to a contagious aetiology for ophthalmia and they instead attributed it to the intense light of the sun, the damp of the night and other climatic and atmospheric changes. After a slow start in Cairo, the epidemic of ophthalmia accelerated and spread and, by September 1798, General Reynier, in command to the east, reported that the disease had reduced all his battalions from around 350 to 125 men. Ophthalmic soldiers with eyes completely blinded by the swelling of the lids had to be employed to man the trenches, their muskets being pointed at the enemy by commanders whose sight had not been affected. In Upper Egypt, General Desaix defeated the Mamelukes but was unable to follow the beaten enemy as ophthalmia had rendered 1,400 men incapable of service. Desaix himself suffered from the disorder and was confined to his tent. 'We were,' says Captain Savary, 'more like a hospital being evacuated than troops on the march ... There were more blind men than there were healthy. Every soldier who was able to see or had just one eye served as a guide to several blind comrades who had, however, to carry their arms and baggage.' Ophthalmia sufferers at the temporary hospitals at Manssurah were massacred by the local population whilst the more fortunate were evacuated to the special military ophthalmia hospital at Gaza. Ophthalmia subsided in the summer of 1799 but again blighted the French Army during 1801 with outbreaks in Alexandria and Cairo.

A number of French military surgeons wrote accounts of the disease. One typical treatment suggested by a surgeon called Assalini was copious bleeding from the arm, feet, neck and temples, leeches, scarification of the skin, purgations and the application of a solution of verdigris to the eyes. This can hardly have helped and Bonaparte was obliged to dispatch several convoys of blind soldiers back to France throughout the course of the campaign. Larrey notes that several French grenadiers committed suicide in Egypt because they had lost their eyesight. For those who could bear the immediate distress of blindness, the future was not entirely bleak as a number of invalids who returned to France eventually recovered their vision either spontaneously or after eye surgery. Ophthalmia never again attacked Napoleon's armies as viciously as in Egypt although it is mentioned in accounts of the Russian campaign. Heinrich Roos recalls blind men being led along by their comrades as the retreating army approached the Berezina.[23]

Napoleon's men were as vulnerable to disease in Europe as in the Tropics or the Orient. It was only the nature of the epidemics that changed. Disease was depressingly omnipresent although it fluctuated in incidence and severity according to the season and the degree of overcrowding. Figures provided by Intendant General Daru for 1807 show that only one in four men admitted to hospital at Warsaw in Poland were wounded.

Over half had a fever and the rest either venereal or skin disease. Official figures may underestimate the impact of disease. Whereas Daru listed 19,500 French sick around this time, other sources suggest that Davout's corps had at least 45,000 men in hospital and that some regiments, such as the 31ᵉ *léger*, had been reduced to a tenth of their normal strength within a month.[24] In Italy in the summer of 1807, it was commonplace for disease to have reduced regiments from their full strength of 1,800 to only 400 fit men. In Spain, disease struck Junot's invading force and in a short time 8,000 of his 26,000 men were in hospital, an outcome blamed on 'the wine, the debauchery and the unhealthy garrisons'. Napoleon's unfortunate Iberian armies were never to escape its clutches with overall sick rates up to 30% and individual divisions, for instance Morlot's division of 3ᵉ corps in 1808, having over half their men hospitalised.[25] These few examples make the point that high levels of morbidity were routine during the *Grande Armée*'s European campaigns. The diseases were a mixture of infections and disorders secondary to exposure and deprivation. We will never have accurate disease statistics for the wars but we can say with confidence that the two greatest killers in the European theatre were typhus and dysentery.

In the early 19th century, typhus was an inevitable companion of war; no encampment, no besieged city or campaigning army could expect to escape it. This dreadful infectious disease is caused by bacteria-like organisms called 'Rickettsia' which are transmitted to humans by the body louse. War provides the perfect conditions of filth and overcrowding in which lice thrive and typhus epidemics proliferate. Outbreaks of typhus punctuate the history of conflict from the Peloponnesian War of 420 BC to the Second World War. Once infected, soldiers develop a high fever and variable additional symptoms including headache, breathing difficulties and mental confusion. Red eruptions (petechiae) may appear in the skin and gangrene develops in the extremities. In epidemic conditions the mortality can be frighteningly high, even approaching 100%. Contemporary descriptions of typhus accord well with our modern definition of the disease with frequent references to the characteristic 'red spots'. The presence of these petechiae and the relatively short duration of the illness (around three weeks) enable us to distinguish typhus from typhoid fever, another infection thriving in unsanitary conditions.[26] The potentially fulminant course of typhus is well illustrated by Physician Gilbert's account of the affliction in a colleague in Poland in 1807.

Monsieur Grösse, age 26 years, a physician employed at the hospital at Thorn, was serving in the army for the first time after having spent his life in civilian medicine. He worked for two months with an exemplary assiduity and zeal, his talents distinguishing a poor local hospital containing 200 fever cases. He appeared delicate with a feeble constitution. He was struck by diarrhoea which he controlled with large doses of opium. This malady passed, returned and then relapsed several times. He did not stop working despite my attempts to dissuade him. He came to see me one evening, asking me to feel his pulse, saying that he believed he was lost. I was frightened. The pulse was very weak, quick and irregular. The same evening, he was admitted to the officers' hospital and spent the night tranquilly enough; the next day he died. I had never seen, not even with yellow fever in Saint Domingo, so striking an example of a quick death. This was caused by typhus.[27]

There was no effective medical treatment for the disease. Percy criticised the use of aggressive medicines and purging and it was common experience that bleeding simply hastened death. Conversely, fresh air and cold came to be viewed as beneficial as physicians noted that men transported through a freezing winter were more likely to survive than those packed together in warm hospitals. Cold was more deliberately applied in the form of cold water baths and douches. The contemporary attempts to manage established typhus cases now seem pathetic in the context of the relentless progress of the disease. The campaigns of Napoleonic France and army life itself were perfect catalysts for its spread. As large bodies of men moved, the disease followed them. Spanish prisoners of war carried it from their homeland across the Pyrenees into France and, ultimately, all the way to Paris. There was no doubt as to its highly contagious nature as the disease suddenly appeared wherever the prisoners halted. At one *Charité* hospital, the nuns, medical students, attendants, night-watchmen, porters, gendarmes, chaplain and casual visitors all contracted typhus and many died.

After the Russian campaign in 1812, the typhus-ridden remnants of the retreating *Grande Armée* spread the infection along the military roads of Poland and Germany. In late 1813 and 1814 the defeated French brought the blight back to their own villages. Attempts to limit dissemination of typhus were hindered by ignorance and well-meaning medical advice could exacerbate the situation. A German staff surgeon commented in 1812, 'people think that they can prevent the disease from spreading by congregating and isolating the patients but, as a matter of fact, this has the opposite effect'. There were clues as to the mode of disease transmission but they were difficult to decipher without knowledge of infectious organisms or disease vectors. It was known that the clothes and other effects of people who had died from typhus were highly infectious. Those soldiers and civilians who acquired cheap lice-infested garments in this manner often paid a heavy penalty. Similarly, it was clear that the disease increased during periods of bad weather when men were forced to group together in houses and bathing was infrequent. Military hospitals were always implicated in typhus outbreaks, one *officier de santé* unequivocally referring to them as *'centres de contagion'*.[28]

In the years 1805–14, typhus took a heavy toll on the manpower of the *Grande Armée*. After the Battle of Austerlitz, the 18,000 typhus deaths in the hospitals eclipsed the losses in the actual fighting. In the war of 1806–7, typhus broke out in the provinces of East Prussia and very severe epidemics attacked the French forces in Spain and Portugal between 1808 and 1814. In Russia, typhus can be easily identified in the eyewitness accounts of an army which lost perhaps over 200,000 soldiers solely from disease. This was predictable as lice were everywhere; Sergeant Bourgogne remembers:

> I had slept for an hour when I felt an unbearable tingling over all of my body … and to my horror discovered that I was covered with vermin! I jumped up and in less than two minutes was as naked as a new-born babe, having thrown my shirt and trousers into the fire. The crackling they made was like a brisk firing.[29]

It may be thought that typhus had done its worst in 1812 but in the following year an influx of green young recruits from France met the routed remnants of the *Grande Armée* in Saxony and the disease exploded, only eventually petering out in Paris in late 1814. A lengthy book would be required to fully detail the suffering of Napoleon's army from this single disease in the last few years of the Empire. Outbreaks particularly occurred after the battles of Bautzen, Lützen and Leipzig and in all the French garrison towns. The best estimate is that around 200,000 to 300,000 soldiers and civilians died from typhus with up to a tenth of the whole German population becoming infected. The mortality rates were probably very variable with the highest death rates in the military hospitals. One account of typhus in Russia states that half of those contracting it died, but in more favourable circumstances the chance of death was probably lower at around one in ten.[30]

Dysentery favoured similar conditions to typhus. This bowel disease is caused by either bacteria or parasites. It is likely that most outbreaks in Europe were of the bacterial type, whereas the dysentery that struck Bonaparte's army in Egypt was probably the parasitic (amoebic) form. Milder cases of dysentery are difficult to distinguish from the many other causes of diarrhoea but in severe cases the soldiers developed the characteristic symptoms of the painful passage of bloody stools with colicky abdominal pain and fever and dehydration. Dysentery alone could cause death but there was a tendency for the disorder to complicate other diseases (particularly typhus) and also to debilitate men, making them more vulnerable to the prevalent fevers. Treatments were typically antiphlogistic. Desgenettes believed many of the 'inveterate' Egyptian forms to be incurable but he found opiates helpful in milder attacks – these are constipating and may have relieved the diarrhoea.[31] Percy also used the emetic ipecacuanha, rhubarb, and rice water and Gilbert advocated wines, laudanum, the application of ointment to the abdomen and various diets.

Less dramatic in its presentation than other types of fever, dysentery was the most common affliction in the *Grande Armée* in the winter of 1806/7. The distressing symptoms of the disease were a further indignity for the troops in 1812. Heinrich Roos points out that the relatively good health of the Russian army compared with the French could be ascertained by the stink from the latter's camp sites. On the march, the affected men suddenly clutched their stomachs and made quick dashes to the side of the road to drop their pants. 'On some stretches of the road I had to hold my breath in order not to bring up liver and lungs and even to lie down until the need to vomit had died down,' wrote Franz Roeder, a Hessian life guard officer. The extreme cold increased the agonies of dysentery. At Smorgonie, Lieutenant Colonel Le Roy saw '… several soldiers and officers unable to do their trousers up. I myself helped one of these unfortunates to put his ---- back and button himself up. He was crying like a child. With my own eyes I saw a major make a hole in the seat of his trousers so as not to have to undress to relieve himself. He wasn't the only one to take this disgusting precaution.'[32]

The combination of several infectious diseases both confused the army's doctors and caused exceptionally high death rates. A classic example of this occurred on the Island of Walcheren off the Dutch coast where a mysterious disease called 'Walcheren fever' or 'Flushing sickness' created havoc among occupying French and British troops in both the Revolutionary and Napoleonic wars. The future Marshal MacDonald visited the island in 1795 and over 80% of his men went down with fever. He was relieved to escape back to Paris with only a mild version of the disease which eventually remitted. When the British invaded the Scheldt area in 1809, over 40% of the force developed Walcheren fever and around 4,000 men died from the disease compared with only about a hundred killed in sporadic fighting. French descriptions of this campaign are scarce but, taken in conjunction with the more numerous British accounts, they support the view that Walcheren fever was not a new disorder but a lethal combination of malaria, dysentery, typhus and typhoid. Jean-Baptiste Trésal, a military physician at the hospital in the capital Middelburg, documents intermittent fevers, which were probably malaria, but also an 'adynamic' fever with petechiae which was most likely typhus. A similar phenomenon occurred in the French garrison of Torgau in Saxony which was besieged by the Prussians after the Battle of Leipzig. A pestilence took hold turning the city into a 'large overcrowded lazaret' and in the period September 1813 to January 1814 between 20,000 and 30,000 French soldiers died. A detailed contemporary description of the disease by Richter, a Prussian army physician, leaves little doubt that dysentery, typhus and typhoid combined to cause a level of devastation that the doctor believed, 'had scarcely a parallel in the history of the world'.[33]

In the Russian campaign, many soldiers of the *Grande Armée* undoubt-edly perished more from the effects of cold and hunger than from any specific disease. Certainly, Larrey quotes these factors as the commonest cause of death on parts of the retreat. There are countless descriptions of the damage inflicted by the brutal Russian climate. The following was written by Colonel Louis-François Lejeune.

> We were all covered with ice. Our breath, looking like thick smoke, froze as it left our mouths and hung in icicles from our hair, eyebrows, mous-taches and beards, sometimes quite blinding us. General Haxo, in break-ing off the icicles which were bothering me, noticed that my cheeks and nose were discoloured. They looked like wax and he informed me that they were frozen. He was right for all sensation was gone from them.

Lejeune vigorously rubbed his face with snow and painfully restored the circulation. Not all were so fortunate. Larrey noted that frostbite was more likely at the stage of the subsequent thaw than at the time of maximum cold. This happened not only in Russia but also after the Battle of Eylau five years earlier. Rapid heating of frozen limbs at bivouac fires led to extensive tissue damage.[34]

Where death followed cold exposure, Larrey says that it was often pre-ceded by a period of 'imbecility', difficulty in speaking and loss of sight. This mental state is confirmed by Chirurgien-Major René Bourgeois.

> A great many were in a state of real dementia, plunged into a kind of stupor with haggard eyes and a fixed and dazed stare; one could single them out in the crowd, in the midst of which they walked like automata in profound silence. If one hailed them one could get only disjointed and incoherent answers; they had entirely lost the use of their senses and were impervious to everything – the insults and even the blows they received could not move them or bring them out of this state of idiocy.

Such men would eventually sink to the ground and die. Larrey regarded this demise from cold as 'not a cruel death' but Bourgeois disagreed, invoking the contortion of the dying men's faces as evidence of great pain.[35]

Men were less likely to survive the Russian cold if they were also severely malnourished. Hunger was a common accompaniment of campaigning but on the retreat from Moscow the troops starved. Ségur remembers that the desperate food shortages turned men into savages, '… hunger, raven-ous, devouring hunger had killed everything in those unfortunate beings but the instinct of self-preservation'. Soldiers resorted to eating dead birds and horseflesh. Heinrich Roos saw men eating from fallen animals when they were still alive. There are enough accounts of cannibalism for there to be little doubt as to their veracity. Lieutenant Roman Soltyk of the Polish Lancers walked up to a group of men standing around a steaming pot at Orsa on the retreat. He bargained for a share: 'But hardly had I swallowed the first spoonful that I was gripped by irrepressible disgust and I asked them whether it was horsemeat that they had used to make it. They coolly replied that it was human meat and that the liver, which was still in the pot, was the best part to eat.'[36]

Of the particular diseases arising directly out of malnutrition, scurvy, caused by a shortage of vitamin C, was best understood. This is more associated with sailors but there were several outbreaks in the French Army, notably in Russia and Egypt. In the Orient, the disease was brought on by a diet of dry vegetables and salted meat, lacking in fresh fruit and vegetables. Larrey had no appreciation of vitamin C deficiency but he followed the lead of British doctors in encouraging the consumption of fresh foods. Unfortunately, these were in short supply and, in April 1801 180 out of 626 sick men in the hospitals were suffering from scurvy. Larrey graphically describes the characteristic ulceration and bleeding of the gums with looseness of the teeth. As the disorder progressed the limbs swelled up with black spots in the skin and the patient became febrile and prostrate. 'The last stage of the scurvy is really dreadful to the spectator.' Despite the army's doctors best efforts to improve the diet of their men the disease continued at epidemic levels; between July and October 1801, 3,500 troops entered the hospitals at Alexandria with scurvy and 270 died.[37]

Venereal and skin diseases were less life-threatening than many infections attacking the *Grande Armée*, but the need for specialist hospitals to house patients with these disorders is testimony to the attritional effect they had on the army's manpower. During the Revolutionary Wars, officers and medical men pleaded with the Convention to do something about 'the scourge of women and girls who followed the army'. The women were accused of causing the loss of more men than the enemy's missiles, cannon and bayonets. The situation was unchanged under the Consulate and Empire. Where Napoleon's soldiers were deprived of the attentions of these camp-followers they had recourse to the local women. François Lavaux, a soldier in the 100e line regiment, alleges that the girls of the Tyrol who made themselves available to the soldiers all had venereal diseases, 'when they bend down their private parts are all revealed'. The two major diseases were syphilis and gonorrhoea but there was considerable confusion between the two with various syndromes receiving pithy descriptions such as '*le mal de Naples*' (probably syphilis) and '*la chaude-lance*' (gonorrhoea). Treatment relied on applications of mercury although many other approaches were tried including purgation and an assortment of baths.[38] Percy's favoured tactic of bleeding from the dorsal vein of the penis at least reduced the chance of a further dose of the disease.

Perhaps the most frequent of all the *Grande Armée*'s maladies was a skin complaint called '*la gale*' by the doctors and '*la charmante*' (literally 'charming') by the soldiers as it guaranteed them some rest in hospital. In 1800 it was cited as having removed a tenth of men from their corps and, in Spain in 1809, Surgeon Lagneau had an astonishing 900 cases in his 1,600 soldiers. Contemporary accounts of itching and pustules between the fingers suggest that most cases were scabies, a contagious skin infection caused by a mite. As for venereal diseases, all sorts of remedies were attempted, the most effective being a sulphur based ointment invented by a *chirurgien-major* called Helmerich in 1813.[39] For both venereal and skin diseases, prevention was both more feasible and effective than cure – a theme to which we will return at the end of this chapter.

Other infectious diseases can be more briefly reviewed. Typhoid fever, caused by a species of salmonella, is often difficult to distinguish from typhus. As it was endemic in many European cities in the early 19th century, we can assume that many soldiers died from it. The term was commonly used by doctors and soldiers during the wars; for instance, Lejeune refers to 'typhoid fever' raging in the military hospitals of Germany in 1813. Smallpox was a murderous disease but it appears to have made relatively little impact on the French armies of the period. Outbreaks in Egypt in 1800 and 1801 carried off 150,000 local people but affected Bonaparte's expeditionary force remarkably little. This was probably due more to the significant levels of natural immunity among the troops than to any introduction of vaccination. A study of almost a thousand French conscripts in 1811 suggests that over a third had signs of a previous milder form of the infection (variola minor) which gave some protection against the more serious strain of the disease (variola major).[40]

Not all the disease entities of the wars are recognisable today. Several doctors and soldiers describe a strange disorder called 'Polish plica' in which the hair on the head became matted together and formed a painful mass resembling a cap. Polish physicians maintained that this was the culmination of a general chronic disease but Larrey concluded that the plica was more the result of laziness and dirt. 'Madrid colic' was another self-induced disease well described by Larrey. Unlike plica, this syndrome attacked a significant number of French troops, among them Murat who had to be invalided back to France because of it. The abdominal pains were very likely due to lead poisoning which, in turn, was caused by over consumption of the local Spanish wines which were contaminated by the metal. Alcohol abuse was commonplace both in civilian life and in the armies of the Napoleonic era. In 1794 there were a total of 1,685 cafes and wine-shops in Paris (as compared to 724 bakers' shops, 562 butchers' shops and 1,091 grocers). The people of the city consumed prodigious amounts of low quality wines. When they entered the army they had an even greater incentive to drink to relieve stress and create amnesia for the lost pleasures of home. A young soldier in Spain in 1810 confessed that any coins they laid their hands on were likely to end up in the nearest inn. 'We are afraid to hold on to them till the following day lest we die a sudden death during the night. So we spend them on drink the day we receive them.' Pharmacist Fée witnessed the overindulgence of the French soldiers in the Peninsula. On one occasion,

> ... the drummers could not hold their drumsticks or the soldiers their rifles. They were singing at the top of their voices and showing an extraordinary tenderness towards their officers ... It was necessary to wait for them to recover on the road where the wine fumes dispersed. Fifty armed men could have skinned them all and us with them.

There were identical scenes in Russia where the discovery of stores of brandy and rum frequently proved fatal for men already debilitated by disease and cold. Doctors tried to limit these excesses. Percy noted that the wines in Spain caused not only drunkenness but also vomiting and diarrhoea. In Poland, in 1807, he urged the troops to shirk the local schnapps and to instead drink vinegared water provided by the army. Larrey perceptively noted the connection between constant heavy drinking and diseases of the liver. Smaller degrees of consumption were actually encouraged. Percy acknowledged to the Emperor that it was better to drink a little alcohol than consume stinking water and Desgenettes noted that brandy taken in large quantities 'did as much harm as a modest amount does good'.[41]

Napoleon's soldiers suffered from diseases of the mind just as men in other wars. Frank psychoses were probably quite rare although Hussar De Rocca describes the bizarre actions of two 'madmen' of his regiment in Spain. The most prevalent mental disease of the army was a disorder termed 'nostalgia' or *'mal de pays'* which was defined at the time as 'an exaggerated melancholic state arising from the removal of the sufferer from the familiar environment in which they have lived and accompanied by an irresistible desire to return there'. This extreme form of homesickness led to the symptoms and signs of severe depression and those afflicted were unusually vulnerable to what would normally have been minor physical ailments. The syndrome probably overlapped with the 'shellshock' of the Great War and what we might now term 'post-traumatic stress disorder'. It was ever-present but it became particularly widespread and dangerous in the army of the Moselle in 1793–4, in the Egyptian campaigns of 1798–9, in the Army of the Alps in the same year, and in 1813 and 1814 when the Empire was declining and morale was generally low.[42]

Affected soldiers expressed their fears of alienation and isolation in their correspondence with their distant families; one young man in his first letter home from campaign complained that he felt 'like a tree that has been uprooted'. Demoralised soldiers were easy prey for the epidemic diseases that pursued them. In 1793 Percy observed that nostalgia much aggravated the dysentery which raged in the hospitals. For most sufferers, the best cure was a quick return home and desertion was rife. The army's doctors and officers tried to distract affected men with games and other diversions but nostalgia was considered as much a physical as a mental disorder and there were attempts to treat it with antiphlogistic strategies including purgatives, spirits and quinine. Those who escaped the complicating fevers could fall to the temptation of suicide. This was especially common in Egypt. Moved by an unusually tragic case, Napoleon issued an order of the day in May 1802 decrying the taking of one's own life which he described as 'abandoning the battlefield before having been beaten'.[43]

More trivial mental disorders merged almost imperceptibly into frank malingering. Was the soldier with inexplicable physical and psychological symptoms a mild case of 'nostalgia' or was he simply aiming for an early discharge from the army? Many were unwilling participants caught by the '*levée en masse*'. When faced with the harsh reality of military life, men inevitably saw disability and illness as a quick way out. Well before Larrey's investigation of the alleged self-mutilations of 1813, it was widely accepted that soldiers commonly harmed themselves to escape duty. Indeed, Percy suggested using hundreds of these men as *infirmiers*. He concluded that their injuries were self-induced as the affected men, mostly young conscripts, always refused an 'operation' he had offered them which 'made the lost fingers grow back'. Percy's rather cynical management of perceived malingerers was the rule. Elzéar Blaze says of his comrades who feigned illness: 'The doctors recognise them at first glance, they give them several doses of an emetic and one or two purgatives and put them on a very strict diet; very soon our fine fellows, facing starvation, decided to behave themselves.'[44]

We can only estimate the number of soldiers of the Revolutionary armies and *Grande Armée* who died of disease between 1792 and 1815. The commonly quoted figure of 2.5 million taken from Garrison's *Notes on the History of Military Medicine* may be an exaggeration but the scale of the losses in the Iberian Peninsula and in central Europe in the years 1812–14 suggest a seven figure total. This mortality was not evenly spread through the armies. New recruits were always the first to fall sick and hardy veterans, the *grognards*, the last. Of 1,500 young Frenchmen sent to Italy in July 1807, there were only 300 fit for duty by September. In an even more striking example from the Russian campaign, the 6th *chasseurs à cheval* received 250 recruits from the depot in northern Italy but their delicacy and lack of immunity to the prevailing diseases ensured that none survived. Differences in mortality between corps reflected varying levels of durability of the troops, quality of accommodation and discipline. In Spain, the sickness rates in 1808 varied between 3% in the regiments of the

Old Guard and 35% in the two Swiss Corps. Officers fared better than the rank and file. They may have been less vulnerable due to a combination of better nutrition and less exposure to overcrowding. In Russia, a marked imbalance developed with many regiments having 'too many officers'. Ney's twelve Württemberger battalions lost so many men that they were reformed as only three and yet there were hardly any officers missing. Overall sickness rates in the *Grande Armée* were broadly comparable to those in other armies of the period but there were differences. Figures from the Peninsular War for the period 1808–14 suggest that average French sick rates were 13–14%, a little lower than the British figure of 21%. This may reflect the more continuous and arduous nature of campaigning for the much smaller British force compared with the patchy involvement of the more widely disseminated French troops in Portugal and Spain.[45]

Napoleon was sceptical of most medical interventions and advocated prevention over cure. He was justified in this view as most medical treatments of the period, both in civilian and army life, now appear archaic and useless. The *officiers de santé* and a few more progressive military officers of the *Grande Armée* did make well-reasoned efforts to prevent the development and spread of disease and it is appropriate to complete this chapter with a description of the strategies they used. The first step was to keep sick men out of the army. In the Revolutionary period it was stipulated that a conscript had to be of a certain standard of physical strength and fitness. There were significant geographic variations in the frequency of disease but the local records are mostly depressing reading. In the Cantal in southern France in 1798, only three young men out of fifty-seven passed a basic medical examination. Their problems included deafness, epilepsy, septic wounds, respiratory disorders (probably tuberculosis), ulcers, unexplained lumps and untreated fractures.[46]

Once a man was admitted to the ranks, the considerable challenge was to keep him well. The seminal French work of the late 18th century on 'military hygiene' was Colombier's *Préceptes sur la Santé des Gens de Guerre*. Colombier was inspired by his British counterparts, John Pringle and Richard Brocklesby, and he recommended common sense measures to maintain a soldier's health such as ventilation of barracks, scrupulous cleanliness, strict discipline and provision of good food and clean water. The Revolutionary politicians and doctors tried hard to follow these dictums and, in 1793 the Committee of Public Safety distributed a pamphlet to all *officiers de santé* instructing that their hospitals were to be kept as clean as possible, beds were to be widely spaced and patients regularly washed. In the following year, the committee ordered the beds of patients with communicable diseases to be retained for hospital use only. The word 'hospital' was to be burnt into the bedstead and all sheets and mattresses were to be similarly marked.[47] The issue of such sophisticated and detailed healthcare advice so early in the era underlines the fact that the subsequent frequent failures to prevent rampant infectious disease were more often due to a lack of will or resources rather than to ignorance of the necessary measures.

The most successful prophylactic regime of the period was instituted during the Egyptian campaign where, despite the outbreak of plague, fewer men died from disease than from wounds. Here, Desgenettes, Larrey and other senior doctors were well supported by Bonaparte in the creation both of a general infrastructure and the development of specific measures to limit cases of infectious disease. All legislation relating to maintenance of the health of the army was overseen and enforced by groups of doctors and military officers. There was a general '*commission de santé*' and other bodies with more specific responsibilities such as supervision of the hospitals. Preventative actions included screening of troops, assiduous attention to the soldier's uniform, provision of clean water and fresh food, encouragement of personal hygiene, cleaning of accommodation, and careful placement of camps away from excreta. Where plague appeared, the affected men were quarantined and their clothes burnt. These plague hospitals or 'lazarets' were regularly disinfected.[48]

The success of prophylactic measures in Egypt was dependent on the support lent by the General in Chief. Doctors had limited authority and troops were always likely to be healthier when a senior military officer took a keen interest in them. Marshal Davout was just such a man and the health preservation measures taken in his corps in Germany between 1810 and 1812 are a model of their type. They are recorded in a register of orders of the 48^e regiment in Friant's division – this small book was left in Moscow at the time of the retreat and was later recovered and kept by the regiment. Much of the advice given to troops in Egypt is repeated and there is also explicit instruction as to exercise, indulgence in alcohol, filtering of drinking water, the lighting of fires and the type and quality of rations. Venereal diseases were discouraged by keeping *cantinières* and *vivandières* and 'man hunters' out of the camps. An order of May 1810 recommending the vaccination of soldiers who had not derived immunity from cowpox (*la petite vériole*) is a reminder that this new scientific discovery was potentially available to Napoleonic soldiers. It was actively supported by Napoleon and medical figures such as Coste and Percy but large-scale vaccination was never achieved. At the start of 1807, only 2,000 soldiers of the *Grande Armée* had received the vaccine and this figure probably only tripled by the end of the wars. A laudable initiative to vaccinate all the new conscripts of 1813 remained another paper exercise.[49]

Notes

1. Horne, A, *Seven Ages of Paris*, pp. 215, 185; Robiquet, J, *Daily Life in France under Napoleon*, p. 65.
2. Tulard, J, *Dictionnaire Napoléon*, Vol. II, pp. 250–1.
3. Prinzing, F, *Epidemics resulting from Wars*, p. 93.
4. Vess, D M, *Medical Revolution in France 1789–1796*, pp. 138–9, 142–3; Brice, Docteur and Bottet, Capitaine, *Le Corps de Santé Militaire en France*, p. 83.
5. Ackerknecht, E H, *Medicine at the Paris Hospital 1794–1848*, p. 49; Larrey, D J, *Mémoires de Chirurgie Militaire et Campagnes 1787–1840*, p. 371.
6. Vess, p. 139; Larrey, p. 325; Desgenettes, R, *Histoire Médicale de l'Armée d'Orient*, Vol. I, pp. 58, 248; Lixon, L J M, *Médecin à l'armée d'Espagne en 1808 1809 et 1810*, p. 93; Gilbert, N P, *Tableau historique des maladies internes de mauvais caractère qui ont affligé la Grande Armée dans la campagne de Prussie et de Pologne*, p. 33; Percy, Baron, *Journal des Campagnes de Baron Percy*, pp. 115, 392.
7. Percy, p. 277.
8. Lixon, p. 92.
9. Gilbert, pp. 50–1; Weiner, D B, *French Doctors Face War 1792–1815*, pp. 64–5; Desgenettes, Vol. II, p. 248; Larrey, p.162; Smith, D, *The Prisoners of Cabrera. Napoleon's forgotten soldiers 1809–1814*, p. 53.
10. Howard, M, *Wellington's Doctors. The British Army Medical Services in the Napoleonic Wars*, pp. 162–4; Vess, p. 139.
11. Larrey, p. 605.
12. Vess, p. 84; Desgenettes, Vol. I, p.160; Ducoulombier, H, *Le Baron P-F Percy. Un chirurgien de la Grande Armée*, p. 255.
13. Fenech, E, *Mémoires d'un Officier de Santé Maltais dans l'Armée Française (1786–1839)*, p. 28; Roos, H de, *Avec Napoléon en Russie*, pp. 41, 51.
14. Laurillard-Fallot, S-L, *Souvenirs d'un Médecin Hollandais sous les Aigles Françaises 1807–1833*, p. 60; Blaze, E, *Military Life under Napoleon. The Memoirs of Captain Elzéar Blaze*; Elting, J R, *Swords around a Throne. Napoleon's Grande Armée*, p. 129.
15. Weiner, pp. 63–4; de Jonnès, A M, *Adventures in Wars of the Republic and Consulate 1791–1805*, p. 270.
16. Weiner, p. 64; Peterson, R K D, *Insects disease and military history: the Napoleonic campaigns and historical perceptions*.
17. Brandt von, H, *In the Legions of Napoleon. The memoirs of a Polish Officer in Spain and Russia 1808–1813*, p. 146.
18. Marcel, N, *Campagnes en Espagne et au Portugal 1808–1814*, pp. 118–19.
19. Milleliri, J-M, *Médecins et Soldats pendant l'expédition d'Égypte (1798–1799)*, p. 198.
20. Larrey, pp. 174, 176; Desgenettes, Vol. I, pp. 78–9; Moiret, Captain J-M, *Memoirs of Napoleon's Egyptian Expedition 1798–1801*, p. 84; Fenech, p. 178.
21. Larrey, p. 183; Moiret, p. 22; Desgenettes, Vol. I, p. 138.

22. Desgenettes, Vol. I, pp. 50, 88; Bertrand, General, *Napoleon at St. Helena. Memoirs of General Bertrand Grand Marshal to the Palace*, p. 115.

23. Meyerhof, M, *A short history of ophthalmia during the Egyptian Campaigns of 1798–1807*, pp. 131–50; Roos, p. 192.

24. Sokolov, O, *L'Armée de Napoléon*, p.508; Morvan, J, *Le Soldat Impérial*, Vol. II, p. 320.

25. Morvan, Vol. II, pp. 310–11, 325; Brice, Bottet, p. 216.

26. Prinzing, pp. 112–13.

27. Gilbert, pp. 102–3.

28. Prinzing, pp. 102, 120–4, 153–6, 110, 108–11.

29. Bourgogne, Sergeant, *Memoirs of Sergeant Bourgogne (1812–1813)*, p. 66.

30. Prinzing, pp. 128, 162–3; Rose, A, *Napoleon's Campaign in Russia Anno 1812: medico-historical*, p. 184.

31. Desgenettes, Vol. II, p. 23, Vol. I, p. 131.

32. Roos, p. 62; Zamoyski, A, *1812. Napoleon's fatal march on Moscow*, p. 188; Austin, P B, *1812, The Great Retreat*, p. 358.

33. MacDonald, Marshal, *Recollections of Marshal MacDonald*, pp. 47–8; Howard, p. 173; Trésal, J B, *Essai sur la fièvre adynamique qui a régné dans l'île de Walcheren dans l'année 1809*, p. 21; Prinzing, pp. 314–16.

34. Lejeune, Baron, *Memoirs of Baron Lejeune Aide-de-Camp to Marshals Berthier, Davout and Oudinot*, Vol. II, p. 245; Dible, J H, *Napoleon's Surgeon*, p. 198.

35. Zamoyski, pp. 494, 505.

36. Ségur, Count P-P de, *Napoleon's Russian Campaign*, p. 256; Roos, p. 166; Zamoyski, pp. 484–5.

37. Larrey, p. 342; Milleliri, p. 194.

38. Vess, p. 87; Forrest, A, *Napoleon's Men. The soldiers of the Revolution and Empire*, p. 141; Brice, Bottet, p. 142.

39. Lagneau, L-V, *Journal d'un Chirurgien de la Grande Armée 1803–1815*, p. 124; Ducoulombier, p. 184; Brice, Bottet, p. 43.

40. Lejeune, Vol. II, p. 297; Barblan, M-A, *La variole dans le Département du Léman en 1811*, p. 197.

41. Dible, pp. 78, 98; Cobb, R, *Reactions to the French Revolution*, pp. 171–2; Forrest, *Napoleon's Men*, p. 138; Brice, Bottet, pp. 211–12; Bade, Margrave de, *La Campagne de 1812. Mémoires du Margrave de Bade*, p.175; Fezensac, Lieut-General de, *A Journal of the Russian Campaign of 1812*, p. 164; Percy, pp. lxxxvi, 417; Larrey, p. 226; Desgenettes, Vol. I, p. 184.

42. Rocca de, A J M, *In the Peninsula with a French Hussar*, pp. 170–1; Evrard, E, *La Nostalgie: un malade qui se meurt sa signification dans l'histoire de la médecine militaire*, p. 21.

43. Forrest, p. 170; Evrard, pp. 24–5; Tulard, Vol. II, p. 352.

44. Forrest, A, *Conscriptors and Deserters. The army and French society during the Revolution and Empire*; Lemaire, J-F, *Napoléon et la Médecine*, p. 207; Blaze, p. 145.

45. Garrison, F H, *Notes on the History of Military Medicine*, pp. 169–70; Morvan, Vol. II, pp. 303, 328; Zamoyski, p. 418; Austin, P B, *The March*

on Moscow, p. 250; Hodge, W B, *On the mortality arising from military operations*, pp. 247–8.
46. Forrest, *Conscript and Deserters*, p. 45.
47. Milleliri, p. 75; Vess, pp. 144, 158.
48. Milleliri, pp. 79–157; 195–217.
49. Brice, Bottet, pp. 232–6; Tulard, Vol. II, p. 912.

CHAPTER X

Campaigning: On the Road with Napoleon

The journals, memoirs and letters of the *officiers de santé* of the *Grande Armée* are as much about the elation and despair of a soldier's life as they are about medicine and surgery. Their authors were doctors but they were also men trying their best to survive and prosper on campaign. Many had mixed feelings regarding their strange new life in Napoleon's military machine. Pharmacist Pierre-Irénée Jacob wrote the following in his journal on 3 October 1812 as he marched towards Russia.

> Passing through woods and crossing fields, usually not knowing where I was going to find a house to pass the night or a piece of bread to restore my energy, I had some serious reflections on this singular manner of travelling with the army. No longer one's own guide and judge, and in some ways no longer a man; marching or stopping according to the will of some invisible directing power; such is the life of a soldier and it is a life to which I have not been able to entirely get used to. And yet this artificial life, contrary to natural law, is not without a certain gentleness which compensates for the loss of liberty. Happy events seem to have been sent directly by Providence; difficult moments can be supported more patiently because they are simply caused by circumstances; it is not as in normal life when one has to reproach oneself for bad judgement, poor calculations or a lack of initiative.[1]

Pharmacist François Duriau also committed his innermost thoughts to his journal which he kept on the road in 1805–6 and again in 1809. He bemoans the endless marches through mud and rain at the tail of the columns and the grim sight of convoys of wounded stamping in the snow. More happily, he also remembers the unexpected warm billet, the furtive kiss in the stable with the daughter of the host, the 'fanciful dreams' of deep sleep on a river bank, a table or the back of an ambulance. His life,

Duriau concludes, was 'the complete opposite of Imperial glory', it was rather a mixture of simple joys and trivial miseries.[2]

All hardships were more cheerfully tolerated in the close-knit community of the *Grande Armée*, especially in the early years. Surgeon Jean-Baptiste d'Héralde enjoyed his familiarity with the military officers of his regiment. In his memoirs, he describes the bivouacs of the Prussian campaign of 1806.

> The colonels ate the mess soup with a wooden or bone spoon. This soup was prepared by the sappers of the 1er *peloton* for the colonel, the commandant, the adjutant-major, the chirurgien-major and his aide who, when in bivouac, ate and slept near to the colonel under a shelter built by the sappers. At this time every man was equal. The colonel, the commandant and adjutant major would often say; 'when I was a grenadier ...' The discipline was no less severe but it was fair. It is there that I learnt to be sober: who would dare to get drunk in front of his colonel! All the officers had carried the haversack and respected those who still carried it. The generals knew that the soldiers and colonels slept at the bivouac and tried to spare them this. When they were there, they went there themselves to pass on the orders they had received from the marshals. In the campaigns of 1805, 1806 and 1807 I have often seen General Suchet come to our bivouac while waiting for the marshal's orders. There he ate potatoes with the grenadiers and chatted with them about their needs, their fatigues and their wounds. He called our sous-officers by their first names.[3]

Military life was a serious business but the army's doctors were often sustained by a lively sense of humour and an enjoyment of the unexpected. Typical was Maltese *officier de santé* Eugene Fenech who had some comic moments in the hell-hole of the Peninsula. In one characteristic episode during the evacuation from Coimbra in 1810, he galloped over a bridge and inadvertently covered two pedestrians with mud. Stopping to commiserate with the disgruntled pair, he realised that it was Marshal Masséna and his mistress who had temporarily descended from their luxurious carriage. Fenech quickly weighed up his options, dug his spurs into his horse and, with a final spray of mud, galloped over an adjacent hill to conceal himself behind some houses.[4]

We can gain some impression of the appearance of Napoleon's doctors on campaign by scrutinising contemporary plates and reading the uniform regulations. Legislation of 1796 stipulated that *officiers de santé* should wear a tricorn hat and a grey blue coat with distinctive collar and facings; black for physicians, crimson for surgeons and green for pharmacists. The ranks within the medical subspecialties were distinguished by different embroideries and buttons. New regulations appeared throughout the period but these were mostly minor and not worthy of detailed description, not least because they probably bore little relation to the actual dress of many doctors in the field. At the commencement of a campaign, their original uniform may have been largely intact. Twenty-three-year-old Sous-Aide Pierre Bénard set off towards Spain in his new surgeon's kit and felt himself to be 'in fancy dress'. However, this regulation appearance was usually short-lived as Pharmacist Fée relates:

> I was scarcely twenty years old. I took pride in my youthful moustache which, helped by a large sword, gave me a marshal and imposing air. A hat, protected from the rain by a piece of oilskin, was held on my head by a piece of string tied under the chin. An enormous overcoat made up of a large sheet and supplemented by the coat of the uniform withstood the cold of the mountains and December's north wind. Some saddlebags placed by the side of my pistol holsters contained my provisions and a few books. Never, during this time, was any attention paid to the uniform or the equipment of the *officiers de santé*. My sword was a parade sword and my pistols could not have sent a ball ten paces. Nearly all my colleagues were on foot.

Six months after Fée entered Spain, all he retained of his uniform was his hat, '... of all the head-dresses ever invented by the capricious genius of man this was the most inconvenient and grotesque.' He and his friends were reduced to wearing the coats and trousers of the locals.[5]

Fée relates that most of his fellow *officiers de santé* had no means of transport. The battles of the period were sporadic short bursts of activity and the doctors, like most of the *Grande Armée*, spent much of their time trudging along the roads of Europe. When, in October 1805, a young captain of artillery complained to Napoleon that his mission to collect 300,000 pairs of shoes had removed him from the theatre of operations, the Emperor was quick to put him in his place: 'Child! You do not understand the service you have just rendered; shoes are needed for marching and marching wins battles.' The infantry which left Boulogne in April 1805 reached Spire towards the end of September having covered 700 kilometres on foot. The greatest single march by a unit of the *Grande Armée* was probably that of Friant's division of Davout's corps between Leopoldsdorf and Gross Raygern in the same year; 125 kilometres over frozen ground in less than forty-eight hours with only five halts of half an hour each. Unsurprisingly, such efforts left a long trail of stragglers along the way, most of whom eventually rejoined their units.[6]

Such feats are all the more incredible when one considers the state of the roads. Percy's journal contains numerous complaints on the subject, for instance in Spain in January 1809: 'There have never been more dreadful roads; the carts and the horses are dying; we can't move forward; we can scarcely cover two leagues [six miles] per day. We took a turn a little too far to the right and lost contact for two hours. What a day!' Other accounts leave little doubt that the ordinary army doctors spent many of their days on foot; Chirurgien-Major Jérôme Dumas up to his knees in mud returning to France in 1806, Chirurgien-Major Louis-Vivant Lagneau marching along frozen roads to Warsaw in 1807, and Physician Laurillard-Fallot walking from Valladolid to Salamanca in 1810.[7]

Officiers de santé were not strictly entitled to horses. An official directive dated July 1807 addressed very specifically the question of whether an army doctor returning alone to his regiment after escorting a convoy of wounded was allowed to received an allowance for an animal. The administration concluded that the *officier de santé* in this situation should be treated no differently from his colleagues. He would only be refunded for a horse if he was over 50 years of age. In reality, the serious shortage of horses in the later years of the wars meant that doctors of any age were unlikely to receive one gratis. Many used their own funds to purchase a suitable animal and then struggled to feed it. A horse was a valuable commodity. In Sébastien Blaze's words, 'My first care was for my horse. One must always start there when one is on a journey.' Physician Tyrbas de Chamberet discovered his previously lost steed grazing in a Spanish meadow, paid an 'exorbitant' sum to have it re-shoed and led it back across the Pyrenees. When the dashing surgeon Urbain Fardeau was reunited with his lost horse in Italy, he thanked God, '... I liked to believe that my horse was equally pleased to see me'. Not all *officiers de santé* were natural horsemen. Astonishingly, Monsieur Sue, chief physician of the Guard's hospital, had never sat on a horse in his life. His reluctance to follow the army on campaign in 1812 is understandable.[8]

Other modes of transport included carriages, country carts and sledges. Rickety vehicles on rutted roads added to the perils of war. Percy recounts several accidents. Near Danzig in 1807, the driver of his carriage fell asleep causing the vehicle to roll down a slope into a shallow stream. Percy escaped with only a cut finger but suffered the indignity of being soaked in vinegar and brandy from broken bottles in the baggage – he was able to see the comical side of this: 'I was in a worse state than a gherkin.' Not all such incidents were so cheerfully borne. In a similar accident in Poland, Percy had to step in to prevent several surgeons who had narrowly escaped serious injury manhandling the officer of a train of artillery whom they believed responsible for the mishap.[9]

As the day wore on, the thoughts of the army's soldiers and doctors turned to their likely accommodation for the night. If the *Grande Armée* was a safe distance from the enemy and a town was close by then the men might be accommodated in the buildings, either billeted in the houses of locals or in public buildings such as churches. Percy has left several detailed descriptions of his billets with the bad ones always outnumbering the good. In Osterode, he slept on a little straw on a wooden floor which smelt strongly of the excrement of the previous incumbents, a hundred Russian prisoners. In Burgos, he was relieved to find a pigsty to give shelter from the fog and the cold. A night in the Eylau campaign is well captured by his pen.

> We are lodged in a large house which, like all the others, has been pillaged and devastated. I lay down for eight hours but only slept until midnight. The snoring of twenty people sleeping in the same room, the excessive heat of the stove, the fleas and the bugs, all kept me awake. I had a tongue as dry as a piece of wood; I drank some water and, not able to get back to sleep, I got up to write these miserable lines by the light of a small cheap candle. I have looked over the multitude of my room-mates; to the right nine surgeons sleeping on straw and, to the left, twelve people of the house, stretched out on the wooden floorboards and snoring loudly.

It could be much more pleasurable. Whilst in Danzig, he occupied one of the best houses in the town and in Ostoroch, also in Poland, he and six fellow surgeons spent a charming evening in the house of a friendly local family, eating well and sleeping on warm straw. In Russia, Heinrich Roos enjoyed a night in a cosy hayloft, eating the eggs, butter and bread generously provided by the farmer's wife.[10]

Not all locals shared their homes so easily or willingly. Pharmacist Jacob sensed that he was making a considerable imposition on his impoverished hosts in Ulm in 1806.

> It has always been very uncomfortable for me to be, in their eyes, a blight, a tax of war, and to be a trouble-maker in their families. I have always done all that I could to be the least inconvenience possible and, more than once, this has been amply recognised by my hosts.

A reluctance to provide shelter for the French army's doctors was understandable. Eugene Fenech was careful not to reveal his occupation to the locals in Cologne in 1813 as they were hesitant to house *officiers de santé* who worked in the typhus ridden hospitals. Even the most comfortable billets could have hidden dangers for the unwary. Surgeon Urbain Fardeau describes stretching himself 'voluptuously' onto some straw, crushed by fatigue and cold, not realising that he was lying on a cache of shells and powder. These were only discovered when a soldier's pipe set fire to the straw and the lucky doctor and his companions made a hasty escape. Two doctors who overslept in their billet in Spain were the cause of heated discussions between military and civil authorities before the stragglers were returned shamefully to their units. According to Heinrich von Brandt, 'the general placed them under arrest for a week to teach them how to sleep a little more lightly in future.'[11]

Oversleeping was less likely when the army was forced to bivouac in the open air. Here, the troops generally slept in battalions circled around the fire using straw, sleeping bags and their coats to give themselves some protection from the ground and the elements. Tents were regarded as unhealthy by Napoleon and were infrequently used although Surgeon Lagneau provided himself with one for the Russian campaign. Bivouacs were often opportunistic and disorganised, a fact emphasised by Lagneau.

> It is difficult to comprehend the degree of confusion produced by thousands of men who don't know where they are to sleep or where to find water for their soup and wood and straw for themselves and their horses, particularly if they arrive in heavy rain which persists through the night. It is a hellish noise with cries and struggles without equal or end.[12]

Percy spoke for many when he confessed that he 'feared nothing more than a bivouac'. Miserable though a wet campsite could be, it is the cold that the *Grande Armée*'s veterans remember. In Egypt, where Bonaparte's men were subjected to extremes of temperature, Physician Barbès notes that they were normally woken by the cold about an hour after midnight and were then forced to move around and relight the fires to restore themselves. Similar nocturnal scenes occurred in the campaigns of central Europe and Russia. Pierre-Irénée Jacob bivouacked near the Berezina river on the retreat from Moscow.

> We had made about five leagues that day and we stopped in a forest to bivouac. We were not able to make ourselves a shelter; we had no straw and it was with great difficulty that we lit a fire of green wood on the snow ... The cold was intense and it was impossible to sleep. I got up twice and took a useless axe into the forest to cut more wood. A soldier who we had allowed to pass the night with us near to our fire was found dead the following morning ... we thought he had died of cold and fatigue.

Heinrich Roos remembers that the severe cold, frost and dew froze the straw so that in the morning he had to break out of an envelope of ice. The most experienced campaigners became inured to the unpleasantness of the bivouac. When Physician Tyrbas de Chamberet returned to France from the Peninsular War in 1813 he found lodgings in a small inn at Saint-Jean-Pied-de Port. After futile attempts at repose in the warm comfortable bed he slept soundly on the hard wooden floor.[13]

Doctors frequently employed servants to assist them in their routine domestic tasks, the number dependent on their seniority and finances. Percy started out on the Jena campaign with three '*domestiques*' but it was more common for an ordinary *officier de santé* to have a single helper.

Chirurgien-Major Lagneau had a servant captured in Russia in 1812. He replaced him in June 1813 with a young man from the Meurthe region of north-east France to whom he paid twenty francs per month. He notes that this amount would have to be doubled when they returned to France as the servant would then no longer be able to live off his own army rations. Servitude often arose out of personal misfortune. Physician Laurillard-Fallot employed a German officer who had been made a prisoner of war at Wagram and who took the post as a means of escaping captivity.[14]

The appalling consequences of starvation have been discussed in the previous chapter. When food was more plentiful it was a source of solace for the soldiers and considerable time and effort was invested in making it as interesting and palatable as possible. In theory, each soldier was supposed to receive a daily ration – typically 300–700g of bread, 300g of meat, vegetables, and half a bottle of wine or beer – but in practice the distribution was irregular and even when it was sustained, for instance at the outset of the Peninsular War, the troops were inclined to supplement it with the fruits of their own pillage. One officer claimed to have served in eight campaigns of the Empire and to have not once received a ration from the army's magazines. Napoleon believed that a soldier exposed to the hardships and exertions of campaigning needed four times as much to eat as he would in a more sedentary life in his home town. Perhaps this explains why so many *Grande Armée* memoirs, including those of the doctors, are peppered with accounts of scavenging and haggling for the next meal. Percy's journal entry for 18 May 1807 outside Danzig:

> The weather is wonderful and the countryside blooming. I have caught around forty gudgeon which we have shared with others; we have here only what we can get with our own efforts or with money; a Jew has just sold us eggs, butter, wine and white bread. The Polish soldiers, a rude and famished race, have stolen from the market at Ohra and have scattered the small village traders on which we rely so much.

Percy and his colleagues had to think not only of themselves but also of the needs of their wounded. In Poland, we find him paying some men of the Imperial Guard to slaughter a cow to make soup for the patients in his care.[15]

Local food was often sampled but not always enjoyed. Percy describes Spanish offerings made of 'stinking oil' and pungently seasoned with pepper. Pharmacist Blaze shared his distaste. 'The Spanish are almost entirely lacking in the culinary art ... with the exception of a few people of very elevated rank, all the other classes of society live and eat in a mean-minded and parsimonious manner.' He was also unimpressed with the local markets which, he asserted, had neither the abundance nor luxury of those of his native France. Under the circumstances, many preferred to prepare their own food from acquired ingredients. French memoirs of the wars differ from the British accounts in the attention given to the quality of food – both Percy's and Tyrbas de Chamberet's writings contain recipes recorded in sufficient detail to reproduce the dish two hundred years later. Food was always part of the equation; Chirurgien-Major d'Héralde in Andalusia in 1810:

> The 1er brigade marched and fought at Aracena where the 28e *leger* was actively engaged. Its colonel and several officers were wounded. No deaths in action but four fractures of the hip of which three proved fatal at Seville where we returned loaded up with the excellent hams of Aracena which are the best I have eaten in my life.

Clean drinking water was precious. When Percy discovers a fresh local spring in Germany, his joy is undisguised: 'What a delight! It is a long time since I have drunk such good water.' Thirst was a particular problem in Egypt and Spain. During the Egyptian campaign, camels carried water from the Nile and the wells were kept under military surveillance. Each infantry soldier was provided with a can for one day's ration of water and the cavalrymen carried larger amounts of fluid in goatskins and water bags. Spain, according to Pharmacist Blaze, was a country without streams or fountains and water was only available from occasional wells at the side of the road which had often been deliberately polluted by the locals. As was the case for food, the *officiers de santé* had the double difficulty of finding water for themselves and their patients. In the hospital at Talavera in 1810, Tyrbas de Chamberet admits to being overwhelmed by the desperate requests of the sick for water which he was unable to dispense because of the shortage of jugs.[16]

It is clear that food and other basic necessities of life could often only be procured with money. *Officiers de santé* were entitled to remuneration according to formal pay scales. In the later years of the Revolutionary Wars the salaries were relatively generous. In 1799 inspector generals received an annual wage of 8,000 francs, *officiers en chef* 4,000 francs and physicians 3,000 francs. The pay of surgeons and pharmacists was determined by their grade and location. For surgeons and pharmacists of the first, second and third class in the hospitals, the annual pay was 2,000, 1,500 and 1,100 francs respectively. For those serving with the army, the pay was greater at 3,000, 2,250 and 1,200 francs.

The effective amount of pay was less before 1797 as it was received in the form of *assignats*. These bank notes of the French Revolution were commonly refused by local shops, especially where the troops were on foreign soil.[17] After 1797 all army officers, including the doctors, were paid in cash. This period of relative affluence was not to last. At the end of 1799, the Minister of War suddenly cut off the pay of the *officiers de santé*.

Percy was enraged and wrote to Berthier, the *Grande Armée*'s chief of staff, in January 1800.

> For four months you have suspended the pay of the *officiers de santé* of the army. They are in extreme distress and yet they remain zealous and altruistic. As a witness to their misery and the voice of their understandable feelings, I pray, citizen-minister, that you stop all the delays and obstacles preventing the assistance and justice owed to these employees, perhaps the most useful and certainly the most unfortunate in the army. All seems to predict that the ministry of the *officiers de santé* will again be needed by the army this year. It is necessary to encourage and retain them.[18]

This had the desired effect although, for many, the glory of Marengo was to be followed by dismissal.

It is of interest to compare the rates of pay of *officiers de santé*, specified by regulations of 1803, with the salaries of other army officers and doctors in civil life. At this time, the remuneration of those working in the military hospitals was partly dictated by seniority, the maximum annual salary of 2,700 francs being received by doctors who had served for thirty years or more. More humble posts, such as that of *sous-pharmacien*, would attract around 800 francs per year. In the army corps, regimental *chirurgiens-majors* earned between 2,200 and 2,700 francs with *aides-majors* receiving 1,000 francs and *sous-aides* 800 francs. For military officers, the annual rates were 5,500 francs for a colonel, 4,300 francs for a major, 2,400 francs for a captain of the first class and 1,000 francs for a junior lieutenant. Comparisons with medical earnings in civilian life are more difficult as outside the army the better qualified doctors might have aspired to a lucrative practice in a major city whilst others would have been simple *officiers de santé* living in penury in the provinces. The army's most senior doctors were making a financial as well as a personal sacrifice in following the *Grande Armée*'s legions across Europe. In one of his frequent conversations with Napoleon, Percy made this point, although in suitably reverential terms.

> 'What is your pay in the army?' asked the Emperor.
> 'Sire, my colleague Desgenettes and myself are paid less with the army than in Paris because, being absent, we earn little from the School and we lose our consulting rights; Monsieur Desgenettes has lost a fine clientele which could have made him a rich man in a few years but we do not look at it like this and, although our pay with the army scarcely covers our expenses, we are always ready to march when Your Majesty himself marches.'

Napoleon then asked about the earnings of the regimental surgeons and Percy stressed their low pay, comparing it with the expense of their education and their potential wealth in their home towns. However, again he was careful to add that they served not out of self-interest but only out of loyalty to the Emperor.[19]

The explicit salary scales of the regulations disguise both complexities and shortcomings in the pay of soldiers and doctors. Just as they received *assignats* in the years of the Revolution, the army's doctors might still be given token money of doubtful value. In Spain in 1808, Chirurgien Sous-Aide Eugene Fenech obtained his salary at Lisbon in the form of '*vales*' or '*bons*', paper bills which were worth only two thirds of their nominal value. The government undertook to make up the difference but he and his fellow soldiers were at the mercy of the local money changers. At the time of the peace of Tilsit in 1807, pay had been owed to the army for more than six months, whilst in 1810 it was estimated that the pay of French troops in Spain was twelve million francs in arrears. This led to real hardships. Joseph Tyrbas de Chamberet battled against a murderous epidemic of dysentery at the hospital at Treviso in Italy in 1809. Despite being surrounded by disease and death, he says that he would have been happy if it had not been for his extreme poverty. For the previous five or six weeks, he had had insufficient money to buy food.

> The money which I had brought from Paris had been all spent despite every possible economy. I had not been handed a single centime during my four months in Italy. My father, informed of my distress, had sent me 400 francs but I had not received this because there was disorder and corruption of the post just as in the other branches of the army's administration.

Many of Tyrbas de Chamberet's colleagues resorted to eating food intended for the sick. Others were denied their rightful rewards by the army's red tape. Each soldier carried a *livret*, a parchment bound notebook containing details such as his name, company, battalion, service numbers, physical description, place of origin and parents. Doctor André Guilmot, serving in St Domingo in 1802, became parted from his and was unable to receive any pay until its return.[20]

There were periods of relative plenty and for the more lucky or astute of the *officiers de santé* war brought its own opportunities. At the end of the Spanish campaign in May 1812, Eugene Fenech was able to reflect on his financial affairs with some satisfaction. By buying and selling his mules and horses he had contrived to make a profit of 1,800 francs. Added to the savings he had derived from his *sous-aide*'s salary he had, tucked in his belt, more than 6,600 francs in gold. He was also owed seven months back pay.[21]

If an *officier de santé* was to do anything more than survive on campaign it was crucial to try and get along with the locals. Language was an obvious barrier. Physician Tyrbas de Chamberet expresses his frustration at being unable to properly thank a welcoming family in Valladolid because of his near complete ignorance of Catalan. On the other hand, doctors were often well educated and intelligent men and most made great efforts to learn something of the language and dialects of the countries through which they passed. In August 1807 Percy methodically translates a few simple Polish words and phrases into his journal; 'bread', 'water', 'immediately', 'I do not understand', 'that's fine'. Others were more ambitious and became skilled linguists. Chirurgien-Major Lagneau could converse in Latin, Italian and Spanish. His grasp of the latter language was such that when serving with the Old Guard in the Peninsula he acted as an interpreter and intermediary between the villagers and the colonel of his regiment. This was not unique. At a ball in Madrid, Eugene Fenech translated the words of the local ladies for Marshal Masséna so proficiently that he was asked if he was Spanish.[22]

The attitudes of the local population to French invasion varied enormously. There are innumerable anecdotes of kindness. The Germans were notably solicitous towards the French wounded in the years 1805 to 1814, their contribution often compensating for the deficiencies of the *service de santé*. Local women provided dressings and German doctors greatly outnumbered their French military counterparts in the hospitals. At Eylau, Percy contradicts the propaganda of his country's press, stating that the French wounded were well treated by the Russian troops in the nearby towns. In the rear, there were eight French *chirurgiens-majors* and sixty-four Polish surgeons to tend the *Grande Armée*'s wounded. There was some generosity in Spain. D'Héralde relates that the people of Estremadura were generally hospitable and that they preferred the French to the British who were viewed as less sociable and more demanding. Lagneau describes a friendly billet at Ocana and Percy was well treated by the peasants in northern Spain. 'We spent the whole evening surrounded by thirty Spaniards, in the middle of whom we felt not the least fear.' He says that the men were simple farm labourers and bore no grudge against the French soldiers. The guerrilla bands were greatly feared but not always merciless. A hospital employee seized on the road to Toledo was well treated by his captors, although this may have been largely because they were nervous of the surrounding French forces.[23]

If these incidents reveal a gentler aspect of the wars, there was also widespread animosity towards the French coupled with a deep distrust. Nowhere was this more so than in Spain where the apparently friendly local could suddenly become a worst enemy. Percy believed that many of the more educated Spanish were ambivalent towards the French but that in the common mass there were 'wild' and 'maniacal' elements who would stop at nothing. Pharmacist Blaze witnessed the people of Seville, whom his comrades had viewed as friends and 'trusted blindly', quickly turn on the remaining French troops when the main force left the area. This fickleness is confirmed by Surgeon Lagneau who during his campaign in Spain was under constant fear of attack by local gangs of guerrillas made up of villagers and often led by priests and other local dignitaries.

French doctors' accounts of the Peninsular War contain much anecdotal evidence of the profound hatred felt by many Spanish. When Percy arrived at Irun, the first town in Spain, in 1808, the local mayor received him coldly and did not offer him a drink. It was the first of many rebuffs. These encounters could be more menacing. Eugene Fenech, travelling alone near Toledo, asked a local shepherd for directions. 'He replied to me in a Castilian dialect, "You have eaten more bread than me in Castile". I said to him, "Show me the way or you will see what I am capable of doing"'. The shepherd's bluff was called and the doctor proceeded on his journey. When Tyrbas de Chamberet offered some sweets to the young girl of a family with whom he was billeted in Segovia, she recoiled from him. 'Leave me alone monsieur. I hate you and I want to see all the French have their throats cut in front of my eyes.' In this climate, it is of little surprise that the French wounded received scant sympathy. Captain Charles François was insulted and stoned by the local inhabitants of Andalusia when they saw that he was wounded. 'I cannot describe how much I cursed my fate.'[24]

Despite this mixed reception, many doctors were sympathetic to the local people whose lives were destroyed by French conquest. Percy retained his compassion through the most miserable of campaigns. In Poland, he came across an old woman clothed in rags and starving who had been abandoned by her family. After gradually winning her trust, he gave her bread and wine. Near Danzig, a few months later, he took pity on the homeless inhabitants of the devastated countryside and shared his meal with a young peasant woman. Although the doctors were perhaps, because of their professional ethos, more empathetic with the 'enemy' than their military compatriots, it was not always wise to disclose this. In Spain in 1810, Tyrbas de Chamberet was outraged when a belligerent French soldier ruined a peasant's crops and then abused him when he legitimately complained.

> Indignant at this act of vandalism, I made to move forward to expose the truth and argue in favour of this innocent, when an old surgeon, standing next to me, pulled me back by the arm, saying, 'Nothing you say will save this unfortunate family man and you will only compromise yourself with these maniacs and imbeciles. I have experience of this, believe me! Don't get yourself involved in it'.[25]

The French had their prejudices regarding their continental enemies. According to Percy, the Prussians were 'detested as braggarts' whilst the

Russians were relatively favoured. The surgeon had few good words for the 'English', although he had to acknowledge that their behaviour in the Peninsula was no worse than that of his own army. The Spanish receive a poor press. Sébastien Blaze's claim that they were lazy was widely echoed. The ill feelings between French and Spanish can hardly have been improved by the contempt shown by the *Grande Armée*'s soldiers towards their southern neighbours. Tyrbas de Chamberet, who appears able to view the war in an unusually objective manner, was appalled by two young officers who repaid their compliant Spanish hosts by leaving excrement in their previously clean beds.[26]

The frequency of venereal disease in Napoleon's armies is testimony to the interest that the men took in the local women. Not all pretended that their own involvement was entirely 'scientific' as did Dominique Larrey who included a visit to a women's baths in his exhaustive study of the Egyptian way of life. Bonaparte's chief surgeon viewed proceedings through a small hole in the wall. There are many references in the journals and diaries of *officiers de santé* to beautiful women but there is also much critical comment. Percy was unsparing in his judgements; in Poland, a young lady was so fat that she weighed at least as much as him, in Spain two young sisters with the largest noses he had ever seen ('larger than that of Charles IV'), whilst elsewhere in the Peninsula, the women were 'as ugly and dirty as Hottentots'. Many soldiers were less discriminating and surprised at the easy availability of local women. One officer of the 17e *leger* expressed bewilderment that German women were superficially very religious but, in reality, had few morals. Surgeon Lagneau notes that the women of Leipzig were not particularly attractive but they were 'friendly and easy to approach. They have got used to the French ...'[27]

Some local liaisons developed into full blown romance. Physician Laurillard-Fallot fell in love with a beautiful Andalusian girl, a daughter of the local postmaster. Like many of her countrywomen, she was deeply antagonistic to the French and the forlorn physician had to admire her from afar, not least because she carried a well sharpened dagger. Fortunately, Mariquita's younger sister developed an abscess in her armpit which caused her great suffering and necessitated regular visits by the altruistic army doctor. He eventually won over Mariquita and, 'mad with love', risked his life by riding alone in the countryside around Ciudad Rodrigo to meet with her. She thought him to be wealthy and, not wanting to disabuse her of this opinion, he eventually slipped away to follow the army. 'It is fifteen years since these events and I still write these lines with emotion.' Sébastien Blaze recounts a similar interlude where he flirted outrageously with the daughter of his Spanish hosts, furtively communicating with her under the dining table. Not all approaches were so welcome. Laurillard-Fallot recalls an awkward episode later in the Spanish campaign, when he was pestered by the sister of the village pharmacist.

She promised him wealth, a good local clientele, and wrote him letters, 'of great originality with lively passions mixed with quotations of Goethe, of Schiller etc.'[28]

The *Grande Armée* was not a peculiarly male preserve. Heinrich Roos says that the Poles and the Russians were 'much astonished' at the number of women and children who accompanied the French forces. In addition to the women legitimately following the soldiers, those selling useful items (*vivandières*) and the laundrywomen (*blanchisseuses*), there were also a large number of hangers on who lived parasitically on the military machine. Sébastien Blaze saw them in Spain.

> This army of women marched behind us, all of them from a marchioness to a gypsy rushing to come with us … And what will become of them? – They will do what they can; on campaign there is little thought of the future and it is the least of their concerns and yet it is easy to predict. Those who are married will share good and bad fortune with their husbands and the others will stay with their lovers or move on. Thus, the mistress of a general will become that of a captain and later that of a sergeant; it is very rare for these women to advance a grade. The same fate awaits them all on our return to France. They will be abandoned.

It was unusual for doctors to take their wives on campaign. In his account of the Egyptian expedition, Desgenettes briefly mentions a wife nursing her young physician husband at Alexandria but there are few other examples.[29]

Not all found the solace of female company. In Moscow, Marie-François Shaken, a 19-year-old surgeon in Davout's corps, wrote home to his sister: 'Find me a pretty little mistress for my return, for there are none here … Tell her I will love her very much.' He must have been unusually reticent or fussy for prostitution was rife in the Russian capital and there were always plenty of prostitutes in the wake of the *Grande Armée*. At the camp of Boulogne in 1805, a special barracks was created for them and named the *'quartier général du beau sexe militaire de Boulogne et de sa banlieue'*. The users of this facility were quaintly referred to as *'l'état major des troupes légères du sentiment'*. In occupied countries, prostitution was routine. In Prussia, Percy says that young boys ran after the soldiers to offer them women, whilst Pharmacist Cadet de Gassicourt reports that the prostitution in Vienna was 'more immoral and less scandalous than in Paris'.[30]

It is clear that women were often at the bottom of the army's food chain. There is less evidence that they played a significant professional role in nursing the sick and wounded. Where 'nurses' appear, they are mostly local women acting for reasons of self-preservation or with genuine goodwill. We must presume that the 'five or six pretty women' who nursed Aide-de Camp Lejeune's wounded brother after Friedland were Polish and not French. There are scattered references to female employees in the *service de santé*. Of the 340 women entitled to accompany the Egyptian expedition in 1798, ten were attached to the hospitals. However, it is difficult to make any case for women having fulfilled a routine nursing role in the hospitals or on the battlefield. Thus, when Heinrich Roos saw some young Bavarian women accompanying the troops into Russia to care for the sick and wounded, he comments, 'my astonishment was extreme'. That is not to say that wounded and sick men never received assistance from the army's women. *Vivandières* and officer's wives won respect for their practical help behind the lines. In Syria, General Verdier's wife was famous for her kindness to the wounded, giving them food and water, the use of her horse, and her own clothes for dressings.[31]

Campaigning was not all action and the army's doctors commonly found themselves billeted in a small country town or village far from home with time on their hands. Reading was a popular distraction from the anxieties and tediousness of military life and their choice was eclectic and often historical. Pierre-Irénée Jacob spent a night near the Berezina leafing through *The Confessions of Jean-Jacques*, a book he had found during the day. 'Unfortunately, my dream was short-lived. Sad reality soon returned me to a French bivouac 500 leagues from home under a glacial Russian sky.' Percy overcame boredom in Poland by reading the memoirs of Frederick II, whilst in Spain Sébastien Blaze bemoaned the fact that the libraries of the houses contained only multiple copies of Don Quixote. Writing was also popular and many *officiers de santé* kept daily journals. Typical is that of Chirurgien-Major Dumas who methodically noted all his billets and bivouacs of 1805 and 1806 in a leather notebook small enough to slip into his pocket. Like many of these very personal records of a soldier's life it was discovered a hundred years later and published in the famous French military periodical *Carnet de la Sabretache*.[32]

Many a hard day on campaign was brought to a close with the obligatory diary entry; for instance, Percy in Spain in 1809: 'I have arranged a dirty mattress and some woollen blankets on the wooden floor near to the fire; I am laid down and am writing, my eyes nearly shut, the lines above.' Others kept a less regular record but used a lull in the fighting to scratch their military memoirs with an improvised pen and ink. Sébastien Blaze wrote his in a farm at the foot of the Pyrenees. He later reflected: 'Written fifteen years ago, these memoirs were meant to be read only by family and a few friends ... my brother suggested that we throw them into the whirlwind of books of this type which are offered every day to the publishers ... I let myself be seduced ... I have braved the English cavalry and I tremble at exposing myself to that of the critics.'

Writing home and receiving mail was much more than a way of passing the time. Letters were the only link with family, a powerful antidote to the 'nostalgia' of campaign. In the best conditions, a letter sent from Paris would reach the environs of Moscow in two to three weeks. More typically, Percy's letters to his wife from Spain took around two months. *Officiers de santé*, like other literate military men, came to rely on this trickle of information from their families and home towns and they became indignant if the letters dried up. Chirurgien-Aide-Major Pierre Darrigade to his older brother from northern France in 1793:

> I have not received a letter from you for a long time. I do not understand, my brother, the reason for you not writing to me. There is not a notorious town in the department of the Ardennes, the Nord, and the Somme through which I have not travelled since my return to France and from which I have not written to you. And you have not had the decency to reply. I do not pretend to give you a lesson in politeness but I believe I can allow myself to call you to order.

Physician Laurillard-Fallot was keen to stress to his family that he could not presume that no news was good news. From Dresden, September 1813:

> Why do I not receive any more news? It is more than a month since I have received anything from you. My spirit, which is only too susceptible to gloomy impressions, sees in this silence only some new misfortune. I tremble at the prospect of learning something dreadful.

He continues in a similar vein, listing several possible catastrophes which might have befallen his relatives in his absence. For illiterate soldiers, the great majority of the rank and file, and those very far from their homeland, there was no prospect of regular communication. Heinrich Roos's letters from Russia failed to reach his parents and his homecoming caused consternation as his regimental colleagues had previously assured them that he was dead, even describing his final resting place on the side of the road near Vilna.[33]

Remarkably, at least a few *officiers de santé* retained their broader intellectual and cultural interests whilst on campaign. Percy's passion for collecting armour has been alluded to. He was also a keen gardener and easily distracted by a fine tree or plant. In Madrid in 1809, he finds a beautiful garden and documents the types of flowers in his journal. French army doctors immersed themselves in the local Spanish culture which they were eager to compare with what was available at home. Pharmacist Blaze thought the Spanish theatre to be 'lacking in delicacy', the locals allegedly preferring quantity to quality. As for bullfighting, 'The passion of Spain for this type of diversion is proof of the barbarity and ferocity of this uncultured nation.' Travel could be an endless slog through bland countryside but the prospect of entering a new city brought a rush of excitement. After Austerlitz, Surgeon Dumas spent an enjoyable week playing the tourist in Vienna, visiting the library, the museum, the arsenal and the theatre. The latter was running a German farce and Dumas compared it poorly with the theatres of Paris. When Surgeon Lagneau learned, in the same campaign, that he was not to go to Milan as originally ordered, he and his comrades were 'bitterly disappointed' at not being able to view the famed Italian city.[34]

Between these pleasant interludes, there was much work to be done and the *officiers de santé* played their full part. It is obvious that both Larrey and Percy drove themselves relentlessly, often to the point of complete exhaustion. In Egypt, Larrey showed the capacity for work that he was to sustain throughout the wars. At the siege of Acre, he remembers: 'I did not enjoy a moment's rest. I was incessantly in the ambulances or running from the camp to the trenches and from the trenches to the hospitals or busied in going through the divisions …' At Eylau, he admitted to his wife that he was physically worn out. The army's senior doctors had to cope with unrelenting administrative tasks in addition to their immediate medical duties. In the Eylau campaign, Percy complains that he is crushed by these demands.

> I have worked all day and have sent out more than fifty letters or parcels; I have received 280 ministerial commissions … I have seen nobody for three days; I am up to my armpits in papers; when others rest, I continue to suffer … I would well like to tear up and burn the papers which are always making a new pile on my desk.

The more junior *officiers de santé* were also afflicted by periods of extreme over-work. Of the Egyptian campaign, Larrey simply states, 'It is almost impossible to describe the fatigues which the army surgeons underwent at this time.' Eugene Fenech worked eighteen hours a day to help organise the hospitals in Astorga in 1809 and diagnosed himself as having a scurvy-like disease brought on by his fatigue and unhealthy diet. When Physician Laurillard-Fallot campaigned in France in 1814, he became so exhausted as to sleep soundly on his horse and to worry that he might fall onto the bayonets of the surrounding soldiers. Percy had sympathy for his junior colleagues, often mentioning their personal difficulties and privations in his journal. In 1799 the 'poor surgeons' are very fatigued and after Eylau they are 'exhausted and harassed'. He attributes the death of a *chirurgien-major* at Preuss-Eylau to the excessive surgical workload that had resulted from the battle.[35] Early 19th-century army life always had the potential to be hard and miserable, but most complaints by French soldiers relate specifically to the campaigns in Spain, Poland and Russia. The war in the Peninsula had a unique character well summed up by Laurillard-Fallot.

> Everywhere poor billets; between Burgos and Dunas some bivouacs; nothing from the inhabitants who hold us to ransom; an infinite amount of dirty vermin which devour us; endlessly surrounded by enemies who watch out for the moment to kill us with impunity.

He could not wait to leave Spain, a sentiment shared by most of his friends. Joseph Tyrbas de Chamberet shudders at the memory of bivouacs in the forests near Salamanca where they were forced to eat raw acorns under the leafy shelter of the oaks. Percy's journal for 31 December 1808:

> The weather is foggy and cold. What a shame to be in such a country on the last day of the year, far from all that we hold dear in France! But we have to accept our fate. They have lent me a shirt whilst mine is washed.

In Poland, everything seemed to be coated in mud. Soldiers died at the side of the road who, according to Percy, could have been saved by a glass of water or wine. The surgeons were hungry and dejected. On the retreat from Russia, Larrey claimed that the doctors were particularly unfortunate as their commitment to their patients meant that they had little time to scavenge for their own needs. Eugene Labaume concurs with this view, '... none were to be more pitied than the physicians, and especially the surgeons, who, without hope of advancement, exposed themselves like the common soldiers by dressing the wounded on the field of battle'. He relates a grim anecdote of a young surgeon driven back by a mob in his efforts to obtain a small amount of bread. The *officiers de santé* who did survive 1812 must have been tough and determined in equal measure. Pharmacist Gannal escaped from the clutches of the Russians at Vilna and travelled alone on foot through Lithuania, the Grand Duchy of Warsaw, Silesia, Bohemia and Saxony, only moving at night and hiding in woods during the day. He later made a great reputation in Paris as an embalmer. Pharmacist Jacob improved his chances of survival by forming a small club of six doctors who each vowed to help each other in time of need.[36]

Larrey believed, surprisingly, that men from the south of France best tolerated the Russian climate but Physician Roos asserted that it was less a matter of nationality than of experience and acclimatisation. He noted that it was the veterans who won through as the youngsters fell away. This durability came at a price; in Percy's words:

> No pity in the armies, no sensitivity ... One must not expect to find a man there. It is only among the surgeons that compassion, philanthropy, the love of his fellow man, is retained.

However, as early as 1799, Percy was concerned that he too was becoming inured to the human cost of war.

> We see here the dead and the dying; we hear the cries and the moans of those who are suffering and the yells of those who are being operated on; but it is as if we do not hear them. We come and go, each thinking of his own safety and his own business.[37]

Officiers de santé falling into the hands of the enemy were exposed to many of the same indignities as other prisoners of war. Rough rules of treatment for captured soldiers were gradually emerging but much still depended on the humanity of the captors. Officers were usually treated considerably better than the common man. Elzéar Blaze claimed that, of the 'civilised nations', the French treated prisoners of war with the greatest kindness. In his opinion, the Russians banished their captives to Siberia, the English treated them as enemies and were spiteful and the Spanish were the cruellest. His brother, Sébastien, broadly agreed although he reserved his bitterest invective for the British. 'The pontoons of Plymouth were places of torture, tombs a hundred times more dreadful than the floating prisons of Cádiz.' A considerable number of French doctors were captured during the Russian campaign. Of course, we only have the accounts of the survivors – men such as Physician Heinrich Roos, Chirurgien-Major La Flize, Chirurgien Sous-Aide Désiré Fuzellier – but it seems that they were often able to gain favourable treatment by using their medical skills. La Flize was asked to act as regimental surgeon for the Russian unit which had captured him and Fuzellier built a good reputation among the local peasants for his free medical treatments, '… after having cured several chronic ophthalmias and ulcers, my renown extended so far that they brought me sick from Simbirsk and even Kazan'. It may be an exaggeration to say that he thrived in Russia but Heinrich Roos followed a period of service in the Russian army by becoming a physician at the hospital at Schutzkow where he had a sizeable clientele among the local nobility and army officers.[38]

The best medical account of the grim conditions in the Spanish prison ships has been left by Chirurgien-Major Chapuis who was captured at the Battle of Baylen and incarcerated with a thousand other prisoners in one of the eleven vessels at Cádiz.

> The excessive heat, the poor quality of the food, the frequent lack of drinking water, the vermin, the filth, the contaminated air and the general atmosphere of deep depression all contributed to the propagation of disease; a bilious putrid fever made frightening ravages on all the ships. There was no help and we were only able to quench the thirst of the unfortunates who were dying. The Spanish physician responsible for us visited only once every eight days and then only took to the hospital on land those sick in which death appeared almost certain. The space we had to sleep in was so small that the dead and dying touched each other and often when a prisoner awoke in the morning he found his comrades dead at his side. There were 36 to 40 deaths per day on the ships; they immediately threw them into the sea to get rid of them and, at each tide, one could see the bodies they had thrown in several days before floating around the ships.[39]

The British prison ships were not, as Sébastien Blaze alleges, much worse than the Spanish but they were not much better either. Physician Laurillard-Fallot was captured by the British at Coimbra and was taken to Lisbon and then by sea to Portsmouth where he was shut up in an ancient ship of war crudely converted into a prison.

> We boarded the *San Damaso* in the evening. When they opened the hatch to make us descend into the compartment which awaited us, there came up a suffocating stench. It was revolting. I will not attempt to describe my emotions as I saw myself being thrown into a world so new, strange and without any precedent; in the middle of a mixture of repulsive faces and indescribable costumes!

With the help of his fellow prisoners, the young physician survived his month afloat and was then transferred onto the mainland where he spent time at Bishops Waltham in Hampshire and Whitchurch in Shropshire. In these country towns he was much better treated as he was lodged with local people and became friendly with the English general practitioners.[40]

The camaraderie of the *Grande Armée* was all the more important in times of adversity. Many close friendships were formed on the long stages en route to the corners of the Empire. On the march to Spain, junior physician Léon Dufour was delighted to meet a young lieutenant of infantry of his own age who came from a neighbouring village. The friendship lasted and when the doctor later taught medicine at Rouen he was able to litter his lectures with references to his old friend 'Marshal Bugeaud'. There was also goodwill between the soldiers of different nations. At Tilsit in 1807, the French, Russians and Prussians mingled freely together. Because of the frequent hardships, these good times on campaign were all the more appreciated. Percy's journal provides a unique insight into the brutality of war in the Napoleonic era but, in stark contrast, there are days when he extols the beauty of the countryside and quality of birdsong. A spirit of optimism often emerges in the most torrid circumstances. In Russia, Heinrich Roos saw with dismay that the men were dying from hunger and he wondered if the same fate awaited him. 'Suddenly, I saw an elegant wooden spoon on the road at my feet; I picked it up and, at that moment, considered it an omen that I would never die of hunger; my spirits lifted.'[41]

The greatest joy was still that of homecoming. When Sébastien Blaze, returning from the campaign of Spain, saw the large words *'premier village français'* written on a wall he burst into tears. This elation could be short-lived as the end of the fighting at the two Restorations inevitably brought the likelihood of dismissal from the army and the uncertainty of a new life in civilian practice. Any pension received depended on rank, length of service and wounds and disabilities. The regulations of 1800 stipulated that, after thirty years of service, an officer would receive an annual pension equal to half his pay and that this would increase incrementally to a maximum amount paid out after an improbable fifty years' service.[42] The army's most distinguished doctors were mostly able to integrate back into civil life although the transition was not necessarily painless. Old loyalties and allegiances were not quickly forgotten. At the second Restoration, Percy was watched by the secret police and informers in an atmosphere of paranoia. His quaint collection of antique armour was suspected as a potential arsenal. Eventually, Louis XVIII personally intervened to stop the groundless persecution. At this time, Larrey also suffered social ostracism and his scientific publications were treated with caution. His rehabilitation started in 1818 when the government restored his pension and praised his humanity.[43]

The final fall of Napoleon brought mixed emotions and fortunes for the ordinary doctors of the *Grande Armée*. The more able among them did transfer successfully into the army of the post-Napoleonic state or into civilian medicine. In some ways the army was the more difficult choice of the two. Jean Baptiste d'Héralde rejoined the service in January 1816 but old soldiers of the Empire were distrusted and he had little doubt that he was under close surveillance by the police. Louis-Vivant Lagneau was not a great admirer of Napoleon but he admitted that he and his brother were broken-hearted to see the victorious Prussians marching through Paris in July 1815. His yearning for the *Grande Armée* may have been fanned by a letter that he had just received from twenty-three officers of his old regiment thanking him for his kindness and devotion. He gradually found his feet in the capital.

> I still had a number of old clients and I found some more among families of our acquaintance connected with the Guard and the army. I also had some new civilian clients because, having been away for eleven years, I was able to do surgery and obstetrics as well as medicine and, in all, I was busy enough not to be bored and to be able to meet my expenses.

Lagneau joined medical societies in Paris which were frequented by old army comrades and his civilian practice thrived. Within five years, a combination of hard work and useful army connections had increased his annual earnings from 2,000 to 18,000 francs. In his own words, '... each day brings me more work and more prosperity'. With their superior education, many of the army's physicians also returned successfully to private practice. Joseph Tyrbas de Chamberet was penniless when he was laid off in 1815 but, in the following year, he was named by the Minister of War as assistant professor of medicine in Lille.[44]

The ease with which many army doctors re-entered civilian life is not so surprising as, in the decades after Waterloo, French, and particularly

Parisian medicine was still dominated by men who had served in the *Grande Armée*. This list of eminent ex-army doctors is lengthy but we may quote René Théophilus Laennec, the inventor of the stethoscope, who was a humble *médecine-sous-aide* of the third class, the great surgeon Alexis Boyer who served with the Peninsular army, and François Broussais, the leader of Paris medicine, who was a physician in Napoleon's armies in Holland, Germany, Austria, Italy and Spain between 1803 and 1814. Broussais was typical of many of these successful doctors in that he had retained some of the manners of the old Napoleonic soldier, the *grognard*. His academic lectures were likely to be interrupted by anecdotes of a previous life when, for more than ten years, he had marched with the all-conquering armies of Napoleon. His bitter antagonism towards British medicine was based not on any intellectual objection but on hostility against the country which had exiled his hero. At his funeral, the cortege halted at the foot of the Napoleonic monument in the *Place Vendôme*. Broussais would have fervently agreed with the parting words of Chirurgien-Major Lagneau.

I have spent many earlier years which are dear to me and which give me joy in my old age. It is always with pride that I think of my journeys across Europe with my dear companions in arms in the footsteps of the Emperor.[45]

Notes

1. Jacob, P-I, *Le Journal Inédit d'un pharmacien de la Grande Armée*, pp. 200–1.
2. Lemaire, J-F, *Napoléon et la Médecine*, pp. 219–20.
3. d'Héralde, J-B, *Mémoires d'un Chirurgien de la Grande Armée*, pp. 97–8.
4. Fenech, E, *Mémoires d'un Officier de Santé Maltais dans l'Armée Française (1786–1839)*, p. 52.
5. Pigeard, A, *Le Service de Santé de la Révolution au 1er Empire 1792–1815*, pp. 47–58; Lemaire, p. 220; Brice, Docteur and Bottet, Capitaine, *Le Corps de Santé Militaire en France*, p. 188.
6. Quennevat, J-C, *Les vrais soldats de Napoléon*, pp. 161–7.
7. *Journeaux et Souvenirs sur la Campagne de 1805*, p. 78; Lagneau, L-V, *Journal d'un Chirurgien de la Grande Armée 1803–1815*, p. 83; Laurillard-Fallot, S-L, *Souvenirs d'un Médecin Hollandais sous les Aigles Françaises 1807–1833*, p. 50.
8. Lemaire, J-F, *Coste: Premier Médecin des Armées de Napoléon*, p. 297; Blaze, S, *Mémoires d'un apothicaire sur la guerre d'Espagne*, Vol. II, p. 201; Fardeau, U, *Urbain Fardeau. Mémoires d'un Saumurois chirurgien-sabreur*, p. 160; Lemaire, *Napoléon et la Médecine*, p. 97.
9. Percy, Baron, *Journal des Campagnes de Baron Percy*, pp. 233, 275.
10. Percy, pp. 152, 187, 413, 112, 257; Roos, H de, *Avec Napoléon en Russie*, p. 113.

11. Jacob, p.89; Fenech, pp. 92–3; Fardeau, p. 181; Brandt, H von, *In the Legions of Napoleon. The memoirs of a Polish Officer in Spain and Russia 1808–1813*, p. 89.
12. Lagneau, p. 93.
13. Percy, p. 425; Milleliri, J-M, *Médecins et Soldats pendant l'expédition d'Égypte (1798–1799)*, p. 129; Jacob, p. 252; Roos, p. 125; Tyrbas de Chamberet, J, *Mémoires d'un Médecin Militaire*, p. 137.
14. Lagneau, p. 163; Laurillard-Fallot, p. 38.
15. Quennevat, p. 136; Percy, pp. 302, 177.
16. Blaze, Vol. II, pp. 64, 150, 260; d'Héralde, p. 132; Percy, p. 378; Milleliri, pp. 110–14; Tyrbas de Chamberet, p. 99.
17. Forrest, A, *Soldiers of the French Revolution*, p. 175.
18. Brice, Bottet, p. 90.
19. Brice, Bottet, p. 127; Pigeard, A, *Dictionnaire de la Grande Armée*, p. 540; Percy, pp. 471–2.
20. Fenech, p. 31; Elting, J R, *Swords around a Throne. Napoleon's Grande Armée*, p. 583; Tyrbas de Chamberet, p. 68; Guilmot, A N J, *Journal de Voyage d'un officier de santé à Saint-Domingue (1802)*, p. 91.
21. Fenech, p. 68.
22. Tyrbas de Chamberet, p. 84; Percy, p. 380; Lagneau, p. 122; Fenech, p. 66.
23. Quennevat, p. 205; Percy, pp. 200, 450; d'Héralde, p. 165; Blaze, Vol. II, p. 94.
24. Percy, p. 431; Blaze, Vol. II, p. 294; Lagneau, p. 109; Fenech, p. 27; Tyrbas de Chamberet, p. 86; François, C, *From Valmy to Waterloo. Extracts from the diary of Capt. Charles François a soldier of the Revolution and the Empire*, pp. 191–2.
25. Percy, pp. 150, 277; Tyrbas de Chamberet, p. 82.
26. Percy, pp. 307, 452; Blaze, Vol. II, p. 16; Tyrbas de Chamberet, p. 87.
27. Larrey, D J, *Mémoires de Chirurgie Militaire et Campagnes 1787–1840*, p. 310; Percy, pp. 382, 444, 482; Quennevat, p. 95; Lagneau, p. 80.
28. Laurillard-Fallot, pp. 56–7, 98; Blaze, Vol. II, p. 156.
29. Roos, p.242; Quennevat, p. 155; Blaze, Vol. II, pp. 254–5; Desgenettes, R, *Histoire Médicale de l'Armée d'Orient*, Vol. I, p. 152.
30. Zamoyski, A, *1812 Napoleon's fatal march on Moscow*, p. 339; Percy, p. 385; Pigeard, *Dictionnaire de la Grande Armée*, p. 486.
31. Lejeune, Baron, *Memoirs of Baron Lejeune Aide-de-Camp to Marshals Berthier, Davout and Oudinot*, Vol. I, p. 67; Milleliri, p. 85; Roos, p. 22; Desgenettes, Vol. I, pp. 103–4.
32. Jacob, p. 204; Percy, p. 214; Blaze, Vol. II, p. 344; *Journeaux*, pp. 49–86.
33. Percy, p. 481; Blaze, Vol. II, p. 378; Quennevat, p. 125; Duliere, A, *Pierre Darrigade Chirurgien aux armées de la Révolution*, p. 21; Laurillard-Fallot, pp. 93–4; Roos, p. 273.
34. Percy, p. 496; Blaze, Vol. II, pp. 16, 57; *Journeaux*, p. 76; Lagneau, p. 59.
35. Larrey, pp. 168, 193; Percy, pp. 310–12, 28, 176, 209; Fenech, p. 46; Laurillard-Fallot, p. 101.
36. Laurillard-Fallot, p. 53; Tyrbas de Chamberet, p. 22; Percy, pp. 446, 137, 189; Labaume, E, *A circumstantial account of the campaign in Russia*, p. 349; Jacob, pp. 253, 263.

37. Roos, p. 266; Percy, pp. 171, 31.
38. Smith, D, *The Prisoners of Cabrera. Napoleon's forgotten soldiers 1809–1814*, pp. 18, 180; Blaze, E, *Military Life under Napoleon. The memoirs of Captain Elzéar Blaze*, p. 194; Blaze, S, Vol. II, p. 388; Zamoyski, p. 531; Fuzellier, D, *Journal de captivité en Russie 1813–1814*, p. 167; Roos, p. 236.
39. *Pontons et Prisons sous le Premier Empire*, pp. 10–12.
40. Laurillard-Fallot, pp. 69–82.
41. Lemaire, J-F, *Napoléon et la Médecine*, p. 220; Percy, pp. 322, 366; Roos, pp. 157–8.
42. Blaze, S, Vol. II, p.369; Pigeard, *Dictionnnaire de la Grande Armée*, p. 513.
43. Percy, p. lxi; Richardson, R, *Larrey. Surgeon to Napoleon's Imperial Guard*, p. 226.
44. d'Héralde, p. 222; Lagneau, pp. 192–203; Tyrbas de Chamberet, pp. 171–5.
45. Ackerknecht, E H, *Medicine at the Paris Hospital 1794–1848*, pp. 76–7; Lagneau, p. 203.

Appendices

Appendix I

Number of Officiers de Santé *employed with the French Army 1800–1812*

Designation	1800	1801	1802	1803	1804	1805/6	1807	1808	1809	1810	1811	1812
Inspector-Generals	3	3	3	3	6	6	6	6	6	6	7	7
Inspecteurs en chef	17	13	7	17	33	40	46	52	75	82	70	55
Physicians	210	133	62	75	94	122	170	196	256	288	158	277
Pharmacists	540	337	171	200	306	395	462	601	721	957	888	1011
Surgeons in hospitals	1036	565	327	441	152	408	517	904	1050	1412	1153	1704
Surgeons with army	629	609	515	501	899	1015	1095	1230	1730	1804	1572	2058
TOTAL	2435	1660	1085	1237	1490	1986	2296	2989	3838	4549	3848	5112

From: Brice, Docteur and Bottet, Capitaine, *Le Corps de Santé Militaire en France*, p.171.

Appendix II

Fate of a group of soldiers of Napoleon's Army enlisted in 1805–1812*

	Infantry (4,890)	Cavalry (2,645)	Artillery (896)	Whole Army
Retired	8.5	5.7	5.4	7.9
Invalided out	6.0	9.8	7.5	6.7
Became veterans	0.7	0.5	0.5	0.6
Erased from record for long absence	3.7	3.8	3.8	3.7
Erased for long absence in hospital	11.3	2.0	2.6	9.4
Killed	2.9	3.2	3.3	3.0
Died from wounds	4.2	5.6	2.0	4.3
Died from disease	17.0	7.9	17.2	15.5
Presumed taken prisoner	12.2	19.8	11.7	13.4
Remained in rear	1.0	7.6	7.0	2.3
Deserted	8.5	9.3	8.0	8.6
Disappeared in 1812	6.4	0	0	5.0
Promoted to officer	0.6	0.4	0	0.6
Moved to other units	11.5	10.9	14.0	11.5
Remained active in the army in 1814	5.5	13.3	17.0	7.3

* Figures are percentages and are probably very approximate with overlap of categories. Soldiers from the Guard or foreign regiments are excluded. From: Sokolov, O, *L'Armée de Napoléon*, p.64.

Bibliography

Ackerknecht, E H, *Medicine at the Paris Hospital 1794–1848*, Baltimore, 1967.

Almanach Impérial pour l'Année M.DCCC.XI, Paris, 1811.

Austin, P B, *1812, The Great Retreat, London*, 1996.

Austin, P B, *1812, The March on Moscow*, London, 1993.

Bade, Margrave de, *La Campagne de 1812. Mémoires du Margrave de Bade* (ed. A Chuquet), Paris, 1812.

Baldet, M, *La Vie Quotidienne dans les Armées de Napoléon*, Paris, 1964.

Barblan, M-A, *La variole dans le Département du Léman en 1811 (d'apres les registres de la conscription napoléonienne)*, Gesnerus (1974), Vol.31, pp. 193–220.

Barrès, J-B, *Memoirs of a French Napoleonic Officer*, London, 1988.

Bégin, L-J, *Études sur le service de santé en France*, Paris, 1822.

Bellot de Kergorre, A, *Journal d'un Commissaire des Guerres pendant le Premier Empire (1806–1821)*, Paris, 1997.

Bertrand, General, *Napoleon at St. Helena. Memoirs of General Bertrand Grand Marshal to the Palace*, London, 1953.

Blaze, E, *Military life under Napoleon. The memoirs of Captain Elzéar Blaze.* Chicago, 1995.

Blaze, S, *Mémoires d'un apothicaire sur la guerre d'Espagne*, 2 Vols., Paris, 1828.

Blond, G, *La Grande Armée*, London, 1995.

Bourgeois, R, *Tableau de la campagne de Moscou en 1812*, Paris, 1814.

Bourgogne, Sergeant, *Memoirs of Sergeant Bourgogne (1812–1813)*, London, 1926.

Bowden, S, *Napoleon's Grande Armée of 1813*, Chicago, 1990.

Brandt von, H, *In the Legions of Napoleon. The memoirs of a Polish Officer in Spain and Russia 1808–1813* (ed. J North), London, 1999.

Brett-James, A, *Europe against Napoleon, The Leipzig Campaign 1813*, London, 1970.

Brett-James, A, *1812, Eye-witness accounts of Napoleon's defeat in Russia*, London, 1967.

Brett-James, A, *The Hundred Days. Napoleon's Last Campaign*, Cambridge, 1989.

Brice, Docteur and Bottet, Capitaine, *Le Corps de Santé Militaire en France*, Paris, 1907.

Briot, P-F, *Histoire de l'état et de progress de la chirurgie militaire en France pendant les guerres de la Révolution*, Besançon, 1817.

Bugeaud, Col., *Memoirs of Colonel Bugeaud 1784–1815* (ed. C M Yonge), Felling, 1998.

Cabanès, A, *Chirurgiens et Blessés à travers l'Histoire*, Paris, 1918.

Cadet de Gassicourt, C-L, *Voyage en Autriche en Moravie et en Bavière fait à la suite de l'armée française pendant la campagne de 1809*, Paris, 1818.

Campagne de Saxe à la Campagne de France, Lettres et Souvenirs (1813–1814), Paris, 2000.

Cartwright, F E and Biddiss, M, *Disease and History*, Stroud, 2000.

Caulaincourt, General de, *With Napoleon in Russia. The memoirs of General de Caulaincourt Duke of Vicenza*, New York, 1935.

Chandler, D, *The Campaigns of Napoleon*, London, 1966.

Charles-Roux, F, *Bonaparte: Governor of Egypt*, London, 1937.

Chlapowski, D, *Memoirs of a Polish Lancer*, Chicago, 1992.

Cilleuls, J des, *Le service de santé militaire de ses origines à nos jours*, Paris, 1961.

Clausewitz, General Carl von, *The Campaign of 1812 in Russia*, London, 1992.

Cobb, R, *Reactions to the French Revolution*, London, 1972.

Coignet, Captain, *The narrative of Captain Coignet 1766–1850* (ed. L Larchey), New York, 1890.

Combats et captivité en Russie. Memoires et lettres de soldats français, Paris, 1999.

Connelly, O, *Blundering to Glory. Napoleon's Military Campaigns*, Wilmington, 1990.

Coste, J F and Percy, Baron, *De la santé des troupes de la Grande Armée*, Strasbourg, 1806.

Damamme, J-C, *Les Soldats de la Grande Armée*, Paris, 2002.

Davidov, D, *In the Service of the Tsar against Napoleon. The Memoirs of Denis Davidov 1806–1814* (ed. G Troubetzkoy), London, 1999.

Desgenettes, R, *Histoire Médicale de l'Armée d'Orient*, 2 Vols., Paris, 1802.

Desgenettes, R, *Souvenirs d'un médecin de l'expédition d'Égypte*, Paris, 1893.

D'Héralde, J-B, *Mémoires d'un Chirurgien de la Grande Armée*, Paris, 2002.

Dible, J H, *Napoleon's Surgeon*, London, 1970.

Ducoulombier, H, *Le Baron P-F Percy. Un chirurgien de la Grande Armée*, Paris, 2004.

Duliere, A, *Pierre Darrigade Chirugien aux armées de la Révolution*, Dinant, 1972.

Dunbar, RG, 'The introduction of the practice of vaccination into Napoleonic France,' *Bulletin of the History of Medicine* (1941), Vol. 10, pp. 635–50.

Elting J R, *Swords around a Throne. Napoleon's Grande Armée*, London, 1988.

Esdaile, C, *The Peninsular War. A new history*, London, 2002.

Evrard, E, 'La nostalgie: une malade qui se meurt, sa signification dans l'histoire de la médecine militaire,' *Annales Medécine Militaire Belgium* (1994), Vol.8, pp. 21–9.

Exteberria, F, 'Surgery in the Spanish War of Independence (1807–1813); between Desault and Lister,' *Journal of Paleopathology* (1999), Vol.11, pp. 25–40.

Fardeau, U, *Urbain Fardeau. Mémoires d'un Saumurois chirurgien-sabreur*, Grasse, 1999.

Faure, R, *Souvenirs du Nord ou la Guerre, la Russie et les Russes ou l'esclavage*, Paris, 1821.

Fée, A-L-A, *Souvenirs de la Guerre d'Espagne dite de l'indépendance (1809–1813)*, Paris, 1856.

Fenech, E. *Mémoires d'un Officier de Santé Maltais dans l'Armée Française (1786–1839)*, Paris, 2001.

Fezensac, Lieut-General de, *A Journal of the Russian Campaign of 1812*, Cambridge, 1988.

Fleischman, T, *En écoutant parler les grognards de Napoléon*, Brussels, 1962.

Forrest, A, *Conscript and Deserters. The army and French society during the Revolution and Empire*, Oxford, 1989.

Forrest, A, *Napoleon's Men. The soldiers of the Revolution and Empire*, London, 2002.

Forrest, A, *Soldiers of the French Revolution*, Durham, 1990.

Forrest, A, *The French Revolution and the Poor*, Oxford, 1981.

François, C, *From Valmy to Waterloo. Extracts from the diary of Capt. Charles François a soldier of the Revolution and the Empire*, Felling, 1991.

Fuzellier, D, *Journal de captivité en Russie 1813–1814*, Montreuil, 2004.

Gabbay, J, 'Clinical Medicine in Revolution,' *British Medical Journal* (1989), Vol. 299, pp. 106–9, 166–9.

Gallaher, J G, *The Iron Marshal. A biography of Louis N. Davout*, London, 2000.

Gama, J-F, *Esquisse historique du service de santé militaire en general et specialement du service chirurgical depuis l'établissement de hôpitaux militaires en France*, Paris, 1841.

Garrison,F H , *Notes on the History of Military Medicine*, Washington, 1922.

Gawande, A, *Casualties of War – Military care for the wounded from Iraq and Afghanistan*, New England Journal of Medicine (2004), Vol. 351, pp. 2471–5.

Genty, M, *Avec Napoléon en Russie. Souvenirs d'un médecin wurtembourgeois*, Esculape, 1813.

Geyl, P, *Napoleon for and against*, London, 1982.

Gilbert, N P, *Tableau historique des maladies internes de mauvais caractère qui ont affligé la Grande Armée dans la campagne de Prusse et de Pologne*, Berlin, 1808.

Goddard, J C, *The Navy surgeon's chest: Surgical instruments of the Royal Navy during the Napoleonic War*, Journal of the Royal Society of Medicine (2004), Vol. 97, pp. 191–7.

Gonneville, Colonel de, *Recollections of Colonel de Gonneville* (ed. C M Yonge), 2 Vols., Felling, 1988.

Griffith, P, *The Art of War in Revolutionary France 1789–1802*, London, 1998.

Guilmot, A N J, *Journal de Voyage d'un officier de santé à Saint-Domingue (1802)*, Paris, 1997.

Hapdé, J B A, *Les Sépulcres de la Grande Armée*, Paris, 1814.

Hausmann, F J, *A soldier for Napoleon. The campaigns of Lieutenant Franz Joseph Hausmann 7th Bavarian Infantry* (ed. J H Gill), London, 1998.

Heller, R, 'Officiers de Santé: the second-class doctors of nineteenth-century France', *Medical History* (1978), Vol.22, pp. 25–43.

Herold, J C, *Bonaparte in Egypt*, London, 1963.

Histoire de la médicine aux armées, 3 Vols., Paris, 1982–8.

Hodge, W B, 'On the mortality arising from military operations', *Journal of the Royal Statistical Society* (1856), Vol.19, pp. 219–71.

Horácková, L and Vargová, L, 'Bone remains from a common grave pit from the Battle of Austerlitz', *Journal of Paleopathology* (1999), Vol.11, pp. 5–13.

Horne, A, *Seven Ages of Paris*, London, 2002.

Howard, J E, *Letters and Documents of Napoleon, The Rise to Power*, London, 1961.

Howard, M, 'Walcheren 1809: A medical catastrophe', *British Medical Journal* (1999), Vol.319, pp. 1642–5.

Howard, M, *Wellington's Doctors. The British Army Medical Services in the Napoleonic Wars*, Staplehurst, 2002.

Huard, P, *Sciences Médecine Pharmacie de la Révolution à l'Empire (1789–1815)*, Paris, 1970.

Hughes, Major General BP, *Firepower. Weapons effectiveness on the battlefield 1630–1850*, London, 1974.

Jacob, P-I, 'Le Journal Inédit d'un pharmacien de la Grande Armée', *Bulletin de la Société D'Histoire de la Pharmacie* (1966), Vol. 18, pp. 1–18, 81–96, 187–204, 251–64.

Jonnès, A M de, *Adventures in Wars of the Republic and Consulate, 1791–1805*, London, 1920.

Journeaux et Souvenirs sur la Campagne de 1805, Paris, 1997.

Kaempfen, A, *Souvenirs du docteur Kaempfen du Brigue*, Vallesia, 1962, pp. 1–120.

Kerkhoves (Kerkhoffs), J R L, *Hygiène militaire ou avis sur les moyens de conserver la santé des troupes*, Maestricht, 1815.

Kerkhoves (Kerkhoffs), J R L, *Observations médicales faites pendant les campagnes de Russie en 1812 et Allemagne en 1813*, Maestricht, 1814.

Kiple, K F, *Plague, Pox and Pestilence*, London, 1997.

Kouchnir, S L L, *Considérations sur l'évolution du service de santé militaire de 1789 à 1814*, Paris, 1955.

Labaume, E, *A circumstantial account of the campaign in Russia*, London, 1815.

Lachouque, H, *Napoleon's Battles*, London, 1966.

La Flize, Dr, *Souvenirs de la Moskowa par un chirurgien de la Garde Impériale*, Feuilles d'histoire (1912), pp. 419–26.

Lagneau, L-V, *Journal d'un Chirurgien de la Grande Armée 1803–1815*, Paris, 2000.

Lamare-Picquot, F-V, *Nos anciens à Corfou. Souvenirs de l'aide-major Lamare-Picquot (1807–1814)*, Paris, 1918.

Larrey, D J, *Mémoires de Chirurgie Militaire et Campagnes 1787–1840*, 2 Vols., Paris, 2004.

Larrey, D J, *Memoirs of Military Surgery and Campaigns of the French Armies*, 2 Vols., Baltimore, 1814.

Laurent, C, *Histoire de la vie et des ouvrages de P.-F. Percy*, Versailles, 1827.

Laurillard-Fallot, S-L, *Souvenirs d'un Médecin Hollandais sous les Aigles Françaises 1807–1833*, Paris, 1997.

Lejeune, Baron, *Memoirs of Baron Lejeune Aide-de-Camp to Marshals Berthier, Davout and Oudinot*, 2 Vols., London, 1897.

Lemaire, J-F, *Coste: Premier Médecin des Armées de Napoléon*, Paris, 1997.

Lemaire, J-F, *La médicine Napoléonniene*, Paris, 2003.

Lemaire, J-F, *Les blessés dans les Armées Napoléoniennes*, Paris, 1999.

Lemaire, J-F, *Napoléon et la Médecine*, Paris, 1992.

Lixon, L J M, *Médecin à l'armée d'Espagne en 1808, 1809 et 1810*, Paris, 1814.

Longmore, T A, *A treatise on the transport of sick and wounded troops*, London, 1868.

Lucas-Dubreton, J, *Les Soldats de Napoléon*, Paris, 1977.

MacDonald, Marshal, *Recollections of Marshal MacDonald* (ed. C Rousset), London, 1893.

Marbot, Baron de, *Mémoires de Général Baron de Marbot*, 3 Vols., Paris, 1891.

Marcel, N, *Campagnes en Espagne et au Portugal 1808–1814*, Paris, 2003.

Marchand L-J, *In Napoleon's Shadow. Being the first English language edition of the complete memoirs of Lois-Joseph Marchand* (ed. P Jones), San Francisco, 1998.

Masson, F, *Aventures de Guerre 1792–1809*, Paris, 2003.

McGrigor, J, *The Autobiography and Services of James McGrigor Bt. Late Director of the Army Medical Department*, London, 1861.

Meyerhof, M, 'A short history of ophthalmia during the Egyptian Campaigns of 1798–1807', *The British Journal of Ophthalmology* (1932), Vol. 16, pp. 129–52.

Milleliri, J-M, *Médecins et Soldats pendant l'expédition d'Égypte (1798–1799)*, Paris, 1999.

Moiret, Captain J-M, *Memoirs of Napoleon's Egyptian Expedition 1798–1801*, London, 2001.

Morvan, J, *Le Soldat Impérial*, 2 Vols., Paris, 1999.

Muir, R, *Tactics and the experience of Battle in the Age of Napoleon*, New Haven, 1998.

Napoléon I, Emperor, *La Correspondance de Napoléon I^{ier}*, 32 Vols., Paris, 1858–70.

Ney, Marshal, *Memoirs of Marshal Ney published by his family*, 2 Vols., London, 1833.

North, J, *Napoleon's Army in Russia. The Illustrated Memoirs of Albrecht Adam 1812*, Barnsley, 2005.

O'Meara, B, *Napoleon in Exile or a voice from St. Helena*, 2 Vols., London, 1827.

Oritz, J M, 'The Revolutionary flying ambulance of Napoleon's surgeon', *US Army Medical Department Journal* (1998), pp. 17–25.

Oudinot, Marshal, *Memoirs of Marshal Oudinot Duc de Reggio*, New York, 1897.

Parquin, C, *Napoleon's Army* (ed. B T Jones), London, 1969.

Pelet, J J, *The French Campaign in Portugal 1810–1811* (ed. D D Horward), Minneapolis, 1973.

Pépé, General, *Memoirs of General Pépé (1783–1815)*, Felling, 1999.

Percy, Baron, *Journal des Campagnes de Baron Percy*, Paris, 2002.

Peterson, R K D, 'Insects, disease and military history: the Napoleonic campaigns and historical perceptions', *American Entomologist* (1995), Vol. 41, pp. 147–60.

Petre, F L, *Napoleon's Campaign in Poland 1806–1807*, London, 2001.

Petre, F L, *Napoleon's last campaign in Germany – 1813*, London, 1974.

Peumery, J-J, 'Les propriétés du froid et la Campagne de Russie, d'apres la thèse du Mauricheau-Beaupré (1817)', *Histoire de Sciences Médicales* (1997), Vol. 31, pp. 261–7.

Phipps, R W, *The Armies of the First French Republic and the Rise of the Marshals of Napoleon I*, 5 Vols., Oxford, 1939.

Pigeard, A, *Dictionnaire de la Grande Armée*, Paris, 2002.

Pigeard, A, *L'Armée de Napoléon*, Paris, 2000.

Pigeard, A, 'Le Service de Santé de la Révolution au 1er Empire 1792–1815', *Tradition*, No.28, 2004.

Pontier, R, *Souvenirs de chirurgien Pontier sur la retraite de Russie*, Brive, 1967. *Pontons et Prisons sous le Premier Empire*, Paris, 1998.

Poumiès de la Siboutie, Doctor, *Recollections of a Parisian (1789–1863)*, New York, 1911.

Prinzing, F, *Epidemics resulting from Wars*, Oxford, 1916.

Quennevat, J-C, *Atlas de la Grande Armée*, Paris, 1966.

Quennevat, J-C, *Les vrais soldats de Napoléon*, Paris, 1968.

Rapp, General Count, *Memoirs of General Count Rapp first aide-de-camp to Napoleon*, London, 1823.

Renoult, A-J, *Souvenirs du docteur Renoult*, Paris, 1862.

Richardson, R, *Larrey. Surgeon to Napoleon's Imperial Guard*, London, 2000.

Rieux, J and Hassenforder, J, *Histoire du Service de Santé Militaire et du Val-de-Grâce*, Paris, 1951.

Robiquet, J, *Daily Life in France under Napoleon*, London, 1962.

Rocca de, A J M, *In the Peninsula with a French Hussar*, London, 1990.

Roeder, Captain, *The ordeal of Captain Roeder* (ed. H Roeder), London, 1960.

Rogers, Col. H C B, *Napoleon's Army*, London, 1974.

Roos, H de, *Avec Napoléon en Russie. Souvenirs de la Campagne de 1812*, Paris, 1913.

Rose, A, *Napoleon's Campaign in Russia Anno 1812: medico-historical*, New York, 1913.

Rosen, G, 'Hospitals, medical care and social policy in the French Revolution', *Bulletin of the History of Medicine* (1956), Vol. 30, pp. 124–49.

Rothenberg, G E, *The Art of Warfare in the Age of Napoleon*, London, 1977.

Ruttiman, B, 'Souvenirs des guerres napoléoniennes: points de vue des blessés et de leurs médecins', *Gesnerus* (1985), Vol. 42, pp. 399–413.

Ryan, E, *Napoleon's shield and guardian. The unconquerable General Daumesnil*, London, 2003.

Ségur, Count P-P de, *Napoleon's Russian Campaign*, London, 1959.

Ségur, General Count de, *An Aide-de-Camp of Napoleon*, London, 1895.

Sèze, V de, *Rapport et Projet de décret sur le service de santé des Armées et des Hôpitaux militaires*, Paris, 1791.

Shoberl, F, *Narrative of the Remarkable Events which occurred in and near Leipzig*, London, 1814.

Simpson, J, *Paris after Waterloo*, Edinburgh, 1853.

Smeaton, W A, 'Pharmacy in Revolutionary and Napoleonic Paris 1789–1815', *Pharmacy History* (1976), Vol. 9, pp. 4–5.

Smith, D, *The Prisoners of Cabrera. Napoleon's forgotten soldiers 1809–1814*, New York, 2001.

Sokolov, O, *L'Armée de Napoléon*, Saint-Germain-en-Laye, 2003.

Soubiran, A, *Le Baron Larey, chirurgien de Napoléon*, Paris, 1966.

Soubiran, A, *Napoléon et un million de morts*, Paris, 1969.

Tascher, M de, *Notes de campagne (1806–1813)*, Châteauroux, 1932.

Thiébault, Baron, *The memoirs of Baron Thiébault late Lieutenant-General in the French Army*, 2 Vols., Felling, 1994.

Thiers, M A, *Histoire du Consulat et de L'Empire*, 21 Vols., Paris, 1843–62.

Tissot, C J, *Observations générales sur l'administration des hôpitaux ambulans et sedentaires des armées*, Paris, 1793.

Trésal, J B, *Essai sur la fièvre adynamique qui a régné dans l'île de Walcheren dans l'année 1809*, Paris, 1815.

Triaire, P, *Dominique Larrey et les campagnes de la Révolution et de l'Empire*, Tours, 1902.

Tulard, J, *Dictionnaire Napoléon*, 2 Vols., Paris, 1999.

Tulard, J, *Nouvelle bibliographie critique des mémoires sur l'époque Napoléonienne*, Geneva, 1991.

Tyrbas de Chamberet, J, *Mémoires d'un Médecin Militaire*, Paris, 2002.

Vachée, Col., *Napoleon at Work*, London, 1914.

Vaidy, J V F, 'Un médecin de la Grande Armée' (ed. P Delaunay), *Bulletin de la Société Française d'histoire de la médecine* (1912), Vol. 11, pp. 463–92.

Vess, D M, *Medical Revolution in France 1789–1796*, Gainesville, 1975.

Vossler, H, *With Napoleon in Russia 1812*, London, 1969.

Walter, J, *The Diary of a Napoleonic Foot Soldier* (ed. M Raeff), Moreton-in-Marsh, 1991.

Watson, S J, *By Command of the Emperor. A life of Marshal Berthier*, London, 1957.

Weiner, D B, *French Doctors Face War 1792–1815*, in Warner, C K (ed.), *From the Ancien Régime to the Popular Front*, New York, 1969.

Wilson, General Sir R, *Narrative of Events during the Invasion of Russia by Napoleon Bonaparte*, London, 1860.

Woloch, I, *The French Veteran from the Revolution to the Restoration*, Chapel Hill, 1979.

Zamoyski, A, *1812. Napoleon's fatal march on Moscow*, London, 2004.

Index